Body Movement:
Coping with the Environment

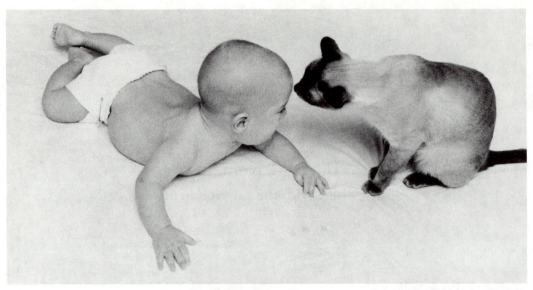

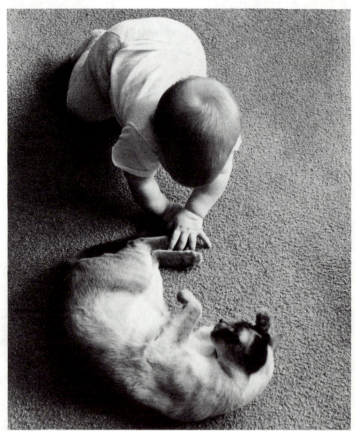

Baby and Cat © Morris H. Jaffe
Communication through
complementary body shaping.
Observe developmental
differences between the younger
and the older infant: the latter
shows clearer relationship to space
and greater complexity of body
shaping.

Body Movement:

Coping with the Environment

by
Irmgard Bartenieff

with
Dori Lewis

GORDON AND BREACH SCIENCE PUBLISHERS
New York   Paris   London

Copyright © 1980 Irmgard Bartenieff and Dori Lewis
All rights reserved

Gordon and Breach, Science Publishers, Inc.
One Park Avenue
New York, New York 10016

Gordon and Breach Science Publishers Limited
42 William IV Street
London WC2N 4DE

Gordon & Breach
58, rue Lhomond
75005 Paris

First published September 1980
Second printing February 1982

Designed by Blaketon-Hall Limited
Typeset by Leaper & Gard Limited, Bristol
Printed in the United States of America

To my sons,

Igor John Barrett and George Bartenieff

and to my mentor,

Rudolf Laban

This book is a triadic collaboration between the genius and inspiration of Rudolf Laban, my total professional experience, and the imagination, insight, and artistry of Dori Lewis, writer, actress, dancer, musician, and analyst who, with vitality and humor, shared her talents to make it happen. The commitment to do the book gave me a new lease on life which I cheerfully renew in this, my eightieth year, to celebrate publication with the hope that new perceptions of ourselves and our world will enhance all our lives.

v

Credits

Thanks and profound appreciation to the two gifted artists whose professionalism persevered through all our demands: Wendy Sarafyan for the elegant anatomical drawings and Laurie Julia for the grace and precision of all the other drawings in the book.

For the photographs beautifully capturing peak moments of movement, we thank Kim Bailey, Suzanne Fields, Bonnie Freer, Morris H. Jaffe, Ann Karlawish, Nana Sue Koch, Stephanie Krebs, Robert Lorenz/Main Street Photography, Leonard Nakahashi, Nat Norman, Popsie, Rehabilitation International, Toby Shimin, Robert Shuster and the Paschal Guzman Downtown Ballet, Liza Stelle, Elizabeth Stopol, Steve Turi, United Nations, UTA French Airlines, Carol Fenner Williams, Bernard P. Wolff, and Judy Van Zile.

Thanks to Irene Politis for the Labanotation autography, to Barbara Gellis for preparation of the Bibliography, and to Henry Engel for the Index.

For permission to reproduce *The Harvesters* by Pieter Breughel the Elder, we thank the Metropolitan Museum of Art, New York.

For permission to reproduce the Suburi exercise illustration from *This is Kendo: the Art of Japanese Fencing* by Junzo Sasamori and Gordon Warner, we thank Charles E. Tuttle Publishers, Rutland, Vermont.

For permission to use a photograph of *Deer and Faun*, an 8th century B.C. Greek sculpture: Museum of Fine Arts, Boston, H.L. Pierce Fund.

For permission to quote from copyright material, we thank the following:

Macdonald and Evans, London: *Choreutics, Principles of Dance and Movement Notation, The Mastery of Movement*, all by Rudolf Laban.

Teachers College Press, Columbia University, New York: *Dance — An Art in Academe*, article by Irmgard Bartenieff and Forrestine Paulay.

Arno Press, New York: *The Gentle Art of Walking*, by Hal Borland.

To the following for permission to quote in the text:

Mayfield Publishing Company, Palo Alto, Ca., and Trudi Schoop: *Won't You Join the Dance?*

Judith S. Kestenberg and Aronson Publishers, New York: *Children and Parents*.

The Dance Notation Bureau, New York: "Fandango," copyright Antony Tudor.

National Institute of Mental Health for observation report.

Suzanne K. Youngerman for excerpts from "Shakers" analysis.

Carol-Lynne Rose for excerpts from "Fairy Tale" and "Mathematics Offers Key to Choreutics."

Diana Schnitt for excerpts from "Duet in Canon."

Alan Lomax for paraphrases from his *Folk Song Style and Culture*, Transaction Books, New Brunswick, N.J., publishers.

Rudolf Arnheim for an excerpt from an address to the LIMS Conference, June 8-10, 1979, to be published in an anthology of dance writings, edited by Professor Curtis Carter of Marquette University.

The four major Laban teaching centers from which numerous branches have also been established are the Laban Centre of Movement and Dance at Goldsmith College, London; The Language of Dance Centre, London; The Dance Notation Bureau, New York City; and the Laban Institute of Movement Studies, New York City.

Acknowledgments

Thanks are, of course, inadequate to express the appreciation I feel for support, inspiration, criticism, and patience of friends and colleagues. To thank you properly would take another book, but, until then, permit me here to acknowledge my gratitude to Margaret Mead, always stimulating and generous, now sorely missed. To Israel Zwerling, who so early saw the promise of dance therapy, thank you for encouraging my participation in it. To Ursula Corning and Margaret Fries, thank you for being my friends in and out of need. To Charles Brainard and Martin Michael, my warm appreciation for understanding legal advice.

For sharing their knowledge with me by sensitive reading and commenting on different versions of the book, thank you to Lisa Ullmann, Marion North, Valerie Preston-Dunlop, Warren Lamb, Martha Davis, Aileen Crow, Kedzie Penfield, Janis Pforsich, Peggy Hackney, and Susan Schickele. For answering special questions about particular material, thank you to Robert Abramson, Rudolf Arnheim, Paul Byers, Pearl Coleman, Norman Cousins, Cecily Dell, Mantle Hood, Ann Hutchinson, Judith Kestenberg, Alan Lomax, Edward Maisel, Forrestine Paulay, Virginia Reed, Carol-Lynne Rose, Claire Schmais, Ella Schwartz, Rosa Shimin, Joan Smallwood, Stephen Smoliar, Muriel Topaz, Bobby Troka, Suzanne Youngerman, Carl Wolz, and Kayla Kazahn Zalk.

To Jody Zacharias and the staff of the Laban Institute of Movement Studies, my thanks for taking on the major responsibility for the Institute which permitted me to work on the book.

For assistance in the infinite numbers of details in gathering materials and preparing them for the manuscript, thank you Carol Hutchinson, Cathy McCoubrey, Eden Graber, Romanie Kramoris, Judy McCusker, and especially Donald Kraus, for the push to the end.

The responsibility for everything in the book I fully assume, but without the help I received there would be no book at all.

I.B.

Preface

This book describes what the body can do, how it does it, how it relates to space, and how the quality of its movement affects function and communication — coping. It addresses itself not only to students of body movement per se, but also to professionals and non-professionals of other disciplines concerned with ways that people attempt to cope with their environment.

The work is based on the perceptions of choreographer/philosopher Rudolf Laban (1879-1958) who, with his colleagues, also developed a notation system for body movement that is analogous to music notation. Labananalysis focuses on the process of movement itself, as related to its goals.

The current play of body-mind relationships as "pop-psych" party games is like fluff brushed off the woven fabrics of serious body movement studies. Such study in the western world can be dated from the publication of Charles Darwin's *The Expression of Emotion in Man and Animals*, with a major impetus coming from the work of psychiatrist Wilhelm Reich and, more recently, the work of anthropologist Ray L. Birdwhistell and many others.

Research has developed with particular psychological, physical, spiritual, cultural, sociological emphases. It ranges, for example, from Birdwhistell's kinesics research (studies of aspects of nonverbal, interpersonal communication with emphasis on cultural interpretations) to the Alexander technique, developed by F.M. Alexander (which emphasizes a specific relationship of head and spine, and conscious inhibition of poor habits so that improved body use follows with its concomitant psychological balance) to Moshe Feldenkrais (who approaches the body as an engineer exploring leverage with specific exercises to improve its usage). It is not within the parameters of this book to discuss the many studies and techniques in body-mind research, but we have tried to include extensive references to such research in the bibliography. In 1978, The Institute for Nonverbal Communication Research was founded in New York by Martha Davis to help researchers keep abreast of the burgeoning research activities. Awareness is now widespread that disciplined attention should be continuously given to the effects of body-mind research because, while it has profound possibility for positive development, it is also potentially dangerous to body and psyche when misinterpreted or misused. The influence of eastern disciplines such as t'ai chi ch'uan and yoga is also becoming increasingly pervasive and also requires careful, responsible attention.

Labananalysis provides a means of perceiving and a vocabulary for describing movement — quantitatively and qualitatively — that is applicable to any body movement research even when there may be differences in interpretation of function and communication. It makes subtle distinctions among a great range of specific components and component constellations inherent in movement process.

One may wish to understand such differences for the personal satisfaction of awareness or to have additional resources for the improvement of functional activity or extension of expressive possibilities. The direct relationship to professions in dance and sports is apparent, and, as Laban's work and its lexicon developed with colleagues and students, it was first applied to the creation, performance, and teaching of dance and physical education.

Now, however, Labananalysis has much wider applications. For psychiatrists, psychologists, anthropologists, ethnologists, sociologists, and related professionals, the nonverbal communication of the body can be incorporated with other research to refine coping distinctions and measure changes. The dance therapist can help patients experience subtle changes in their body movements and understand psychological implications of them. Artists use the Labananalysis techniques as an additional tool in both observation and execution of their crafts. That is, by relating their own bodies to the qualities they perceive in models or images, they can transmit those qualities through their art medium.

Dance is often regarded as such a separate category of movement experiences that it is excluded, unnecessarily, from the training and experience of other disciplines. The framework of Labananalysis does not maintain so sharp a separation. There are differences of intention, choice and degree of body usage, but the components of all body movements are the same. Since dance provides combinations of the components at heightened intensities, any student of body movement for any reason can incorporate the observations from dance analyses.

Schools, colleges, and universities in Australia, England, West Germany, and in twenty-five U.S.A. states have courses of study in some area of Labananalysis, and their graduates are teaching, performing, practicing therapy, and developing important research. The organization, International Council of Kinetography Laban, created to coordinate its vocabulary and theory, has representatives in Belgium, Canada, England, France, Germany, Holland, Hungary, Iceland, Poland, Rhodesia, Spain, Switzerland, U.S.A., and Yugoslavia.

Rudolf Laban was an artist and scientist, architect, choreographer, philosopher, and movement educator, extraordinarily innovative and charismatic. Born in Austria, he traveled widely and participated in the major European artistic activities of his time, especially in the development of modern dance. He was in Germany during the Bauhaus and Expressionist periods, initiating and developing theatrical and recreational dance programs, schools, and publications. In 1936, the Nazis forced him to stop, and he went to England, where he adapted his movement theories to wartime studies of factory workers, helped establish new schools for movement education, and continued to publish his works.

Laban observed movement process in all aspects of life: from the martial arts to spatial patterns in Sufi rug weaving, factory work tasks, rhythmic patterns in folk dances, crafts and the behavior of emotionally disturbed people. It was the process itself that compelled his attention, not just the end points or goals of the action, and he, with his colleagues, refined movement observations into an exquisitely precise method of experiencing, seeing, and recording them so that body movement functional and expressive implications became increasingly apparent.

It was in 1925 that I first encountered Laban not far from my birthplace in Berlin, Germany. I was twenty-five years old. His work was a logical focal point for my background of swings between biology, art, and dance. I studied with him and his colleagues, Dussia Bereska, Ruth Loeser, and Albrecht Knust, and, later, with second-generation colleagues, Warren Lamb, Marion North, and Valerie Preston-Dunlop. Sigurd Leeder, Lisa Ullmann, Sylvia Bodmer, Ann Hutchinson, Martin Gleisner, Kurt Jooss, Geraldine Stephenson, and Laban's daughter, Azra von Laban were all vital participants in the inner circle of Laban's collaborators at different periods, and their contributions to the development of his theories are crucial.

After my marriage to Michail Bartenieff, a Russian Jewish dancer, I taught dance and Labanotation, my husband taught ballet, and we both studied Spanish dance. For a short time, we toured with our own dance company, but in 1936 we fled from Germany to America. In 1938 I was able to go back for our two sons.

In America, with the late Irma Otto-Betz, I introduced Labanotation at the Hanya Holm Studio. I became a physical therapist and gradually rebuilt connections to dance and art. In 1943, I was invited to become a member of the Dance Notation Bureau in New York, and in 1965, with Martha Davis and Forrestine Paulay, started the Effort/Shape department at the Bureau to extend the training in observations of affinities between shaping and dynamic aspects of movement process. In 1978, with the assistance of the Effort/Shape faculty, I founded the Laban Institute of Movement Studies in New York to further develop the work and its applications. We absorb Effort/Shape now in the broader context known as Labananalysis. Fifty years in the field has only strengthened my convictions that Laban's multifaceted approach to the study of human behavior through body movement has a unique contribution to make to the understanding of our world.

ix

The principal objective of this book is to suggest additional modes of perceiving oneself, other people, and relationships to the world around one, using the live body totally — body-mind-feeling — as a key to coping with the environment. In the process of extending the quality and range of one's body movement options, the experience can extend the quality of functional and emotional life as well. The possibility of moving in new ways with less risk strengthens courage to tolerate continuous movement and change with stability and delight. One can learn to recognize where one is caught in private chauvinisms or value judgments that diminish the values of other uniquely dynamic behavior and art.

What is critical to comprehension of these perceptions is that they be understood as a whole — without fragmentation. Change in any aspect changes the whole configuration. Obviously, the experience of self as a whole transcends the consciousness of specific parts, but understanding the parts helps one to recreate the whole, to enliven its mobility, and to play harmoniously with a continuously changing environment.

I.B.
June 28, 1979

Contents

Credits   vi
Acknowledgments   vii
Preface   viii
Introduction   xii

Chapter 1.   Activate and Motivate   1
Chapter 2.   The Body Architecture   17
Chapter 3.   Carving Shapes in Space   23
Chapter 4.   Inner Impulses to Move   49
Chapter 5.   Rhythm and Phrasing   69
Chapter 6.   Affinities of Body, Space and Effort   83
Chapter 7.   Tensions and Countertensions   101
Chapter 8.   Group Interaction   127
Chapter 9.   Dance Therapy   141
Chapter 10.   Ethnic Studies   165
Chapter 11.   Additional Applications   181

Epilogue   215
Appendix A.   Documentation of Observations:
              Notation and Methodology   217
Appendix B.   Bartenieff Fundamentals Exercises   229
Sources of the Quotations   274
Bibliography   275
Index   287

Introduction

We see light etched by shadows, feel joy emerging from sorrow; the present hovers between the past and the future. Between all these opposites, there is a sense of movement that renews the clarity of each experience. Even in apparent stillness, movement variables are active. Nowhere is this more discernible than in the movements of the human body as they fluctuate between stability and mobility. Movement variables enable us to cope with our temperaments and our environment in order to survive. Only in death, perhaps, does the experience of movement cease.

The heart beats, movement flows on the breath. When we are calm, heartbeat, breath and movement are even; when we are healthy or ill, excited or depressed, they change accordingly. Our bodies grow and shrink with the breathing, self-absorbed. We carry our weight, instead of giving in to it.

We reach into space, outside ourselves, gather it and scatter it in the same direction, in different directions, in combinations of directions — with our fingers, our hands, our arms, our toes, our legs, our torsos, separately or in various combinations or all together. Our self-absorption unfolds and incorporates other bodies and things — toys and tools.

We struggle with uprightness. A temptation toward flight or fall is tempered by the body's possibilities. We hold our bodies rigidly as if fearful that some parts might break off; we hold them so loosely that they verge on collapse. Or, we let the parts support each other by using all the subtle internal anatomical mechanisms — rotators and connective kinetic chains — that make for smooth adaptations to infinite varieties of movement. We make different shapes in space and feel all kinds of tensions within those shapes, graceful and grotesque, skillful and clumsy.

We throw ourselves into a task or we approach it gingerly; race through it or bide our time. Sometimes we walk directly to a destination; other times we meander all over space to get there. We move to pick a flower, nurture a child, plant a seed, cut the harvest, lift the fruit, throw a ball, play a piano, row a boat, fight an adversary, grind corn, paint a picture, weave and knit. We stamp in anger, curve in love, retreat in fear and advance in confidence. We make jerky angular progress toward our goal or progress with smooth, rounded symmetrical or asymmetrical phrases and rhythms. We drive ourselves without respite, blind to all but our goal, or we prepare, initiate and move in a particular sequence so that transitions along the way are economical and changes keep us refreshed without waste or losing sight of the goal. Sheer muscle strength is not enough; the real power to fulfill a goal lies in mobility of ordered sequences of movement factors.

What are those movement factors? What happens in the process of going from one place to another? What components of the process can be identified? How do they relate to each other and how do we experience and observe them?

Without analysis, most observers detect differences among their own and other people's movements in a general way. There are days when one is "all thumbs." Other days one has "two left feet." Other days or at another time in the same day, one may feel "all together," graceful, efficient. When observing two people doing the same thing, it is often apparent that, although they handle the same tools toward the same end, they seem almost to be handling different tools for different purposes and there are extreme differences in the results or the time required to achieve similar results. Sometimes there is more similarity between a construction worker and a dancer than there is between two construction workers or between two dancers.

Cultural differences in movement have been observed and recorded. It is possible also to observe subtle differences among the individuals within each culture.

The mentally disturbed or retarded are observed to have distinctive differences in their individual movements. The aged have what are often considered characteristic qualities in their body movements, just as children have recognizable general characteristics, but each individual of either group has distinct differences. The physically handicapped develop individualized movement characteristics associated with their particular handicaps.

Athletes, cooks, cowboys, musicians, carpenters, fighters, lovers, rich and poor, cops and robbers, the grief-stricken and the joyful, drunk or sober — all use their bodies and the space around them in ways that can be analyzed by common components, individually and in interaction.

The central component is, obviously, the body itself. It is this author's contention that a sound knowledge of the physiology of the body is essential to any study related to the use of the body. There is mystery enough in the wonder of its extraordinary creation and operation without creating a mystique of ignorance around what can be known: its parts, their functions, and, most of all, their constant interrelationships with each other and in variations with changing tasks and situations. Bartenieff Fundamentals™ exercises were developed to help, through experience, the understanding of these relationships as configurations.

The second major component in Labananalysis is the space in which the body moves and the resultant shapes that are made in that space. Their tension qualities are determined by intent, preparation, initiation, and developing, changing complexity of the movement process producing them. Laban, strongly influenced by study of survival techniques in the martial arts, organized movement possibilities with reference to geometric shapes and sequences — called scales — of traveling within and around those shapes. By experimenting with different kinds of sequences, exertions and recuperations, phrasing and rhythms, different qualities within the scales and their derivatives are identified, just as in musical scales the same intervals have different qualities in different keys, melodies, and harmonies.

Perhaps the most subtle of the movement components distinguished by Laban are those of Effort. These were developed (though they were embodied in much earlier work) during World War II, when he and a colleague, F.C. Lawrence, were asked to investigate the possibility of more efficient performance among industrial workers. From those studies, the concept of Effort developed as attitudes toward the exertion of energy in flow, space, weight, and time. Different attitudes, conscious or unconscious, can be affined with sequences of spatial paths as being more or less efficient. Each variation is distinctively expressive as well.

All the components of the three major categories — body, space, Effort — are inextricably related to each other in the process of movement and in its functional-expressive content.

There is a recurring body movement theme of scattering and gathering, giving and taking, repulsing and grasping, going toward the environment or toward the body, that is like a metaphor for going toward others or toward self. Each move — a way of coping — has an almost infinite range of possibility from minute to extreme of effectiveness and involvement. Each configuration of moves represents a combination of body, space, and Effort that is definable in some degree through a Labananalysis that can clarify function and/or expressive content. Such configurations are central to this book.

The book is structured in an order of increasing complexity. Chapter 1 is a first person account of the author's early experiences in the practice of Labananalysis, included here because her unusual combination of physical therapy and dance and dance therapy illustrates the functional-expressive links made available by Labananalysis.

Chapters 2, 3, and 4 are discussions of body, space, and Effort in that order. Chapters 5, 6, and 7 discuss the three components' inextricable relationships to each other, in rhythm and phrasing, in affinities to each other, and in tensions and countertensions. Chapter 8 discusses some additional points in group interaction. Chapters 9 and 10 discuss two major areas of Labananalysis application — dance therapy and ethnic studies — in which the author has played an active part. Chapter 11 has additional application observations.

Each chapter is prefaced by photographs with suggested movement observations and each chapter is followed by verbal observation examples. All the examples and photographs are selected to tune the observer into another framework for seeing and experiencing movement as music of the body played on different instruments by different performers in various combinations.

The Appendix includes an introduction to Bartenieff Fundamentals with twelve illustrated exercises and with anatomical drawings of important bone and muscle landmark areas. The Appendix also includes a brief sampling of Labanotation and discussion of methodology. Bibliography and Index follow.

Obviously, in so complex a field, no one book can be totally satisfactory either to its authors or its readers. There has been no intention here to be all-inclusive, but it is hoped that the scope of the material in the observation of both ordinary and extraordinary movement events has been communicated.

It is strongly suggested that the reader try to observe and experience actively, not just intellectually, the movement components and their variations as they are presented. The reading needs to be accompanied by doing. Otherwise, the totality of movement process will be reduced to fragmented, static rhetoric. The vocabulary of Labananalysis only suggests the extensive functional and expressive possibilities that active body, space, Effort participation will fulfill. That participation can provide confirmation of the reader's own observations.

CHAPTER 1

Activate and Motivate

In rhythmic waves regularly spreading, the ether trembles, the small, most minute particles of matter tremble. If there were no movement at all, all things would be lying dead in absolute rigidity and complete apathy. No ray of light, no sound would bring messages from one thing to another.

. . . Movement not only speaks through an object; a living organism owes its final form to it; movement leads to growth and structure . . .

That movement speaks that is about to break out of its form: The weighty power of a rock with its visible potential for impact speaks of the tremendous impetus with which it might plunge into the valley as an avalanche. The grace of a plant speaks of the readiness to move which drives a flower out of its stem from which fruit and new seed will sprout . . . Animal movement speaks of the fine adaptations with which a particular species has immersed itself into its surroundings to fit increasingly finer, more differentially into the workings of nature.

Rudolf Laban

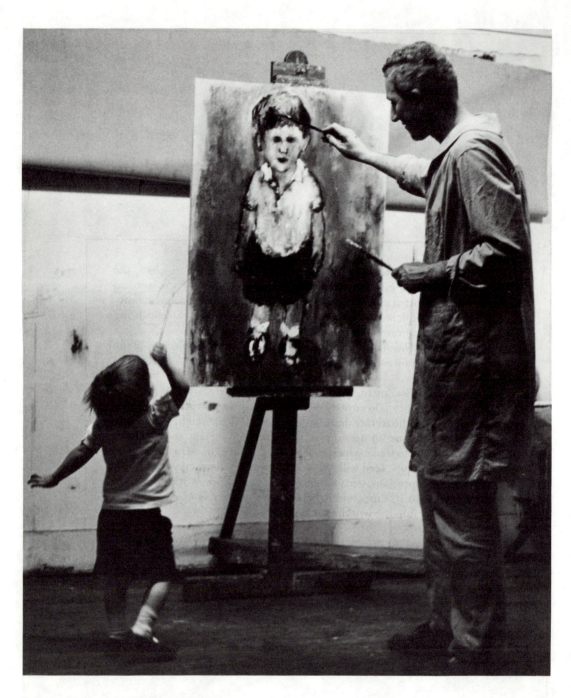

Painters: Child and Adult © Morris H. Jaffe
In contrast to the adult's clear organization of his verticality and Direct/Light Effort combinations, Effort Flow and Shape Flow still dominate in the child.

Activate and Motivate

A short narrative of the author's professional development in the application of Labananalysis to different disciplines is followed by chapters with details of Labananalysis theory and technique. Later chapters include details of other major applications to ethnic studies, anthropology, art and daily life.

Although the emphasis here is on physical and dance therapy, the observations incorporate basic Labananalysis components that can be applied to all movement research. Behavioral differentiations are continuously correlated with differentiated movement process. The observer learns to see, as a continuum, fluctuating ranges between extremes of stability and mobility, common denominators and individual characteristics, constancy and change.

Physical Therapy

My own professional development in the field of physical therapy, always in counterpoint to my training and experience as a dancer and dance teacher, provides points of reference to the intimacy of the relationship between function and expressiveness of the body. It also confirmed, for me, the soundness of Laban's theories of body movement.

Because Laban's focus was always on the body *in movement*, his training crystallized that focus for me when diagnosing both physical and emotional dysfunction. Thus, spatial concepts had to be incorporated into mechanical anatomical activity in order to produce maximal functioning. In physical therapy, that meant thinking in terms of movement *in space*, rather than by just strengthening muscle groups. And, the introduction of the spatial concepts required an awareness of *intent* on the part of the patient that activated his will and thus connected his independent *participation* to his own recovery. There really is no such thing as pure "physical" therapy or pure "mental" therapy. They are continuously interrelated.

Until World War II, physical therapy focused on restoring local function in joints, by the application of heat, massage and passive manipulation. During and after World War II, the focus was expanded to include a more total and active involvement of the patient to achieve optimal function within the limitations of a residual disability, and to rehabilitate him for life activity.

Howard Rusk, chairman of the New York University Institute of Rehabilitation and the late George Deaver, then Head of the Children's Department, developed this approach. They devised an activity training program for the patient comparable to athletic programs. It stressed making the patient as independent as possible of constant reliance on nursing or family care. Programs for the best ways of using crutches, wheelchairs and other mechanical aids were experimented with and developed into teachable techniques.

These programs demanded a new kind of resourcefulness from the physical therapists, a knowledge of and experience with body movement and the possibilities of functional movement which they could transfer to the patient as substitutes for functional losses.

I took the first course given in Physical Therapy and Physical Rehabilitation at New York University under George Deaver. The first set of students was exposed, in field work, directly to wards with chronic and new patients with different degrees of disabilities. The students were encouraged to develop new techniques of dealing with such reduced movement potential.

The polio ward of Willard Parker Hospital in lower Manhattan (at that time the city's hospital for infectious diseases, since torn down) was my first assignment. I stayed there for nearly seven years. My principal guideline was Deaver's slogan: Activate and motivate the patient.

The particular set-up of this hospital, which was lacking in so many technical facilities, was especially conducive to the development of personal ingenuity and responsibility. Every aspect of movement familiar to me through my Laban training and supported by my anatomical training as a physical therapist became a resource. The unity of the functional and expressive aspects of movement behavior became increasingly clarified and led back to the role of dance as a clue to the roots of behavior.

There are three functional, expressive stages to the rehabilitation of movement.

1. The first stage is the realization of sudden loss of function and analysis of its extent.
2. The second stage is an intense effort to restore function or to create an adequate substitute for it.
3. The third stage, with all its technical, personal relationship and career implications, is adjustment to permanent limitation of function, and discovery of new resources.

At Willard Parker Hospital, we had to deal with all three stages.

First, we had to understand, by empathy with the patients, what the presence of partial or widespread loss of function does to all shaping and dynamics as well as to the emotional and mental attitudes of the patient.

Each new patient revealed with striking individuality the impact of being hit with the experience of an inability to move. That reality went far beyond the actual loss through paralysis. The traumatic early stage, this fearsome experience of immobility — whether from stiffness or flaccidity or a combination of both — had to be shortened as quickly as possible.

Mobilization, from the beginning, became more than a problem of the mechanics of function. Fortunately, at the start of my work at the hospital, the influence of Sister Kenny, the Australian nurse, led to the use of special hot packs to replace the immobilizing total body casts. In the early treatment of polio, this was critical to the treatment of stiffness of back and neck, which was frequently coupled with weakness in various parts of the limbs and trunk. Sister Kenny also paved the way for retraining individual muscles by awareness and localization of their functions and she had been successful with this approach even with very young children.

I became more and more aware that every little movement of a patient lying in bed would produce a far-reaching effect on the weight distribution in the patient's whole body. The distribution of muscle contraction and relaxation is affected and results in shifting body shapes. This was borne out by the observation that so-called non-paralytic patients would frequently stay stiff for weeks beyond the early sub-acute stage. In these cases, we found minimal muscle weaknesses, such as a limited inverter of the foot, slight abdominal weakness or shoulder weaknesses. We then started to develop a compromise between rigid positioning and just letting the patient lie unsupervised. This meant frequent changes of the patient's position, cranking up the bed at different angles, and also sitting the patient up at the edge of the bed for a few minutes.

The early stage of immobilization was easier to deal with in the young children (up to 6 years of age). They frequently resented the hot packs, writhing and crying with terror. Instead, they were put into bathtubs — familiar experience — and were allowed to wriggle and, even better, were put into small plastic pools, three or five children at a time, which encouraged communication and created a playful atmosphere. This was followed by placing them, again in a group, on the large exercise mats on the floor, where they could roll around and could make spontaneous moves toward each other and away.

It became clear to me how important it is for therapists to be aware of the patient's image of them — startling as it may sometimes be — and of the other personnel around the patient. That image can be extremely powerful in both positive and negative ways, as the following examples illustrate.

One case was that of a middle-aged major who had lost the use of both legs in an accident and was rehabilitated with long leg braces and crutches. He made some sketches of the process of rehabilitation as the patient sees it. One especially revealing sketch showed the commanding figure of the therapist pointing to a small curbstone and ordering the patient to "Go down." Next to this was the patient, a small, almost dwarflike figure, leaning on his crutches, standing on a wall at least two feet high.

4

Another example was that of a nine-year-old boy who had gone through the agonizing experience of partial loss of the use of his initiating breathing center. He had survived the experience partly because the nurses and the therapist, myself, had been sitting at his bed reminding him to breathe. At the final examination, he suddenly looked at me and said, "When I first saw you, I thought you were a witch. Now," he added reflectively, "I don't understand why I should have thought that."

In our early days at the hospital, it was crucial to sensitize the young nurses and attendants to the nature of the patient's functional loss and the behavior it elicited from the patient. We discouraged punitive attitudes, such as calling a little girl, who was deprived of any arm-hand function, a "bad" girl when she bit the hand of the nurse treating her. Once the nurse understood that the child felt she had no other means of defense, the nurse was able to change the behavior without being punitive.

Only when the hospital personnel made the effort to examine the behavior accompanying functional losses could they understand the totality of the treatment necessary for the loss.

For example, there was an adolescent girl, handicapped in arms, shoulder and lower extremities, who, when put on the exercise mat and left alone even for a couple of minutes, would get hysterical with fear that she might fall or that she could not defend herself or that she would get squashed by someone stepping on her. It had to be recognized that the hysteria had, in fact, realistic foundation because of her particular movement limitation. Then it could be dealt with concretely in terms of reassurances of physical protection and assistance, rather than as an emotional abstraction.

Adults with severe arm disabilities and minimal foot weaknesses often had problems with their walking training because of their inability to ward off danger with the arm or break a fall when out of balance. The feeling was that "my feet are miles away from my head."

These attitudes cannot be fragmented and dismissed as "psychological." They are deeply ingrained attitudinal gestures of defense and of protection realistically based on the actual situation of the patients' being cut off from their environment by the experience of non-functioning. Starting from the reality of the situation, substitutes had to be devised for the loss and different adaptation patterns developed along with constant encouragement to find new ways to do things. In that way motivation and mobilization developed together.

Other experiences with movement intent and motivation confirmed this maturation-mobilization principle. For example, the mechanistic concept of stretching muscles that had become apparently fixed into contraction is to merely lengthen the muscle. In addition to treatment with hot packs and immersion in the warm water of a Hubbard tank,* passive stretching (patient is passive, therapist is active) was one of the early types of treatment.

In stretching the stiff (polio) back, we found that by extending movement possibilities beyond forward flexion of the trunk to include lateral (sideward) flexion and rotation (twisting) we were able to establish full flexibility of the spine in all directions. We therefore moved the trunk passively in a sequence of lateral, rotary, flexion gradually into sitting up.

In the course of stretching the stiff, contracted back into sitting up, the normal length of the back muscles is restored. If there is a muscle weakness in the abdomen and/or the shoulder girdle, secondary tensions might arise, which interfere with the lengthening of the back muscles, and thus the spatial pattern of flexing forward and up. This interference is in the form of "dead weight," experienced by both patient and therapist, which increases the back stiffness. It can be eliminated by careful support of the weak regions and constant encouragement to the patient to focus on the *spatial intent* of forward and up. This sometimes needed additional personnel supporting the weak component, but it paid off in total time for treatment and readied the patient for later intensive active work. (See Bibliography, Bartenieff, "Stretching in Polio.") This experience was to become the cornerstone of what I would later call "Bartenieff Fundamentals."

* *A metal tank widely used in hydrotherapy where patients are almost completely immersed in water during exercise.*

5

During the years of my work at Willard Parker Hospital, Deaver sent us to various wards at Bellevue Hospital to evaluate chronic patients for their potential in rehabilitation. One of the instances in which the Labananalysis evaluation was especially dramatic was the case of David F., a chronic polio patient.

David F. was in the orthopedic ward for children in Bellevue Hospital. He was four years old and small for his age. The previous year he had been afflicted with polio and had been placed in a respirator for a few months. It left him with severe weaknesses in arms and legs, an extremely weak trunk, particularly the back — the latter, a rather rare incident. When I met him, David was lying in a stiff corset, motionless in bed, with greatly weakened legs and some arm weakness.

Drawing on previous experience with dance for young children and experience with neuro-anatomical aspects of reflexes that regulate posture, we began gradually to expose him to all kinds of positions in space, such as holding him upside down with head on floor and tilting the torso, or walking with him, sitting on my arm in such a way that he had to struggle for balance. These activities evoked continuous automatic reactions and reflexes, activating the trunk to balance the body in all positions. We made him float in a Hubbard tank with the same aim.

My focus was on the restoration of shaping possibilities by restoring verticality, and the ability to support body-limb shaping from that verticality. This was in contrast to the more traditional focus on muscular activity without spatial reference.

After a few months, I put him one day in a sitting position in his crib. He did not fall over. His expression at this discovery was unforgettable. With trembling voice, he cried out, while slightly rocking, "I sit. I sit. I sit."

He was very intelligent and sensitive, with a sense of humor and the wisdom of a little old man. From that stage on, he became very cooperative. It took another ten months of work for his trunk to become sufficiently strong to consider bracing his legs for standing. At the end of that second winter, he began to walk with crutches and braces and, with a touching adult quality, he expressed his appreciation with affection and pride.

In the neurological wards of Bellevue Hospital, where I was exposed to neurological pathologies rather than only muscular dysfunction, the problems involved the control of movement patterns rather than the innervation of individual muscles. The appropriate functioning of the controls was visible in the quality of the movement sequences, which could be analyzed in terms of Laban's spatial and dynamic concepts. These identifications lent themselves to a different approach toward rehabilitation.

Total Therapy, Recreation, Learning Program for Children in Hospital

A second major experience in my education in physical and mental rehabilitation occurred when I was asked to reorganize and coordinate the whole program for children (ages 5 to 14 years) living in a hospital. This was at Blythdale Hospital, in Valhalla, N.Y., a small private institution for ortho-pedically and neurologically handicapped children. The medical director was David Gurewitsch, a physiatrist. He gave me the opportunity to develop a program coordinating every aspect of the handicapped child's long period of hospitalization. The concern was to achieve a balance between the therapeutic, the recreational and the learning experience of school. These children came either from other institutions where they had shorter periods of hospitalization or they came from homes where it was not possible to handle their care.

There was one group of boys (7 to 12 years), for example, who were afflicted with a hip bone deterioration that could only be cured by keeping these children off their feet for eighteen to twenty-four months. They had very little discomfort from this condition and no warning pain; they were able to walk, but forbidden to do so. The frustration and rebellion were naturally tremendous and supervision to keep them in bed very difficult.

No treatment was given; their beds were pulled into the schoolroom and the recreation facilities from the wards several times during the day. They were extremely restless and many of them became unable to concentrate on school work or on arts and crafts.

We started to translate active games with balls and baseball bats into sitting games that would, however, give the boys a physical workout. We involved the recreational workers and ambulatory patients. After a while, they began to participate in the art therapy group and began to paint and sculpt.

We also did vigorous bed exercises with dynamic movement sequences, such as thrusts, twists, heavy pulling. Labananalysis suggested subtle changes pinpointed to specific needs.

The younger children presented special problems. The younger they were, the more terrifying the deterioration and regressions: They lost their ability to play with toys or with each other; they could no longer listen to stories — all the things a normal 4- to 6-year-old would do. Instead, they withdrew or became very destructive, breaking toys and other things offered to them.

Gradually, we involved nurses, volunteers who became special friends of individual children, and the art and occupational therapists whose work we helped develop. A variety of stimulating activities was devised, including dancing in bed with props that the children had made themselves. Especially with the younger group, it became apparent that cutting off the possibilities of movement was like cutting off life itself.

Three examples from this young age group are described below. In each case, Labananalysis served as a connection to diagnosis and treatment of the physical and emotional problems.

1. John X. had been afflicted with polio two years before. In addition to severe paralysis in both legs, he had a very severe hearing problem due to a malformation of his outer ear, and, as a result, had inarticulate speech. (In later childhood, that was to be surgically corrected.)

John was five years old when I met him in Blythdale. His afflictions cut him off in many ways from communicating with adults and playmates. He was a passionate, tense, intelligent child, who walked with two long leg braces and crutches, determined to get places.

In the physical therapy treatment room, we would take off the braces, exposing him to the possibility of using his whole body to explore all kinds of ways to get around, using space, his body weight, different dynamics. He was most inventive and determined; he managed to climb a ladder, pulling himself up by his arms. He was, in his determination to move, nearly fearless, using even the trace function (scattered single muscle fiber activity) of his legs.

Again, there was an emphasis on total shaping and total mobility. Even when there is severe disability, with scattered gaps in function, the aim must always be to reorder the fragmented patterns into a new whole from which new potentialities can evolve. The process itself had the clues, not just end positions.

We then exposed him to the playground to try activities with his braces, unlocking the kneelock so he had more freedom with his legs. He climbed in and out of carts, over a fence. With locked braces, he walked up and down steep inclines. He began to be happier and, through speech therapy which he pursued with the same intensity, he was able to make himself better understood and could participate with other children in activities. He formed a close relationship with one of the male recreation workers who supported all this daring activity.

2. Although a very different approach is required in the treatment of spastics, we had the same aim — emphasizing the re-ordering of fragments into a functional whole. At Blythdale, there was a boy four years old, born with mild hemiplegia which moderately affected his coordination on his whole left side. He wore a short leg brace and walked precariously balanced, frequently falling. The challenge here was to make him aware of the whole semiparalyzed body half and to improve hand function as part of a restored sense of the whole body and body image with the awareness of right and left body halves as parts of that whole.

7

He had a restless temperament and was always "on the go." In kindergarten, his attention span was extremely short; when playing with doll house furniture, he would shift from one toy to another, fingering the parts rather aimlessly. When one or two parts dropped to the floor, he would sit down on the floor and continue his chaotic activities.

We found a way to coordinate the two body halves by using a bimanual pulley set, with weights attached to it, fixed to the wall. This set had to be operated by building up total body resistance to it. He had to grasp a handle in each hand and then walk away from the wall pulling the weights while maintaining a regular alternating stepping pattern. He was immediately fascinated by the device and tried it in more than one way, changing the units of weights, letting himself be pulled by the weights without losing his grip with both hands or the connection of his legs to the floor in order to prevent his falling.

We worked his arms with spatial figures-of-8, guiding both arms simultaneously as he was lying on the floor. To my surprise, his interest was sustained and he enjoyed it. It was, he said with a smile, "like dancing."

This introduced the rotary element of his arm socket, not only in the simultaneous symmetrical use of the arms, but also in asymmetrical use. Next we let him use the weak hand for the simple cranks that opened and closed the windows. It took only a few weeks to get him to turn a regular doorknob with the weak hand. His gait had considerably improved.

One of the most dramatic changes with this new awareness of his body and his space was seen in his play. We found him in the playroom with the same set of doll furniture he had been given previously. He now related to the whole set: He placed the table in the middle and arranged chairs around it. He set the doll on one chair and changed the arrangement in various ways, always relating parts to each other.

To summarize: In order to re-awaken awareness of *both* body halves, we concentrated on developing his sense of his own total body weight in motion. The first step was to develop his double grip on the heavy pulleys. In order to pull, he had to walk back, which involved alternating right and left weight shifts, a dynamic use of the impact of his weight throughout his body, and countertensions into the floor — altogether transporting his total body shape. The figure-of-8 exercises with his arms guided by the therapist, developed his sense of the reach space around his body (his kinesphere) and, therefore, new spatial intents could be stimulated. As a result, he had more control over organizing the space around him and the objects he dealt with in space.

3. Another boy, age four, had a spastic paralysis of both lower limbs. He used excessive free flow and was inclined to a passive giving into weight with almost no intent in space. He was actually close to standing and walking with crutches. But he would always collapse after two steps, often with tears, sometimes with hysterical laughter.

When the opportunity to work with him for a few weeks was given to me, I recognized that his problem had more to do with motivation than with function disability. Therefore, a program had to be devised that would, in a sense, distract him from his physical disabilities, by getting him to use his body in ways that were more available to him. His emotional temperament seemed to make him receptive to dramatic play. We played circus where he had, for example, to use a broad stance, a sense of his weight into the floor, controlling flow as well as indulging in flow, and other ranges of dynamics. He was the bear walking on his hind legs, the roaring lion, bouncing and leaping onto his prey, a clown balancing. He got involved with his roles and found his balance; his ability to walk improved on his own initiative. His earlier falls had been partially motivated by a wish to be picked up and supported by the therapist. As, on his own initiative, he discovered new strengths in his physical capabilities, he became increasingly able to let go of the therapist.

All the physical handicaps of these children were additionally affected by the regressive emotional influences of the hospital itself. This was particularly devastating to the lives of the children between four and ten, and especially the age group four to six, which was the youngest in the hospital.

Hospitalization in that early childhood period is particularly traumatic because normally that is such an active period full of new challenges to action. In addition, the young patients felt not only physically, but emotionally torn apart because of their separation from casual interplay with other children and the steady reassurance from family life.

Imagination, initiative, social development was suspended with their movement stasis. The hospital milieu, with the limitations of its emotional and physical quality, exacerbated patients' disabilities.

My task, defined for me by this climate of stasis and regression, was to find ways of keeping alive the movement impulse — the root of all development of a thinking, feeling, acting human being. This problem has continued to remain central to all my work with the emotionally disturbed and dealing with it is the key to dance therapy.

In Blythdale, the problem was particularly difficult because the movement impulse had been damaged by functional disability. Because I had to coordinate total programs for the patients, simultaneous attention had to be directed to both the movement impulse and the emotional climate; their dependence on each other became the most important factor.

It was necessary to find methods to deal with specific physical dysfunction from both anatomical and emotional orientations. The natural action potential involved innate curiosity, a desire to change, the discovery of alternate ways of functioning, relating to others, taking initiative, resisting, asserting — all in both physical and emotional modes — and, especially, enjoying play.

Here, again, the application of Laban's movement process concepts, his vocabulary for observation and his analysis of dance as behavior provided the tools to link the physical and expressive aspects of the problems and treat them as a unity.

Early Dance Therapy
All through my years in physical rehabilitation, I had kept my contact with dance and actors' movement, working individually and in small groups with modern dancers and young acting students.

My introduction into dance therapy was an "accident" similar to those of other pioneering colleagues. I replaced a musician-dancer in the Day Hospital Unit of Jacobi Hospital in the Bronx. The Day Hospital Unit was still in its first year and had already incorporated dance therapy.

Israel Zwerling, a psychiatrist, then the director of the Day Hospital, and at the same time Professor of Social Psychiatry at the Albert Einstein Medical College in the Bronx, was very receptive to further exploration of dance as a therapeutic tool for defusing aggression and anxiety. What particularly reinforced his interest in me was that I brought with me a vocabulary and a notation for recording observations of movement. This became a vital factor in daily observations through the one-way screen, especially of family and therapeutic groups. I stayed for the next six years with the developing Day Hospital.

In the second year, Zwerling brought me my first dance therapy trainee, Martha Davis, then a college student. We collaborated for several years exploring and developing observation techniques and specifically using the Labananalysis vocabulary as a tool. Now a clinical psychologist, Davis has become one of the leading researchers in movement behavior, founding the Institute for Nonverbal Communication Research in 1978.

What excited Zwerling about the Laban vocabulary was its ability to describe many aspects of non-verbal behavior in its own "movement" terms. In fact, like Laban he constantly warned against using psychiatric jargon before this non-verbal level was fully explored.

In collaboration with Martha Davis, working with patients, observing individuals and groups, using Laban concepts, an approach to dance therapy evolved that was both personal and objective.

9

What became increasingly apparent was the value of the inherent structure of dance as a regulating power that could free the patient to express feelings, build relationships, and change attitudes toward living.

Our therapeutic evaluations were implemented as we expanded the focus on the immediate patient-therapist involvement to include observations, through the one-way screen, of the patient's movements in group therapy sessions. In many cases, my own relationship to the patient or group of patients was clarified by this added objective view.

We worked closely with the art therapist, and in weekly staff meetings, we all reported on our work. The art therapist's report complemented our Labananalysis. These reports showed the development during the week in terms of shifting dominances, conflicts between male and female, the specific focus on one particular patient as part of the group. Taking into account individual differences among the patients in their inclinations toward one art form or another, we observed that, during the course of a patient's hospital stay, there were shifts at various stages of their recoveries, toward either art or dance. These shifts would reflect the level of their activity or passivity and were consistent with their behavior in life situations.

Description of Day Hospital Setup

There were never more than twenty-five patients at a time in active therapy. They were all short-term "day" patients (from six weeks to three months). The total population was a mixed group — men and women of greatly varied ages and ethnic backgrounds.

The program stressed all-around activity and was oriented toward patient functioning in the outside community by connecting patient to family and both to the community. It was one of the first groups in New York to encompass school, church, and other training activities in the rehabilitation of the mentally ill. It was also a first training center for family therapy, providing young psychiatrists with family and social orientation programs for patients.

A strong emphasis at the Day Hospital was placed on minimizing the hospital atmosphere. The whole hospital unit was concentrated on one floor of a Public Health building and thus moved away from the central Jacobi Hospital. None of the staff wore uniforms or white coats; they became indistinguishable from the patients, who came in the morning around 9 a.m. and left for home around 5 p.m.

The mid-day meal was brought in from Jacobi Hospital. Nursing staff and patients had this meal together, frequently preparing special dishes and desserts and sharing in all the preparatory activities and cleaning up.

All the rooms on that floor were rather small and used for more than one purpose by the patients. There was an arts and crafts room, used primarily by the art therapist, but also used for some handicrafts activities that were spontaneously and informally developed by the nurses and patients. One room became a beauty parlor, organized by a volunteer grooming expert who was assisted by patients. Because this volunteer was extremely sensitive and observant, she often established close relationships with patients and the "grooming" became a factor in the total therapy. The volunteer came to all the weekly staff meetings and often added significantly to the observations of other staff members. She was an excellent example of the great resources the paraprofessional can bring to the field.

Another small room, used primarily by the men, contained a pool table, record player and a piano. A third room, the so-called "day room," had some chairs and couches and was shared by everyone. It was wide open on three sides, directly accessible to the two elevators, sunny in the morning, and near the smells and clatter of the kitchen. On the other side was a corridor leading to a row of small offices for the doctors and social workers.

This day room was our dance therapy room. Often, it was crowded with the ping-pong table which had to be dismantled before our session. The sessions, once or twice a week, were scheduled between the group therapy and the midday meal. It was the day and hour during which the art therapist would see individual patients; her group mural meetings were scheduled for other mornings.

Because of the informal, "non-hospital" climate of the Day Hospital, art and dance therapy were "open" activities. They were offered; patients were invited, but not forced to come. Since the staff-patient relationships were close, the patients were often persuaded to join. Sometimes patients came out of boredom or curiosity.

The openness of the room, with the elevators spilling any visitor into the area and the general informal atmosphere of the ward, limited intensity of interaction and prevented lying down on the floor. (Later, in other setups, we realized even more how important the floor work is.) In short, the situation here was one that many dance therapists still face when they start dance therapy in a hospital. Gradually, the situation improves as the potentialities of dance therapy are more appreciated by hospital staffs, from administration to doctors.

We, however, did have full cooperation of the entire staff. In spite of the physical limitations of the setup, we were able to develop important aspects of group dance in this experimental situation. And, we encountered the patients informally almost daily.

Dance Therapy Sessions
The sessions lasted about forty-five minutes to an hour.

They began and ended informally, in keeping with the general atmosphere. There may have been some conversation going on in the day room, or individuals sitting and reading, sewing or knitting, when we put a record on the record player. We often selected a waltz or a lively folk tune for the first record.

There was no fixed structure. The therapist had to sense the general mood of the ward or the group that happened to come on a particular day. Eventually, the dance sessions were scheduled after group therapy sessions. Thus, our dance sessions were tuned toward group moods and group cohesiveness. So, also, was the art therapy that worked primarily on group murals.

A "ground rhythm" would often appear in a group mood and the sessions most often seemed to grow from it. This could be communicated in a circle formation, which, in a casual, easy way would mobilize the flow of group rhythm. One or both of the therapists would invite people to join as we started body mobilizing in general within the circle.

Gradually, a theme would be introduced — possibly picked up from a group member — and played with in various ways. It might be built up through group action or by a suggestion, that might also come from a group member, to transform it.

Usually, the circle would remain; it is an almost organic expression of non-aggressive relationship. Everyone sees everyone else and the joining of hands relates people and aids the experience of streams of movement energy spreading from one to the other. Sometimes, the streams would build to a soaring synchrony; sometimes, they would fall apart or divide into subgroups; sometimes, the circle would not be restored.

Some people came with the expectation of social dancing, breaking the circle immediately into couples or, while the circle was kept, one or two couples would dance outside of it. Sometimes, we would surround them and gradually intermix them with the rest of the group, but it could also happen that the whole session turned into a couples dance which reflected the erotic heterosexual tension existing in the whole ward. Other times, we might see the opposite: the males and females splitting and either group seeking domination of the other. Such general group moods might last several weeks until the discharge of one patient or addition of some new patients changed the climate. What we used primarily was the infectiousness of rhythm and the mobilizing elements of movement. Since there were two of us as therapists, who had quite different dynamics, it became possible to work

11

within the group specifically with either a hyperactive or a very depressed, non-moving patient to gradually assimilate him or her into the group.

We seldom talked about the movement experience itself. Instead, we transmitted movement through having one of us direct a particular theme from one patient to another while the second therapist maintained a group rhythm. A session that began this way might end in a tightly woven chain that would dance through the whole ward, picking up whoever they met on the way. These were the roaring endings. There were other sessions where the rhythm energy seemed to completely peter out, where people would leave or wander in and out, where a full unison was never reached.

Although there were some individual sessions, our focus was on the individual in the group. From the dancing together, we picked up subtle and crude clues and they defined the course the session would take as the two dance therapists acted as catalysts and leaders in shifting roles according to the momentary needs of the group.

The dance sessions became a hospital community activity as some of the nursing staff would bring in their most withdrawn or depressed or their most restless patients. The presence of the nurse made these patients feel easier as part of the group, and in some instances, when they were new, the patient's relationship to the nurse could be more easily established. Sometimes, one of the young psychiatrists would bring his patient and move with the group, establishing a different level of relationship outside the psychiatric confrontation.

Case Histories:* Some Crucial Sessions

Case No. 1: A young professional dancer who had had several hospitalizations for "nervous breakdown." She was attracted and repelled by the dance sessions, her moods extremely volatile. After a few sessions of just "being around," she participated.

She danced herself into wild abandon, tears streaming down her delicate face. The wild quality was characterized by highly exaggerated Suddenness (Time Effort) and unlimited acceleration in tempo, abrupt changes from extreme Free Flow (Effort) into short-lived Boundness (Effort).

Though her professional training and her dance talent remained quite recognizable, the exaggerated drive of the Effort elements seemed to fragment the spatial shape of her movement. The high intensity was followed after a short while by near collapse. I had used lively folk music. She was about to collapse when I took hold of her and, supporting her, kept her in the dance circle, repeating over and over: "Keep listening. This rhythm carries you. You can use it to feel calm."

She did stay and began to change the hectic quality of her movement. By the end of the session, she had calmed herself to the extent that she could talk about her fear of losing herself, of going crazy. She said that this had been a good experience. She came to a few more sessions in which this experience repeated itself with lessened exaggeration of Effort and greater cohesiveness of shape.

Many weeks later, after she was discharged, I received a letter from her in which she referred to this experience as a start of a changed attitude toward her dancing and herself.

Case No. 2: A young man in his twenties came to the Day Hospital. He had just gone through a severe catatonic state in another institution. He still showed some of the physical manifestations of the catatonic: The expressionless mask-like face, the peculiar waxen immobility of the limbs and torso which occasionally shifted with amazing radical changes into positions that defied gravity. For instance, when throwing a ball, after the thrust, he would appear to stay suspended mid-air without falling.

I began to move with him without using music — simple movements such as lifting the arms, bending over — and he followed in his sluggish, waxen way. In Labananalysis terms these catatonic

---

* *Case histories will include some Labananalysis vocabulary which is explained in detail in later pages.*

12

manifestations can be described as an almost absolutely Neutral Flow (Effort) with complete absence of fluctuations between Bound and Free and of other clearly defined Effort qualities. The shape and space awareness seem to be reduced to simple flexion and extension movements with no visible intent. Then I made him use a wide stance, spreading the arms at the same time. He seemed to keep on spreading. His wide stance was melting like wax. He was heading for a split on the floor.

Since he weighed more than 180 pounds, I could not support or pull him. I yelled at him while holding his hands: "Charles, stamp, stamp! Charles, stamp, stamp!" And I myself started a stamping rhythm. The percussion of my movement seemed to reach him. He lifted one leg, then the other, and got into a veritable cannonade of stamping the floor, during which he lost the overall waxen quality of his body and, particularly, in his face.

He stopped himself, looked at me with full eye contact, and said, "I see your face for the first time. I am glad."

As the other members of the group came into the room, he joined them, smiling, and finished the session with us. That same afternoon, he was reported to have joined the kitchen crew and other activities of the afternoon. During the next few days he started to talk and to make friends, relating to a number of people in the ward. From time to time, particularly in physical game activities, remnants of the waxy quality could be detected. But the overall improvement continued.

Case No. 3: A discharged patient came to work with me for an individual session. She was a rather unattractive girl, almost masculine in body build and musculature. Originally she was in a hyper-active and excited state but she had calmed down during her several weeks stay and had liked the dance sessions.

On this particular day, she seemed unresponsive and resistive to movement. All of a sudden — and it may not have been all of a sudden, perhaps I just failed to notice the signs — she seized a billiard cue from a table next to her and tried to attack me.

I managed to seize the stick with both hands; we became locked into each other. I began to respond to her pushing, pressing quality by a Sustained (Time Effort), Strong (Weight Effort), Indirect (Space Effort) rhythm, with slight fluctuations in the components. Several minutes passed in this locked, strong encounter.

I had no intention of yanking the stick out of her hands. In a dim way, I held on to the intent of dancing with her. She finally dropped the stick very suddenly on the floor, exclaiming with a broad smile, "That was some workout. I am tired. I feel fine." We parted on friendly terms.

It could seem an almost pointless story, but it, in fact, taught me something crucial about intent and transforming an aggressive tension by gradually dissolving its Effort elements from fighting to indulging qualities.

This principle could be observed in the work of one of the male aides on the ward, who practiced it spontaneously. He was of slight build and had more flexible agility than massive, weighty strength.

Many times he calmed the destructive movements of an excited patient by countering them with a similar but nonaggressive tension and a non-challenging multi-directional shaping rather than with aggressive one-directional poking-type movements. This kind of transformation of tension is at the heart of dance and, through observation training of the Labananalysis components, can be applied to other disciplines.

It is difficult to gauge the effects of such moments of crisis with their after-effects of changed behavior on more than one level. The moments are not always verbally acknowledged (and this should not be forced) by the patient himself, although they appear to create profound impressions. While some verbalization may occur, the integration may be more observable on the non-verbal body level, with accompanying changes in the total response of the organism. With variables on so many levels, one can rarely attribute the patient's condition to a single isolated factor.

13

The critical episodes, which are often spontaneous total responses of the patient, are like moments of truth on the level of the whole organism. Sometimes there are temporary remissions afterward (less often, permanent ones), but if the movements of those moments are appropriately analyzed, they can be restructured — again, in terms of physical movements — in various ways to lead back to the possible near-repetition of the total physical and emotional response.

Family Therapy and Group Therapy Observations
Another aspect of our work at the Day Hospital was to attend family therapy sessions, in addition to the group therapy sessions. Dr. Zwerling was the therapist at these family sessions. He was particularly interested in our explorations of the use of Labananalysis in family therapy research that would relate individual behavior to family process and interactions.

Observations of all participants and the therapist were made through the one-way screen and were recorded with notes and a taped verbal record.

For example, the family of an adolescent boy patient met with the therapist. The boy was completely withdrawn and passive. In the first two sessions, there seemed to be no reaction from him to either of his parents or the therapist.

The doctor felt that the boy seemed to be inaccessible to him. The observers, however, were able to show that, in fact, the boy was reacting to the doctor. The boy appeared completely impassive; the adjustments he made in turning to the therapist seemed to be an indistinguishable Free Flow (Effort) with no other clear dynamics. However, in small hand gestures, addressed to the doctor, Time (Effort) and Weight (Effort) and Bound Flow (Effort) would appear. At the same time, nothing was happening with him in relation to his parents.

These observations alerted the doctor to an aspect of his relationship with the patient that the patient had previously been successful in concealing. By addressing himself, even in these subtle ways, to the doctor, the patient was revealing the beginning of trust. Subsequently, the participation of the boy increased and exposed more of his relationship with the doctor, and, in time, with his parents.

Our research in observations of group behavior developed especially from these early experiences with family therapy. Martha Davis and I gradually evolved a graphic presentation of the trends of interaction during a session. For larger groups, we needed more observers, and with simple, rather crude devices, we became able to reconstruct the main features of the sessions and present a picture of the main exchanges and interrelationships. Other dance therapists, particularly Elissa White and Claire Schmais, assisted us in this; it was an important learning experience for us all. (Later developments in group analysis and dance therapy are discussed in Chapters 8 and 9.)

The Day Hospital Experience: An Evaluation
In retrospect, this experience was a crucial test for the potential of our Labananalysis background. It enabled us to use our skills over wide ranges of adaptations to different therapeutic situations, with clear distinctions of levels of patients' illnesses and differences between individual and group sessions.

For the short-term patients of the Day Hospital already on the way to rejoin the community, our loosely structured groups allowed for different degrees of socially acceptable forms of behavior that could still be compatible in a diversified group. This mobilized the individuals and exposed them to varied dynamics which released feelings and elicited readiness to form relationships.

Many patients coming out of a psychosis will work toward functioning within a structure. Dance therapy reinforced test structures such as links to other family or friendship or work structures. Sometimes, even unsuccessful groups, seemingly fragmented in mood and action, proved to help a patient establish his/her own role in the group structures and to form relationships with other patients and the therapist.

Another important value of the Day Hospital was the opportunity to develop our observation skills as dance therapists. That reinforced our abilities to think and feel in movement, thus reacting to the patient's movement language directly and specifically in the same language, without immediate analysis.

The separate periods of observation — observing and notating simultaneously — heightened our sensitivity to many shades of movement all the time. We learned to recognize and identify behavior quickly — both the patient's and the therapist's. The body exposed resistance, manipulation, ingratiation, persuasion, domination, seduction and control, as well as emotions such as despair or fear, for example, and many of the components of such expressions could be objectively recorded in movement terms with the Labananalysis vocabulary.

Even though the sessions were uneven and unpredictable, the weekly descriptions of them served as very sensitive barometers of the moods of the group during that particular week. In the absence of fixed structures, the therapist had to be very finely attuned to fluctuations of mood in order to make the necessary adaptations to and around them. The therapist's own physical adaptation could precede recognition of the concomitant emotional adaptations. Even during sitting and talking periods, physical adaptations and observations of the body movement could be developed into dance structures revealing deep behavioral roots.

Not all changes that occur through the exposure to dance therapy are of crisis character. Many changes come about gradually; sometimes the immediate effect of the movement response is difficult or impossible to trace. As the observation skills of the therapist become increasingly sophisticated and refined, recognition and adaptations can be made more acutely.

At Bronx State Hospital, there was also the opportunity to develop early applications of Labananalysis to therapy for severely retarded adolescents and adults. Adaptations of Bartenieff Fundamentals provided points of departure for elementary movement experiences that could be adapted to the individual patient's level even in group sessions. Work with the aged was also beginning here.

Today, opportunities for observation are increased by videotaped sessions, where the patient can be observed in a variety of situations and the tapes can be viewed in various comparative sequences. When these observations are communicated through the Labananalysis vocabulary of the movement itself, therapist and doctor can be alerted to patterns of behavior that are not otherwise accessible to them.

Dance therapy in clinical setups is, of course, only a part of the whole framework of therapies — verbal, non-verbal (including arts, music as well as dance). Unless communication between disciplines is well developed, there is rarely a clear picture of the whole process of recovery. It is vital to recognize at any given level of the process, that it is only one aspect of the total multi-level process.

Furthermore, the distinctions between healthy and unhealthy physical and mental behavior have many degrees of gradation and are not necessarily the same for all cultures. For that reason, also, it is important to establish maximum communication between many different disciplines to arrive at reliable assessments of human behavior.

Labananalysis can be approached three ways: through study of the body structure and morphology, through study of the paths and spatial tensions of the movements available to the body, and through study of Effort — the attitudes of the mover in relation to space, weight, time and flow.

The observer needs to have a familiarity with the basic components of all three approaches in order to follow the process of continuously changing interrelationship between them. Distinctions of functional and expressive appropriateness to the intent of the mover are revealed in the process itself rather than in the conclusions (end positions) of movement.

The next chapters will deal with each of the three — body, space, Effort — individually, and then follow with chapters that describe their interdependency.

Body, space, Effort components could all be expressed in Labanotation, which makes it possible to make notes, at shorthand speed, that explicitly identify interrelationships. Because of the training required to read notation, we have chosen to use only verbal descriptions in this book. However, we refer the reader to the Appendix A, Documentation, and to the Bibliography for an indication of how powerfully the notation is woven into the whole of Labananalysis.

CHAPTER 2

The Body Architecture

We should be able to do every imaginable movement and then select those which seem to be the most suitable and desirable for our own nature. These can be found only by each individual himself. For this reason, practice of the free use of kinetic and dynamic possibilities is of the greatest advantage. We should be acquainted both with the general movement capacities of a healthy body and mind and with the specific restrictions and capacities resulting from the individual structure of our own bodies and minds.

Rudolf Laban

Joggers © Bonnie Freer
Man in front: body holding back with Bound Flow.
Unclear spatial intent.
Woman: most clearly sagittal. Clear spatial intent
forward. Free Flow. Postural.
3770: giving in to weight in concave shape with
Neutral Flow, some Bound Flow countertension in
arms. Sagittal inclination. Man to right of 3770:
narrowing of whole body in almost vertical
inclination. Light Weight/Bound Flow.

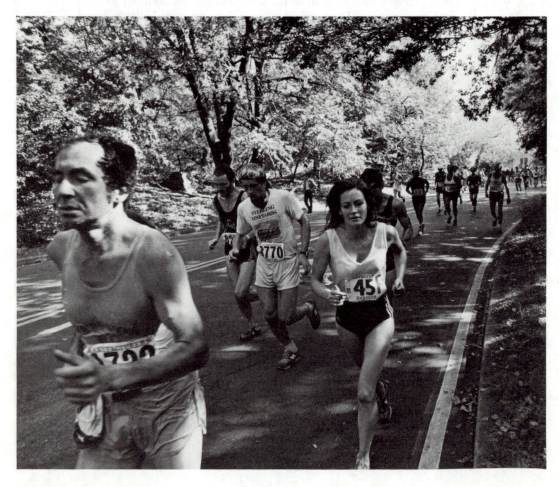

The Body Architecture

Modern living conditions have so reduced the physical demands for survival — even walking is minimally necessary — that the ability to respond fully and instantly to any physical demand has deteriorated to an extreme degree.

As awareness of this impoverishment and its relationship to mental and physical health begins to occur, people rush desperately into all kinds of activity that is sometimes more harmful than helpful because of the mover's basic ignorance of how bodies function and, therefore, how to discriminate among the options that are offered. Important and potentially dangerous aspects of prescribed movements are often overlooked. In general, movement programs are so goal-oriented that the internal and external *processes* of movement are largely ignored. It is one thing to look at all the body parts in an autopsy. Quite another to see them in motion.

Figure 1 will serve as a reminder to the observer of basic components of the body that can be used as reference points in the observation of body movement. More details are shown in the Appendix along with the specific exercises of Bartenieff Fundamentals.

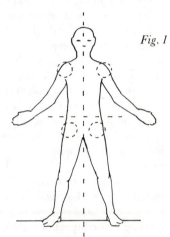

Fig. 1

The lower unit is comprised of
LowerBack/Lower Abdomen
Pelvis/Hip/Thigh/Lower Leg/Foot/Toes
The lower unit, as initiator of the center of weight, essentially serves locomotor activity (the transport of body weight) and postural changes (the support of body weight).

The upper unit is comprised of
Head/Neck
Chest/Upper Spine
Shoulder Joint/Scapula
Arm/Forearm/Wrist/Hand/Fingers

The upper unit essentially serves exploring, manipulating, gesturing activities. It initiates and extends reach space, communicates through spatial gesture, body touch, grasp, enveloping, dispersing, intertwining.

Basic Components of the Body

The observer also sees the body as two halves, right and left and/or as trunk plus segments, and becomes skillful at making fine distinctions about the particular segments involved in a movement.

In the skeleton, the flexibility of the spine is crucial to all torso movement. Also essential to movement and centering is the awareness of the spine's length from the coccyx deep in the pelvic area to the upper (cervical) spinal vertebrae which, to the surprise of many people, go all the way through the neck to the base of the head.

Joints connect the bones. We will deal primarily with two kinds: global (ball and socket) joints which permit movement in all directions and hinge joints which can only move back and forth in one direction. There are two sets of global joints. They connect the limbs to the trunk: one set is where the arms connect to the shoulders and the other set is where the legs connect to the hips (pelvis). All the other joints are hinge joints or modifications of hinge joints. The wrists and ankles are combinations of the two-range joints.

The muscles, connected to the joints, make it possible for the body segments to move around the joints. They always operate in pairs: As one muscle contracts, the other relaxes. The relaxing muscles are like scaffolds; they allow the graded use of the opposing group. There are surface muscles which

19

can be seen and felt externally and there are deep muscles which are not visible. In many cases, there is an overdependence on the external muscles to the neglect of important deep muscles, and this results in limited continuity in the flow of movement that is indicative to the skilled observer of otherwise hidden problems. Continuity is maintained by the relationship of breathing to awareness of muscular connections, not just as mechanical devices, but as kinetic chains, total configurations. In Labananalysis, these are observed with relation to spatial shaping possibilities and the dynamic qualities (Effort) accompanying them.

Bartenieff Fundamentals* were developed to provide exercises for the experience of the body in motion with an awareness of how and why it is moving.

There are six basic exercises and innumerable variations and extensions of them. The six are considered basic because they are applicable to all activity in that they are concerned with the internal support of the body as it develops into uprightness. In that sense, therefore, they are concerned with centering, that is, being able to connect with the source of one's strength (support) even when in motion so that balance is maintained in all activity.

The exercises are deceptively simple. From the starting position of lying on the floor the mover is asked to 1) Lift the thigh and return it to its original position; 2) Lift the hips off the floor, shift the pelvis forward, and return to original position; 3) Lift the hips off the floor, shift the pelvis to the side and return to original position; 4) Keeping flat on floor, bend one side of the body and then the other side; 5a) With knees flexed, feet on floor, drop the knees to one side and then the other; 5b) Repeat 5a and involve arms so that there is a diagonal pull between dropped knee and its opposite arm; 6a) Extend arm movement of No. 5 so that it circles the mover's body on the floor; 6b) Extend 6a with repetitions that build momentum to bring the mover to sitting position.

However, in each case, the action of the exercise is presented in the context of its specific purpose, its desirable experience, notes on possible misinterpretations, and its most obvious functional activity.

The simplest movement involves both ranges of one set of muscles: contraction and expansion in either forward/backward or right/left or twisting in or out movements (technically known, respectively, as flexion/extension, abduction/adduction, internal/external rotation).

Diagonal connections are made by combining in a variety of ways three muscle sets involved in three-dimensional movement.

Diagonal muscular connections in torso/limb movement and the spatial patterns they produce are of primary importance in the understanding of a) upright balance in standing; b) the large shaping patterns in work, sport, dance, etc.; c) how various forms of locomotion affect the rest of the body; d) the degree of involvement of upper vs. lower body in turns around various axes of the body; e) initiation in total body action, whether from upper or lower units or both at once; and f) the role and significance of the rotary element in the arms, legs and their segments, in the torso and in torso/limb combinations as they affect twists, turns, diagonal pathways, circular and rounded shapes.

The most efficient support comes from full use of the outer musculature of the pelvic floor, which is continuously pointed out in the course of the six basic exercises. This is also central to the later exercises that take the mover up from the floor and into increasingly complex uses of his/her body and all the variations possible with other combinations of Effort (attitude toward flow, space, weight, time), spatial paths, and shapes.

The exercises start on the floor close to the state of a newborn baby, who lacks locomotion. The emphasis is on relationship of body parts, awareness of the center of weight and how it relates to the initiation of action. There is a lot of seemingly formless stretching and continuous flexing initiated

---

*   *See Appendix B.*

20

with the inhalation and exhalation of breathing.

The body shape is constantly growing and shrinking; movements flow freely or become tightly patterned. The sensation of body weight is dominant in rolling around, which is the first attempt to transport the heaviest part of the body, the lower part. As the weight shifts, the upper part of the body accommodates the shifts with arms following and gradually beginning to define spatial goals.

Working through exercises on the floor minimizes the struggle with gravity and postpones much of the complex network of acting and reacting to the environment, other people, the space around, and other modifiers of the discharge of energy.

Breathing becomes identified with passage of air through the body's inner cavities — mouth, throat, chest — compressing and expanding the abdomen. The different degrees and ranges of the body's joints are explored and their roles as primary powers of controlling movement range are established.

A sense of the length, width and depth of the body will relate to the spatial patterns that can extend each dimension. The division of the body into upper and lower segments, right and left halves will develop into awareness of tensions and countertensions in their symmetrical and asymmetrical usage. Recognition of kinetic muscular chains — the sequence of muscles used in a movement — diminishes the exclusive dependence on individual muscle strength for movement power.

Bartenieff Fundamentals emphasize the internal connections that are key to dynamic rather than static movement as the newborn's movements develop to adult movements from lying on the floor to uprightness through crawling, sitting, standing, walking and increasingly complex spatial paths.

The anatomical analysis inherent in the development of Fundamentals grew out of the author's rehabilitation work with localized muscle/joint problems of the body. Labananalysis sharpened awareness of the interrelationships of muscle groups, such as hip/pelvis/leg and scapula/shoulder/ arm, because it related their functions to their spatial intents and shapes. Focusing always on constellations of movement elements rather than isolated articular elements led to new solutions of functional and, particularly, coordination problems — all of which directly affected the psycho-logical gestalt.

Many anatomists and movement professionals still define "upright posture" as a static mechanism. Laban defined it as dynamic. The static image is one of piling a series of bricks on top of each other along a vertical axis while being supported by lateral and sagittal forces in a fixed scaffold-like balance. The dynamic image is described by Laban as an ongoing, cohesive, three-dimensional process that creates and recreates a series of relationships of up/down, right/left, forward/backward. In fact, the whole body slightly sways while "standing still" in a figure-of-eight distribution of weight (center, forward, right side, backward, center, forward, left side, backward, center) in continuous subtle fluctuation between stability and mobility to maintain balance. The Fundamentals' concern with centering as the source of support is crucial here.

There are three major Labananalysis concepts that are the core of Bartenieff Fundamentals exercises. First, the emphasis is always on mobility process rather than just muscle strength. Second, in all movement — from the small isolated gesture to a major total action — more than one factor is operating. Third, spatial intent, preparation and initiation in a movement sequence determine the whole course of a sequence and the quality of its function and/or expressiveness.

Connectedness refers to the dynamic alignment of the weight-bearing structure, the skeleton, in movement as well as stillness. It allows the flow, the movement impulse, to pass through the body in such a way that complete activation can be realized most efficiently — without unnecessary exertion and stress. It is obvious enough to say that legs, arms and head are "linked" to the torso, the foot to the lower leg, the arm at the shoulder joint, etc., but their connectedness is more than muscles traveling over the joints to hook up two bones. It is the activated chains, configurations of connections that control the movement process. The detailed exercises and technical descriptions in the

Appendix will specifically illustrate these concepts and the connectedness required to apply them.

The skilled observer will, in preliminary observations, check off the following questions about the body parts in a particular movement:

Which parts are initiating the movement and what is the sequence of those that follow?

Are they initiated from the center or from the peripheral parts of the body?

Which parts are active or held?

To what extent are they involved with other parts?

Are the movements leading toward or away from the body center?

What configurations are formed?

What muscular chains are involved? What has been omitted?

Are the parts used simultaneously or sequentially?

Are they used symmetrically or asymmetrically?

How is the center of weight shifting or holding?

What support systems are operating to maintain centering balance throughout the total process?

How do they relate to the breathing process?

How is the body grounded?

It will be shown that specific research projects such as ethnic studies, for example, require selections from these and other movement observation parameters that are suitable to the project's particular designs. Such selections are, of course, most valuable when made from the context of a wide range of options.

CHAPTER 3

Carving Shapes in Space

Our body is constructed in a manner which enables us to reach certain points of the kinesphere with greater ease than others. An intensive study of the relationship between the architecture of the human body and its pathways in space facilitates the finding of harmonious patterns. Knowing the rules of the harmonic relations in space we can then control and form the flux of our motivity....

It is natural for all living organisms to use the simplest and easiest paths in space when fighting, not only when the fight is a matter of life and death, but also in other activities, since all working is a kind of fighting and struggling with objects and materials. Everywhere economy of effort is in evidence, including all kinds of bodily locomotion.

Rudolf Laban

Right: *Man Casting Net*
© Bonnie Freer
The dynamic action requires
many countertensions to maintain
stability. Almost suspended in
diagonal high/right/forward to
deep/left/back, with arm and leg
in countertension. Weight
counterhold on right knee and
diagonal tension of left arm. Free
Flow/Sudden/Direct Effort.

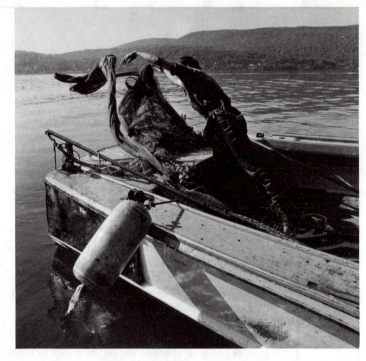

Below: *Face-To-Face* ©
Bonnie Freer
A sagittal contrast. Left advancing
in feet but trunk is rounding in
retreat, Right has total postural
advancing.

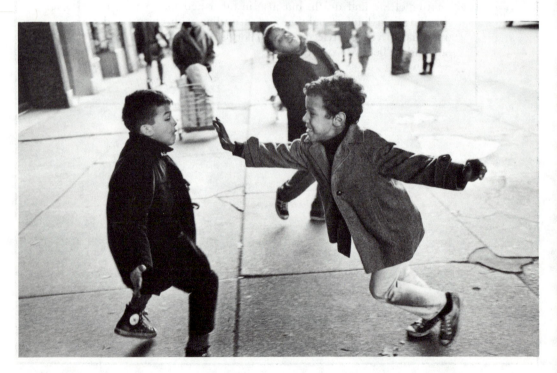

Carving Shapes in Space

The Kinesphere, Body Parts and Spatial Directions

The Kinesphere

The body is a three-dimensional structure. It has length, width, and depth — a length axis, a width axis, and a depth axis.

By extending the farthest reaches of the length, width and depth of the body in the upright position, a sense of the three-dimensional space around it is created. We call that reach space around the body the kinesphere. Gravity exerts the downward, earth pull, and with its opposite, upward, skyward pull, the length dimension along a vertical axis in space can be identified. Maintaining that vertical axis, we can also move forward/backward in the depth dimension along a sagittal axis and we can move limbs to the side or across to the other side in the width dimension along a horizontal axis in space. Each move elicits a particular spatial experience, the feeling of a pull in space that is delineated by its axis.

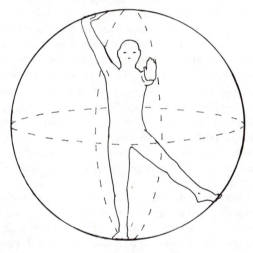

Fig. 2   *The Kinesphere*

Beyond the kinesphere the larger or general space can also be similarly perceived three-dimensionally. This perception of space outside our kinespheres alerts us to where we can transport our kinespheres.

Body Parts, Segments and Spatial Distinctions

The space available to the upright body can be considered as areas around particular body segments. The body segment centers are defined by the joints which link body parts together. Thus, there are large spatial areas around primary body-joint links — shoulders and hips — and smaller areas around finer joint links — elbow and fingers, for example. Articulation makes the space available to the body segments.

The major body segments (as described in the previous chapter) are head, upper limbs (arms) and lower limbs (legs) — all surrounding the torso, which consists of two major segments, the upper (chest and neck) and the lower (abdomen, lumbar region and pelvis).

From a stance (position with support primarily on leg or legs), the space available to a particular segment's movement is considered in two ways: the space available to the segment alone and the space available when other segments are also utilized. From that orientation, it is possible to identify five principal spatial zones of action: those of the head, the two zones of both arms and the two zones of both legs. The torso can also be considered as having its own zone.

When a ballerina, for example, from an upright position with both feet close together, lifts both arms forward and overhead, then spreads them to the side and gradually lowers them back to her starting position, she has delineated the spatial zone of the arms. When she lifts the right leg backward to waist height, then leads it around the body straight to the front, lowers it and places it next to the other foot on the floor, she has used the spatial zone for the right leg. When she simply circles her head around her neck as fully as possible, she has described the spatial zone of the head. When, from a standing position, she circles her torso from the hips as far as possible, she has described the spatial zone of the torso. When she adds any movement of the torso to the limb zones described above, the spatial zones of those limbs are expanded and become super zones.

The observations described in this chapter will deal almost exclusively with the major segments and zones rather than the smaller sub-segments. Smaller movements of sub-segments can, however, be considered as miniature spatial movements in miniature contexts similar to the larger movements. The context of each segment is defined by the range of its joints.

Where and how the body segment moves within its own spatial zone or, with the addition of the torso, into larger zones, is determined first by its structural possibilities and second, by the performer's intent in space.

The limbs, trunk and some segments are capable of bending, stretching, twisting.

Changes in constellations of limbs/trunk in place are position and level changes: lying, sitting, kneeling, standing or their modifications, crouching, squatting, leaning.

Locomotion — moving the kinesphere over a territory or general space — can be rolling, stepping, walking, running, leaping, somersaulting, cartwheeling and modifications such as crawling, creeping, strutting, dashing, sneaking.

The body or its limbs is always handling space in movement by either gathering it toward the body or scattering it away from the body or by some modification of those gestures that gather and scatter — movements of folding and unfolding, possessing and repulsing, sharing and excluding.

In Figure 3, the three levels of space are delineated in the spatial areas through which the body parts might move: High, medium and low.* High refers to the space at the height of the hands when they are raised above the head; medium is at the mid-height (waist) of the body; low is on or near the lower leg and the floor.

---

* *Low refers to level. Deep refers to direction.*

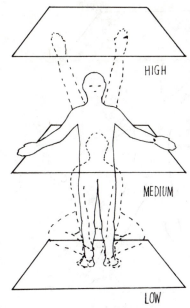

From the body center there are an infinite number of directions to move in. These can be organized according to twenty-six basic directions as follows:

a. Figure 4. On the vertical axis:
    (Up and down through the body center)
    upward direction: high (H)
    downward direction: deep (D)

b. Figure 5. Relating to the horizontal axis:
    (Towards the sides of the body)

Medium Level	**High Level**	**Low Level**
right (R)	right/high (RH)	right/deep (RD)
left (L)	left/high (LH)	left/deep (LD)

Fig. 3　　*Three Levels in Space*

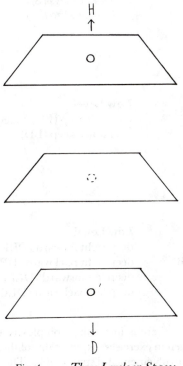

Fig. 4　　*Three Levels in Space: Vertical Directions*

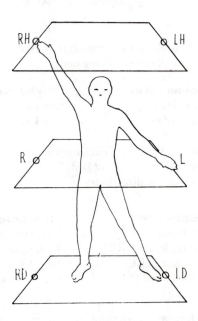

Fig. 5　　*Three Levels in Space: Horizontal Directions*

27

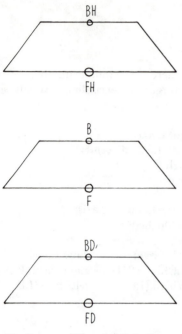

Fig. 6   Three Levels in Space:
            Sagittal Directions

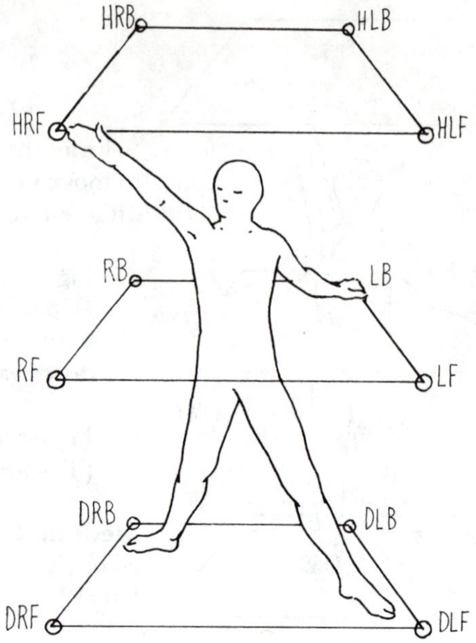

Fig. 7   Three Levels in Space:
            Oblique Directions

c. Figure 6. Relating to the sagittal axis:
    (In front of or behind the body)

Medium Level	**High Level**	**Low Level**
forward (F)	forward/high (FH)	forward/deep (FD)
backward (B)	backward/high (BH)	backward/deep (BD)

d. Figure 7. Relating to diagonal axes:
    (Through the center of body)
    Four oblique directions

Medium Level	**High Level**	**Low Level**
right forward (RF)	high right forward (HRF)	deep right forward (DRF)
right backward (RB)	high right backward (HRB)	deep right backward (DRB)
left forward (LF)	high left forward (HLF)	deep left forward (DLF)
left backward (LB)	high left backward (HLB)	deep left backward (DLB)

When levels and directions are combined in all these ways, there is increasing complexity in the tensions produced to balance their different spatial pulls. Even in exercises, explorations of them are never mechanical; they include the experience of total body involvement and spatial pulls. These will be discussed in greater detail throughout the book.

Spatial Progressions: Space Harmony Scales

Every move of limb-trunk or limbs-trunk or several limbs in space does not just reach an end position or create a static configuration. The moves are processes of radiation into space creating the kinaesthetic experience of spatial tensions. They are not mere lines of different design written into space; they reflect the condensations and expansions of body–muscle–spatial patterns. The shapes sculpted in the space are dependent on the physical structure of the body, especially the global joints connecting the limbs to the trunk, and the spinal mobility peculiar to each of the three dimensions.

"A movement makes sense only if it progresses organically," Laban wrote, "and this means that phases which follow each other in a natural succession must be chosen. It is, therefore, essential to find out the natural characteristics of the single phases which we wish to join together in order to create a sensible sequence."

From that hypothesis, Laban explored the various directional possibilities and organized them into sequences of progressions which he called scales. The ordering process became known as space harmony. The scales serve movement as musical scales serve music. They are structures ordered in time and space as points of reference for mobile shaping processes.

They are important to the movement researcher because they delineate in an ordered way basic options available to the mover. In conjunction with the other Labananalysis components, the observer learns to recognize patterns and variations indicative of appropriate function and distinctive behavior.

Some of the principal scales are illustrated below. Detailed descriptions of them appear later. They are related to geometrical forms which are like maps on which the scales are identified as specific routes.

The One-Dimensional or Defense Scale

The simplest of the scales is called the one-dimensional or defense scale. It is built around the axes of the three dimensions of the body: length, width and depth, and their corresponding axes in the space of the kinesphere: vertical, horizontal and sagittal.

In performing the scale, it is the vertical axis of the upright body experienced as a central pull, to which the horizontal axis is related with its right/left centrality, and the sagittal axis with its forward/backward centrality.

The sequence of the scale is ordered for the easiest shifting from one direction to another within each dimension and from one dimension to another. This is also true of all the different scales and related sequences as they become increasingly complex.

The core of the defense scale is the "cross of axes."

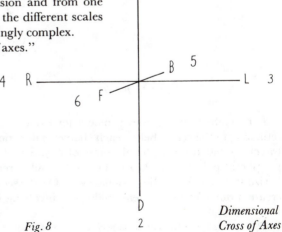

(Performer faces reader.)

Each change of direction is initiated by a return to the center.

Fig. 8

Dimensional Cross of Axes

29

This scale is an ordering of pulling/pushing sequences which change alternately between pushing away from and pulling toward the center of the body. Laban saw this order in training sequences of the ancient traditions in the martial arts of many cultures. Under the stress of survival, great precision in attack and defense actions was developed to protect vulnerable regions of the body in the most effective way. The inward-directed actions shield from attack; the outward-directed actions ward off attack. As weapons were added to the martial arts a more complex use of space was necessary.

The alternation between pushing and pulling goes from one directional range to the other in each dimension. For example, there is a push up and pull down; a push across and pull out; a pull backward and push forward. These are primary movements pulling toward the center or pushing away from the center of the three axes. The pull toward center increases stability; the move away from the center decreases stability, increases mobility in space. Variations of this pulling-pushing appear constantly in most movement tasks and gestures of communication. They can be delicate as well as extreme variations.

Two-Dimensional Movement: Planes and Cycles

Another sequence for using the space around the cross of axes is to move specifically from point to point of its six peripheral points *without* returning to the center. This sequence outlines the form of an octahedron.

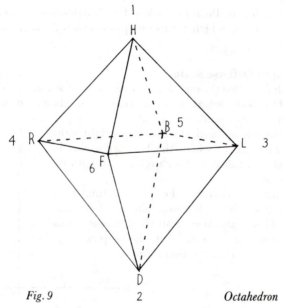

Fig. 9   2   *Octahedron*

The octahedron provides a model for exploring a number of different sequences. Instead of returning to the center before each change of direction, as in the defense scale, the movement might travel around the peripheral points of any two of the axes. For example, the sequence around peripheral points 1, 4, 2, 3 of Figure 9 would create a path, a cycle,* around the vertical and horizontal axes: a two-dimensional cycle. Or, the sequence around peripheral points 6, 4, 5, 3 would create a different two-dimensional cycle, involving horizontal and sagittal axes. Or, the sequence

---

* *The cycles circle around the diamond shape of the octahedron.*

30

around 6, 2, 5, 1 would create still another two-dimensional cycle, involving the sagittal and vertical axes. In the course of the cycle, there are brief moments of one-dimensionality which occur at the specific peripheral axes points 1 through 6. Part of the excitement of performing the cycles is this continuous losing and gaining of two-dimensionality.

Another form of two-dimensional movement is developed as cycles around the three planes available to the body reach from the three axes (see Figure 10). These can be perceived as circling three planes, which are identified as "door" (vertical and horizontal axes); "table" (horizontal and sagittal); "wheel" (sagittal and vertical).

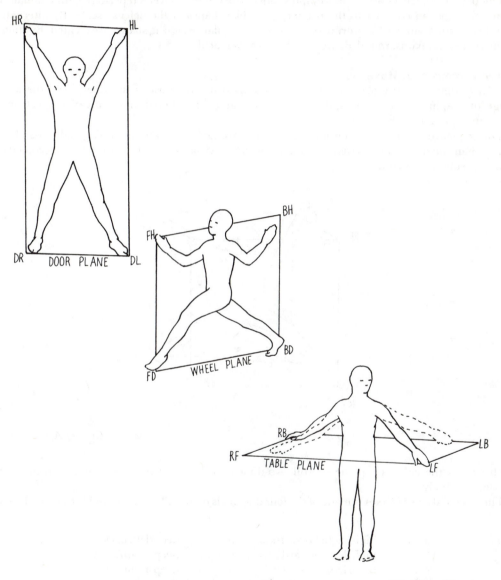

Fig. 10   The Three Planes

31

Because of the differences in flexibility of the spine in different segments and the range of the joints of the limbs, the planes are rectangular and the pull of one of the dimensions in each plane is dominant over the other. Thus, vertical movement is dominant over horizontal in the door plane, horizontal over sagittal in the table plane, and sagittal over vertical in the wheel plane.

These cycles share the excitement of the octahedron cycles in that there are continuously shifting pulls between different degrees of dominance of the two dimensions involved. However, in the octahedron cycle there are fleeting moments when the pulls are equal, but in the cycles developed around the planes, the pulls are never equal.

The planar sequences add more complex movements to the mover's repertoire with angular and rounded shapes in contrast to the primary stick-like shapes of the defense scale. By alternating peripheral paths with paths returning to the center, angular or zig-zag shapes are created. By staying in the peripheral paths, rounded, arc-like shapes are created.

Three-Dimensional Movement

It is three-dimensional movements that offer the most inclusive use of the kinesphere, the widest range of shaping possibilities, and therefore, the largest functional and expressive spectrum of maximum mobility.

The sequences for three-dimensional movement are developed around a diagonal cross of axes rather than the dimensional cross of axes. They can be visualized with relation to the geometrical form of a cube as in Figure 11.

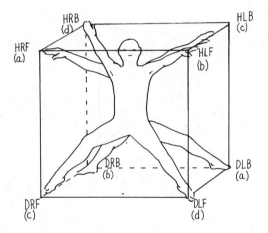

Fig. 11   *Diagonal Cross of Axes in Cube*

Each side of the cube is a plane — still two-dimensional — but now surrounding, rather than dividing the body.

The diagonal cross of axes is made of the four diagonals of the cube. In Figure 11, they can be seen as

a–a:	high/right/forward	to	deep/left/back
b–b:	high/left/forward	to	deep/right/back
c–c:	high/left/back	to	deep/right/forward
d–d:	high/right/back	to	deep/left/forward

32

The Diagonal Scale

By moving through the center of the cube (and the body center) along each of the diagonals in the sequence ordered above, the attempt to perform the diagonal scale can be made. The scale can be started from any corner of the cube. For example, from high/right/forward, the scale could be developed as follows, using diameters of planes as transitions between the diagonals:

high/right/forward — deep/left/back		(diagonal a–a)
deep/left/back — high/left/forward	to	(diameter of plane)
high/left/forward — deep/right/back	to	(diagonal b–b)
deep/right/back — high/left/back	to	(diameter of plane)
high/left/back — deep/right/forward	to	(diagonal c–c)
deep/right/forward — high/right/back	to	(diameter of plane)
high/right/back — deep/left/forward	to	(diagonal d–d)

Other transitions for other ordering of the sequence could also be used.

The structure of the body makes the performance of pure diagonal movements impossible although a skillful mover can give the impression of such movements which appear as extremes of ultimate flight and fall.

Each reach toward a diagonal aim produces a slight twisting, but not a change in basic orientation toward the mover's front. Note that two of the diagonals (a–a & b–b) stress rising forward/falling backward and the other two (c–c & d–d) stress falling forward/rising backward. The tilt of the diagonal cross extends the possibilities of mobility; it can never have the stability of the vertical-horizontal-sagittal cross of axes.

The Icosahedron and Modified Diagonals

Because the body limits the fulfillment of perfect three-dimensional shapes that pure diagonals would offer, most three-dimensional shapes are created through *modified* diagonals in many combinations. These *are* available to the body.

Laban identified the modified diagonals with reference to another polyhedral form, the icosahedron, which can be visualized when the three planes are superimposed on each other and their peripheral points are connected.

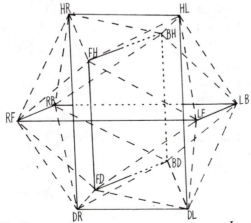

Fig. 12   *Icosahedron Developed from Planes*

The twelve corners define maximal reach possibilities within the kinesphere. Again, the scales are ordered sequences for the most economical and expressive pathways between the peripheral points. Reaching, expanding, twisting, traveling from one point to another, the mover has the possibility of using more of the space in the kinesphere than the other scales allow.

Many sequences are possible for the progression through the twelve points. Each has a distinctive character. Sequences that move *within* the icosahedron are called transverse scales. There are three (each with left arm and right arm versions): "A" scale, "B" scale, which are twelve-cornered scales, and "axis" scale, which is a six-cornered scale. Sequences in all transversal scales move repeatedly from one plane to another in the order of vertical/sagittal/horizontal, although they may start from any one.

"A" and "B" scale sequences are illustrated in Figure 13.

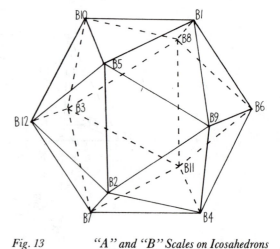

Scale Progression		Plane Equivalent
A1	=	HR — Vertical
A2	=	BD — Sagittal
A3	=	LF — Horizontal
A4	=	DR — Vertical
A5	=	BH — Sagittal
A6	=	RF — Horizontal
A7	=	DL — Vertical
A8	=	FH — Sagittal
A9	=	RB — Horizontal
A10	=	HL — Vertical
A11	=	FD — Sagittal
A12	=	LB — Horizontal
A1	=	HR —

"A" Scale

Scale Progression		Plane Equivalent
B1	=	HL — Vertical
B2	=	FD — Sagittal
B3	=	RB — Horizontal
B4	=	DL — Vertical
B5	=	FH — Sagittal
B6	=	LB — Horizontal
B7	=	DR — Vertical
B8	=	BH — Sagittal
B9	=	LF — Horizontal
B10	=	HR — Vertical
B11	=	BD — Sagittal
B12	=	RF — Horizontal
B1	=	HL —

"B" Scale

Fig. 13   *"A" and "B" Scales on Icosahedrons*

34

If the path moves along the surface of the icosahedron over all twelve points, its sequence describes a peripheral scale called "primary scale." There are four such scales; they are all derived from the axis scale. Sequences in peripheral scales move from one plane to another in the order of vertical/horizontal/sagittal. Other examples are described at the end of this chapter.

The scales can be started from any point. The first two inclinations will establish a quality of either roundedness or angularity in the performance of the scale. The smallest shape units are called volutes and steeples. Volutes are formed when the two inclinations relate to different diagonals; they produce rounded shapes. Steeples are formed when the two inclinations relate to the same diagonal; they produce angular shapes. Thus, the scales could be performed as a series of six volutes or a series of six steeples. The first two steeples and volutes of the "A" scale are illustrated in Figure 14.

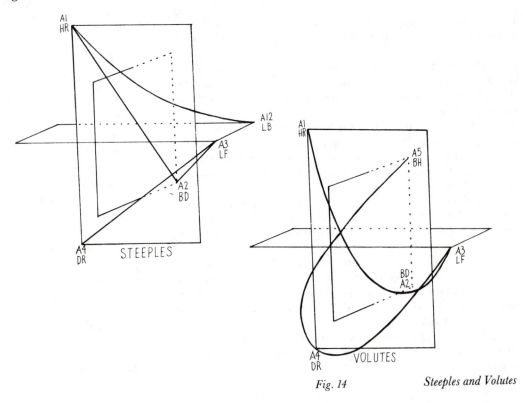

Fig. 14   Steeples and Volutes

This is only a sampling of some of the sequences identified by Laban. Others (axis, peripheral or primary, rings, girdle), are illustrated in the examples at the end of this chapter and in Chapter Five, *Rhythm and Phrasing*.

Although the sequences have been outlined here as primarily total body movements, they are also identifiable in small movements. The skilled observer learns to recognize significant spatial patterns in small and large movements and to question the messages in terms of their relationship to the mover's intent and awareness. It is the process of the movement that is thus observed and the specific changing qualities of its ordered sequence. Later chapters will discuss other attributes of various sequences in terms of their tension variations for functional and expressive distinctions.

35

Examples

Defense Scale

To experience this scale as an ordered progression, try to be aware of each spatial reach and the changes from one to the other. Involve the total body.

Preparation: Stand upright, with arms hanging loosely at sides. To prepare for the first upward push, flex the right arm fully at the side of the upper body, supporting the flexion with a pull toward the body's center.

1.   Maintaining support from the body's center, push the arm vertically up. This protects the head and its vulnerable sense organs.
2.   Pull the right arm-trunk, still supported from the center, strictly downward into squatting, feeling the vertical pull down throughout. This wards off an attack on the right flank between ribs and pelvis.
3.   Push the right arm across the front of the body as you gradually rise from squatting. Let the right shoulder follow the pushing arm toward the left, narrowing the body, with the head inclining in the same direction. This protects the left jugular vein on the side of the neck and/or attacks opponent.
4.   Pull the right arm from the left toward the center and push to the right into full extension of width, as the torso and head straighten. This wards off attack on right jugular vein by attacking as you deflect the opponent's thrust.
5.   Pull the right arm toward the center of the waist, across the body and toward the backward direction as hips and lower trunk also pull backward, hollowing the abdomen. The back is slightly rounded and the head inclined slightly forward. This fends off an attack on left flank.
6.   Reversing, push forward, straightening the trunk and head. This attack shields the abdomen, as it repulses the opponent's frontal attack.

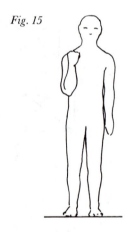

Fig. 15

Defense Scale: Position One

*   *   *   *   *

Two-Dimensional Movements

The spatial reaches in two-dimensional movements will be more complicated than in the defense scale because they have uneven pulls in two directions. Standing in the vertical plane (which includes a horizontal component) — wide stance, both arms spread overhead — is extremely stable, the stability of a wall. The maximal move in the cycle tilts the whole body in the plane so that the body could turn upside down and downside up — as in the cartwheel, Figure 16.

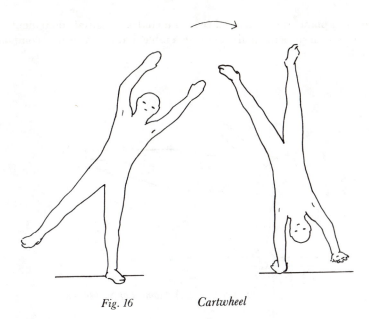

Fig. 16   *Cartwheel*

Standing in the sagittal plane (which includes a vertical component) — feet in a moderate stance with both feet on the same forward/backward line, and one arm raised directly forward of the body with the other arm raised directly behind the head — you are not quite stable even before you move in the cycle. When you move in the cycle you are compelled to progress forward.

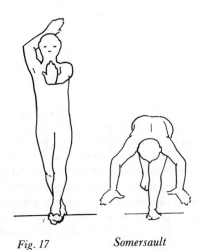

Fig. 17   *Somersault*

It keeps you rolling along as if you are a wheel turning on a very narrow rail. You would only do this on a tightrope or, totally, in a somersault. The necessity to progress forward sends you into walking. It has mobilized you into locomotion.

Finally, in the third plane, the horizontal (which includes a sagittal component), you must lean and spread into space, as if suspended in space over a table. Lacking a vertical component, this plane is the most unstable.

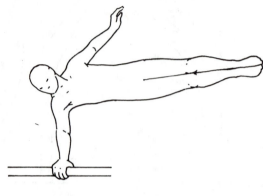

Fig. 18   *A Moment of Suspension*

When you move in its cycle, the forward-sideward combination has a turning, twisting power that tends to lift you off the ground. It would, if possible, suspend you in space in a whirling, circling disc-like drive, which can be seen briefly in acrobatics.

*   *   *   *   *

"A" and "B" Scales*

To trace the differences in "A" and "B" scales we have given the "A" scale sequence the numbers A1–A12 and the "B" scale sequence the numbers B1–B12. In the references below, the sequence in each case is performed by the right arm, supported by the whole body.

Comparing the identifications of the corners of the icosahedron for either of the scales shows that they echo or respond to each other. When two performers face each other and then perform, one a right "A" scale, the other a right "B" scale, they complement each other: up and down is the same for both, but right for one is left for the other and forward for one is backward for the other.

All of the scales relate to the basic diagonals in various ways of dealing with three unequal spatial pulls constantly changing. Each of the two "A" and two "B" scales (each with twelve transversal inclinations) actively involves three of the four diagonals — two that are similar and one opposite. In each scale (using three diagonals), the movement is designed to use modifications of those three diagonals around the fourth — a pure diagonal — which serves as the axis. In each case, one type of diagonal is predominant, as can be seen in the illustration.

* *An attempt to perform the diagonal scale is recommended to precede performance of the "A" and "B" scales. See p. 33 for description.*

In the illustrations below, the "A" scale is developed around the diagonal high/right/back to deep/left/forward. The "B" scale is developed around the diagonal high/left/forward to deep/right/back.

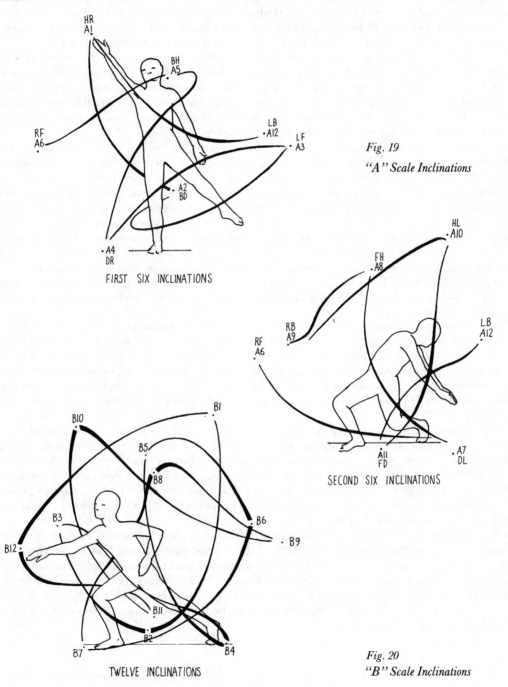

Fig. 19

"A" Scale Inclinations

FIRST SIX INCLINATIONS

SECOND SIX INCLINATIONS

TWELVE INCLINATIONS

Fig. 20

"B" Scale Inclinations

In the "A" and "B" scales, the whole sequence of reaching the twelve corners of the icosahedron is comprised of phrases that move from vertical to sagittal to horizontal planes three times, in each case touching a different corner of each plane. For example, in the "A" scale, A-1 starts on the high/right corner of the vertical plane and moves to A-2, the back/deep corner of the sagittal plane and then to A-3 the left/front corner of the horizontal plane. The next phrase starts again on the vertical plane, but this time on the deep/right corner, A-4, and so on as illustrated in the chart, Figure 13.

The relevance of the planar associations with the scales becomes clear as the experience of changing planar tensions affects the quality of the moves between planes. For example, in the move from A-1 to A-2, the plane change is from vertical plane to sagittal plane. The vertical plane has both vertical and horizontal dimensional tensions; the sagittal plane has both sagittal and vertical dimensional tensions. Since the two planes share the vertical dimensional tensions, the inclination from A-1 to A-2 will be most strongly influenced by those vertical tensions.

In the next move, from A-2 (back/deep) to A-3 (left/forward), the back of A-2 (sagittal plane) and the forward of A-3 (horizontal plane) share the sagittal dimension so the inclination is most strongly influenced by the sagittal tensions. Similar influences can be identified throughout the sequence.

The experience of these sequences evokes distinctive spatial sensations. One of the distinctions that can be made is between steepness, suspension and flatness. Moving from a transversal with a vertical dominance to a transversal with a sagittal dominance (vertical secondary) will have a feeling of steepness. Moving from a transversal with a sagittal dominance to a transversal with a horizontal dominance (sagittal secondary) will have a feeling of being suspended. Moving from a transversal with a horizontal dominance to a transversal with a vertical dominance (horizontal secondary) will have a feeling of flatness. Thus, when up–down is shared, there is a spatial sensation of steepness; when forward–back is shared, there is a spatial sensation of suspension and when side–side is shared, the sensation is of flatness.

The move from one plane to another will be to a plane that has as its major tendency a spatial pull that was weak in the plane you are leaving. For example, in the inclination of the "A" scale from high/right (vertical) to back/deep (sagittal) you start in an off-balance pose which forces you to fall. The sagittal plane into which you fall will include a direction (in this case, forward or backward) that was either missing or little stressed in the previous inclination. The movement between the planes is a part of the recuperation that occurs between the exertion of the previous spatial pull and the exertion of the next pull.

The icosahedron is not a structure fixed in one place. It is a structure one constructs around one's own kinesphere. This is illustrated in the following pictures. On this page, each person leads with right arm. The woman, in her iscosahedron in the upper left picture, is at high/right (A-1) of the vertical plane. In the lower picture, the woman's "B" scale right/back (B-3) is enclosed in the same icosahedron as the man's "A" scale left/forward (A-6). Both are suspended in the horizontal plane. In the upper right picture, the woman is at another corner of the same vertical plane as in the upper left picture, but now she is at deep/left (A-7).

In the second group of pictures, the woman and the frisbee player at the top, each leading with the right arm, are in the forward/deep (A-11) of the sagittal plane. In the bottom set, there are several significant differences between the two: the man is leading with his left arm, while the woman is leading with her right arm; she is in "A" scale (A-12, left/back) position and he is in "B" scale (right/back, B-3) position. If she were leading with left arm, she would be in open position at her point of the scale. If he were leading with right arm, he would be in open position at his point of the scale. Both are in horizontal plane.

Facing page photos: © *Morris H. Jaffe.*

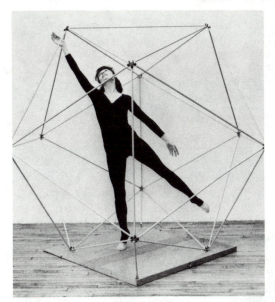
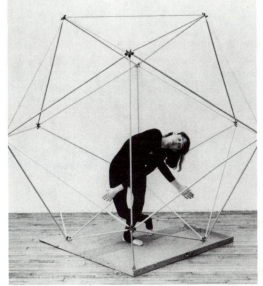

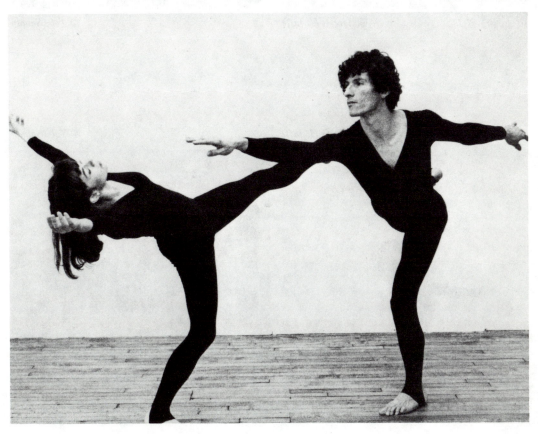

41

"A" and "B" Scale Sequences

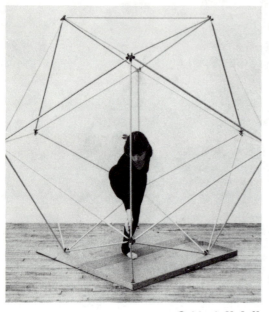

© Morris H. Jaffe

© Toby Shimin

© Morris H. Jaffe

© Toby Shimin

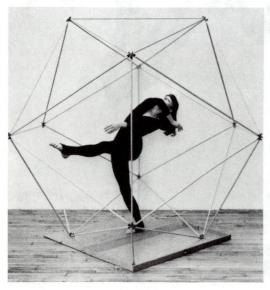

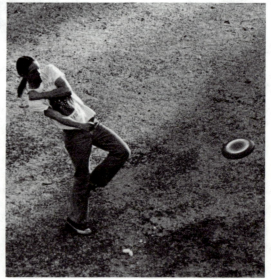

42

Other Sequences Perceived in the Icosahedron

The icosahedron offers a live lexicon of movement potential. Other scales (than the "A" and "B") developed by Laban include four **axis** scales, described on the following page, with six transversal inclinations progressing along only one diagonal, which also serves as the axis of the scale. There are also four **peripheral** scales (also described on the following page) which surround the axis scales along the surface of the icosahedron like the tensile threads of a spider web. The countertension of the peripheral scale is created by the relationship between the diagonal axis and the shaping done on the surface of the icosahedron.

Other sequence forms that can be derived from the icosahedron are transverse or peripheral **rings** (two-, three-, five-, seven-). If, for example, you close a volute by a third transversal inclination, you create a transversal three-ring, with each of its inclinations deflected from a different diagonal. Because there are then movements on three diagonals, the three-ring sequence is dynamically highly mobile, especially when used in turns, jumps and falls. As in all icosahedron sequences, the affinities of spatial direction and Effort are not seen clearly as in the dimensional and diagonal scales where each spatial change has a clear Effort counterpart. Because the inclinations are modified, that is, slightly deflected, diagonals, each spatial component in an inclination has not the same "spatial drive" intensity. This, in turn, affects the Effort components. (See Effort, following chapter.)

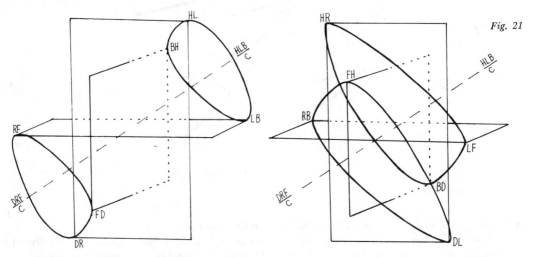

Two Peripheral and Two Transverse Three-Rings Around the Diagonal deep/right/forward to high/left/back.

Two peripheral three-rings around diagonal	**Two transverse three-rings around diagonal**
A10 high/left	A1 high/right
A12 left/back	A2 back/deep
A5 back/high	A3 left/forward
Return to A10	Return to A1
A4 deep/right	A7 deep/left
A6 right/forward	A8 forward/high
A11 forward/deep	A9 right/back
Return to A4	Return to A7

43

The Axis Scale: The monotone of the transversal scales

In the performance of the "A" and "B" scales, you reached the twelve corners of the icosahedron by changing the diagonal inclination in every second transversal using three diagonals in the process.

When you perform a series of transversals that are deflected from the same diagonal, you arrive at four sets (one for each diagonal) of six transversals that return to their starting corners. Each set of six transversals is called an *axis scale*.

This scale, going to and fro in the same diagonal produces a kind of monotone, a repetitious spatial rhythm in a much more limited surrounding action space. You will feel as if you seem to fall into almost the same groove. It is like the movement of a drunk who teeters one way, falls back, makes a new attempt and falls back, etc. The axis scale illustrated in Figure 22 is deflected from the diagonal high/right/forward to deep/left/back (a–a on Figure 11).

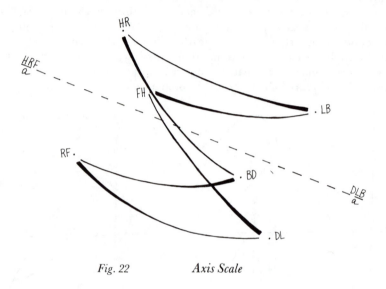

Fig. 22   *Axis Scale*

A Primary Scale: A Peripheral Scale Related to the Axis Scale

From the six transversals of the axis scale, a series of peripheral inclinations can be developed by going along the outer edges of the icosahedron. They wind around the transversals of the axis scale like a winding, looping garland. Because Laban saw this scale in so many communicative gestures and dance forms, he called it the *primary scale*.* To experience the development of these shapes, an example is detailed in Figure 23. Again, the scale is developed around the diagonal: high/right/forward to deep/left/back.

By including a corner of the icosahedron in a transversal's area (for example, the transversal *HR-LB* in Figure 23, includes *BH* in its sequence), the straight transversal is changed into an arc that goes along the edge of the icosahedron, rather than through the inside of the icosahedron. This produces a peripheral scale consisting of twelve peripheral diagonal inclinations — a primary scale.

---

*   *The form of the primary scale can be created around different axes.*

44

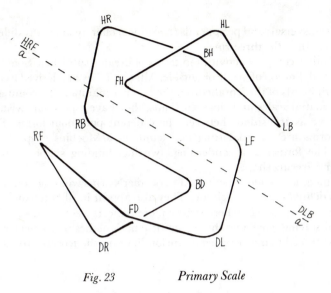

Fig. 23   Primary Scale

The Girdle: A Derivative of the Primary Scale

A sequence of the inserts (back/high, right/back, deep/right, forward/deep, left/forward, high/left) that expands the transversals of an axis scale into peripherals of a primary scale results in another peripheral shape: an equator-like, tilted cycle, going, in this case, around essentially the front and slightly back of the body. This shape is identified as a *girdle*. This process can be repeated in each of the four axis scales. Such girdles can easily be observed in many dances using props such as fans, sticks and ribbons, particularly in dances of the Far East and Southeast Asia (see Ethnic, Chapter 10).

In Figure 24, the girdle is developed around the diagonal high/right/forward to deep/left/back.

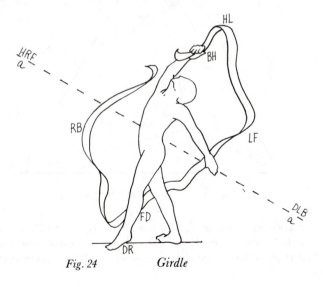

Fig. 24   Girdle

Combinations of transversals and peripherals (two-rings) offer dynamically different, more stable, movement experiences than the three-ring.

Laban identified other complex activities in terms of greater subtleties. Some curves seemed to have no center and no definition of inside or outside. Although they are derived from combinations of transversals and peripherals of the icosahedron, they do not maintain the countertensions with the inner axes that the spatial scales and rings do. Thus, they have a peculiar twisting character that enables them to serve as transitions between the different polygonal forms. Examples of these transitional trace forms are tying/knotting and lemnescata/Moebius strip. They represent two opposite activites: The former is a condensing, twisting, binding shape, while the latter is an unwinding, dissolving, freeing shape.

Laban observed them in the movements of a performer's arms winding and unwinding through· space producing no definable plane or circuit. They also appear in ribbon dances of the Orient and in many group and partner dances where two or more dancers become involved with each other, intermingling and dissolving. He found the geometrical basis of these extremely mobile space curves after he defined and traced many peripheral tension lines on the icosahedron and other complex polygons.

*   *   *   *   *

The Tetrahedron

The tetrahedron is the simplest geometrical form from which all other polyhedra can develop. In body movement, it relates most clearly to certain movements that send the body flying through space, as in a leap forward with arms spread overhead side to side and legs spread forward/backward; the purest — though imperfect — example of the shape may be fulfilled only at the peak of the action.

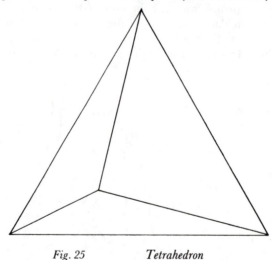

Fig. 25   *Tetrahedron*

Such movements do not relate to the vertical axis. The upper set of limbs forms a horizontal axis and the lower set of limbs forms a sagittal axis. Thus, there is a sagittal tension in countertension with a lateral tension. Movements that relate simultaneously to a lateral and sagittal axis create twisting tension in the body.

In flying leaps, which are supported by the driving force of their twisting countertensions, the shapes are of very short duration so the tensions reflect excited inner dynamics. When the shapes are more stable, the tensions will reflect controlled, measured inner dynamics as can be seen in Figure 26.

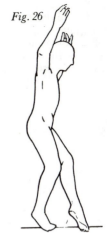
Fig. 26

As with all tension systems, shapes can only be maintained by constant renewal; recuperation is often achieved by moving into the periphery of the model. For example, a sphere can be circumscribed around any tetrahedron. After the pulsating, churning drive of the twisting tensions of the tetrahedral leap, the calming, soothing influences from the periphery of the circumscribed sphere around the tetrahedron can be even more appreciated. When the tetrahedral trace form is repeated several times, one may — perhaps from exhaustion or from giving in to preferred more "comfortable" spatial tensions — give up tetrahedral tension and trail off into the peripheral tensions of the rounded circumference of the sphere.

Twisting Tensions in a Stable Tetrahedron

* * * * *

Fusion of One-Dimensional and Diagonal Grounding

In T'ai Chi Ch'uan training, a high degree of balance between one-dimensional and diagonal tension is developed, which is necessary for the fighting stance. In training exercises, "Push Hands" is used to develop the necessary coordination, flexibility, balance, and sensitivity.

Starting with shoulder, hip and feet in the same vertical line, feet are parallel to each other. Step back with right foot, turning it out diagonally to about a 45 degree angle. Maintain the verticality of the upper body. The toe of the right foot is now in a diagonal relationship to the heel of the left foot. The feet are still separated by shoulder width, hips still facing forward. The body must be relaxed in a readiness for action.

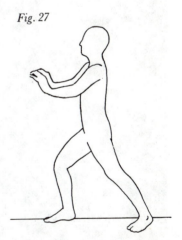
Fig. 27

This combination of one-dimensional and diagonal directions in the feet opens up the body for easy three-dimensional turning away from and towards itself, as well as for pushing/pulling movements in all directions and for cycles in all planes. The body always feels connected to the ground by awareness of the changing distribution of the weight between the two feet. Feet are like roots to the ground with the weight evenly distributed over the whole foot. This provides resiliency for weight shifts: when pushed, weight shifts back and the mover sinks into the back leg. When mover pushes, weight shifts forward to the front leg. In all weight shifts, the total body is involved. The groundedness is coupled with precise use of the upper body parts and the peripheral space.

"Push Hands" Stance in Tai Chi

Thus, the movement of the wrist-forearm leading the spatial patterns of the upper body is not merely a peripheral move. Supported by a central initiation and the groundedness of the foot positions, the performer can maintain balance even as the body weight shifts for a sudden release of high energy through the wrist-forearm that can overthrow the partner when he is slightly off balance.

Right: *Child with Soap Bubble*
© Morris H. Jaffe
Almost a Basic Effort Action:
Float. Light Weight/Indirect
Space/Sustained Time.

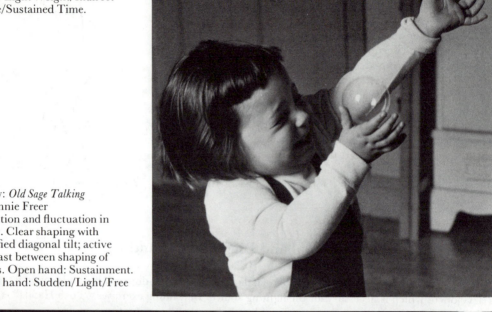

Below: *Old Sage Talking*
© Bonnie Freer
Variation and fluctuation in
Effort. Clear shaping with
modified diagonal tilt; active
contrast between shaping of
hands. Open hand: Sustainment.
Right hand: Sudden/Light/Free
Flow.

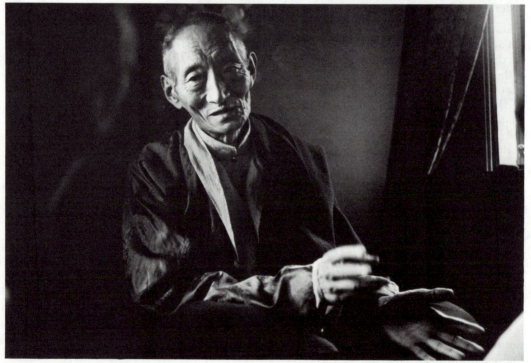

CHAPTER 4

Inner Impulses to Move

Designing trace-forms in the air with only the extremities can lead to a kind of external form-writing.

Rudolf Laban

The source whence perfection and final mastery of movement must flow is the understanding of that part of the inner life of man where movement and action originate. Such an understanding furthers the spontaneous flow of movement, and guarantees effective liveliness. Man's inner urge to movement has to be assimilated to the acquisition of external skill in movement.

Rudolf Laban

Right: *Man Eating Lunch*
© Bonnie Freer
He shows a wide range of potential action. Contrast of powerful frame and attitude with subtle activity. Light Weight, Sudden Time, fine Flow fluctuations, Direct Space.

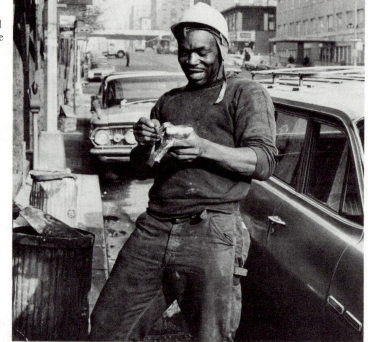

Below: *Man with Wine Bottle*
© Bonnie Freer
Actor and Observer show the contrast of Active and Neutral Effort. Man: Free Flow/Strong Weight/Sudden Time. Postural shaping high and wide with forward deflection. Woman: Bound Flow/Neutral Weight. Neutral verticality.

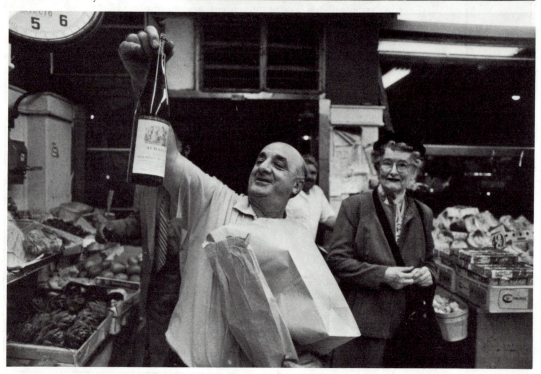

Inner Impulses to Move

When a person takes a leisurely stroll down the street, he appears to just keep going in a continuous flowing progression with no particular urgency or pressing tasks imposed on mind or body. He may see an acquaintance and, without stopping, casually wave to her.

If, however, a couple of children come running, heedlessly, toward him, he immediately prepares himself to meet a threatening impact by somewhat suspending himself in time, controlling the flow of his progress and building up force in his body. He may prepare to meet the impact of two bodies with slow, strong, direct movement warding off the suddenness of the impact.

Even before any visible movement manifestations, there were inner impulses toward these preparations. First, an inner impulse to attention to the space around him and what it included; second, to the sense of his own body weight and the intention of the force of its impact; third, to awareness of time pressing for decision. All of this inner participation interrelated with the flow of his movement whose inner impulses fluctuated between freedom and control. Such inner participation is a combination of kinaesthetic and thought processes that appear to be almost simultaneous at different levels of consciousness.

Laban identified space, weight, time and flow as motion factors toward which performers of movement can have different attitudes depending on temperament, situation, environment and many other variables. The attitudes toward the motion factors he called in German *antrieb*, a combination of *an* (on) and *trieb* (drive), representing the organism's urge to make itself known. In English translation, *antrieb* has become Effort.

The Effort elements, Space, Weight, Time and Flow, are those inner attitudes toward the motion factors of space, weight, time and flow. The quality of the attitudes is identified as Effort elements within the ranges of two extremes: spreading out, expanding, indulging, going with, or condensing, fighting, resisting, struggling against. They communicate the quality of movement — how it is performed. They are usually perceived in combinations and sequences that express dominant characteristics of the mover and that vary for specific intents.

The chart below shows the range of Effort elements for each Effort. The indulging elements offer no resistance to the motion factors of space, weight, time and flow, but they are active qualities. They do not represent limpness. The fighting elements affect, move against, the motion factors. In all cases, their combinations and fluctuations relate to the spatial paths, shapes, and tensions of movements which will be described later.

Effort Elements Continuum

Effort	Indulging	Fighting
Space	Indirect	Direct
Weight	Light	Strong
Time	Sustained	Sudden
Flow	Free	Bound

In the case of the strolling man, the circumstances aroused him into a definite organization of his energy impulses: he controlled his flow, condensed his weight, attended directly to space and sustained his time. That is, in this case, his Flow, Weight and Space were in the resisting range and his Time, in the indulging range. Had he instead combined Free Flow, Light Weight, Indirect Space (all indulging range) and Sudden Time, his movements would have been inappropriate to the event and he could have been knocked down and trampled on.

51

Right: *Singer with Clasped Hands*
© Morris H. Jaffe
Full use of the body's three-dimensionality frees the inner breathing space of the trunk and head. Free Flow/Sustained Time/Strong Weight.

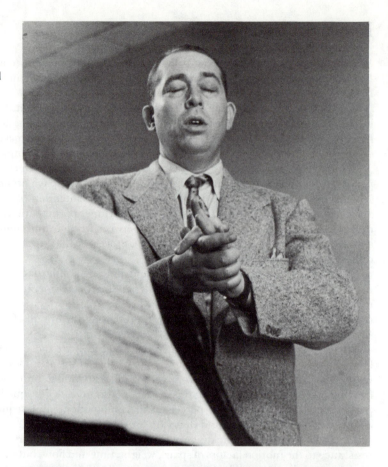

Right: *Woman Playing Tennis*
© Nana Sue Koch
Restricted movement with minimal relationship to space. Shrinking body shape permits only Bound Flow without other differentiated Effort combinations.

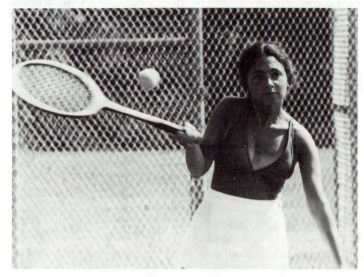

This organization of inner energy impulses is part of all human behavior. Research, especially by the child psychiatrist Judith Kestenberg, describes developmental processes that increasingly confirm Laban's basic distinctions. People constantly utilize and respond to the organization of Effort with or without knowing its components.

When people speak of urging responses, nailing someone down, exploding into action, pressuring others, carefully approaching, they are using metaphors for organizations of Space, Weight, Time and Flow Effort elements. The expressiveness of the Effort elements was described by Laban as indicative of stages of the inner state of mind which prepare the mover for a sequence. He identified — as indications, not absolutes — characteristic qualities of the individual Effort elements as follows:

Effort	**Quality**
Space	**Attention**
In what manner do I approach the space?	Thinking. Orienting, specifically or generally.
Weight	**Intention**
What is my impact?	Asserting. Creating strong or light impact. Sensing my weight, myself.
Time	**Decision**
When do I need to complete the act?	Urgency or non-urgency. Rushing or delaying.
Flow	**Progression**
How do I keep going?	Feeling alive. How to get started and keep going. Freely or carefully.

Most people have predilections for particular Effort elements. Their movements may consistently reflect some more active Effort elements or particular ranges of Effort elements and almost indifference to others. Such predilections define the movement styles of individuals and, consequently, their character traits. In each of the Effort ranges, there are different degrees from neutral to clearly discernible to exaggerated. These lend further shading to practical and non-practical actions.

Every movement has some degree of a Space, Weight, Time and Flow Effort. Although the muscular energy used can be measured, we are not here concerned with its measurable aspects, but with the qualitative aspects — what colors the expressiveness, what stands out — as enumerated below. They are visible signs of the performer's movement quality.

Even in moments of relaxation some Effort is present, although it is greatly reduced in degree of exertion. In all activity, there is a constant play for proportionality among the Effort elements to balance exertions and recuperations for most effective function and expression. Furthermore, the same activity, done by two individuals, may be organized with somewhat different Effort punctuations — Effort rhythms — even though the same elements are being used. When two people do the same thing, it is not the same.

We will discuss below the four Effort elements and their continuum range possibilities. Their combinations and relationships to geometrical forms or spatial shapes and expressiveness will be described throughout the book.

Flow Effort

What is the mover's attitude toward the goingness, the quality of continuity of his/her movement?

Free	or	**Bound**
easy flowing		controlling the flow
streaming out		streaming inward
abandoned		holding back, restrained
ready to go		ready to stop

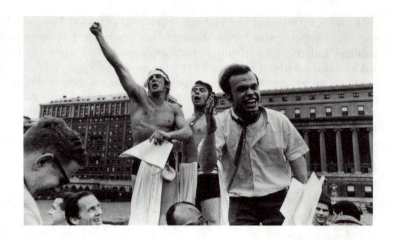

Above: *Columbia University Protest* © Bonnie Freer
Two approaches to arousing a crowd. Left appears demanding, passionate. Right appears persuading. Left is almost Full Effort Action Drive with Bound Flow, Strong Weight, Sudden Time and Direct Space. Right has more fluctuation: Free Flow going toward Neutral; Sudden with Dominant Sustained Time; Dominant Light fluctuating with Strong Weight. Left is posturally lifting: convex shape. Right is slightly rounded, sinking: concave shape.

Below: *Healer at Meeting* ©Bonnie Freer
He shapes with Free Flow, Sustainment, Strong/Light Weight fluctuations. She neutralizes all Effort.

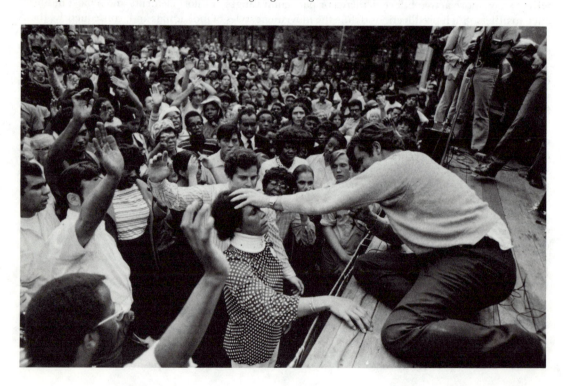

Free Flow can be observed in the swinging of a heavy object before flinging it away. It is also the dominant element in a child's relaxed whirling in delight. Bound Flow can be observed in a gesture of cautious refusal or in the tightening of one's chest in a state of fear.

The contrast between an easy, swinging movement and one in which the mover tries to control all the points of the path illustrates the contrast between Free and Bound Flow. The former movement indulges in the flow motion factor while the latter resists or fights it. Free finger painting is an expression of Free Flow, while careful tracing of a drawing is an expression of Bound Flow. Walking with the wind on a windy day, one has only to use Free Flow to get along with ease, without collapsing. Walking against the wind will be aided by Bound Flow along with elements of Weight and Time Effort. Finding one's way in a totally dark room will elicit Bound Flow.

Flow is the initiator of action. Although it is not necessarily dominant, and may not appear identifiable as Bound or Free, its neutral continuity as flux will still underlie all the other Effort elements. An abundance of Flow Effort is a characteristic of young children; their Space, Weight, Time Efforts become more fully crystallized later.

Space Effort

How does the mover approach space? What is his/her attitude toward exertion in space as it is approached?

Direct　　　　or　　　　**Indirect**
zeroing in　　　　　　　　　encompassing focus
pinpointing　　　　　　　　flexible

The difference between pointing to something specific or making an encompassing reference to the area in which it exists illustrates different ranges of the Space Effort: Direct in the former and Indirect in the latter. If a gesture is used when demanding concentration, it will most likely express a Direct attitude toward space. If, however, the gesture accompanies a request for general consideration of a matter, it will most likely express an Indirect attitude toward space. To crack an egg, the attitude toward space must be Direct, as opposed to the Indirect attitude of folding beaten egg white into a dessert. In all cases, the Direct attitude is a quality of resisting, fighting the space motion factor, and the Indirect attitude is a quality of indulging in the space.

The Space Effort appears to be distinctive from the other three in the degree to which consciousness is involved in its activation.

Weight Effort (Some analysts call this "Force" Effort)

What is the mover's attitude toward the use of his/her body weight? What is the quality of the exertion of weight?

Strong　　　　or　　　　**Light**
impactful　　　　　　　　using fine touch
vigorous　　　　　　　　airy
powerful　　　　　　　　delicate

When an object is smashed with a fist, the attitude toward Weight is Strong, as opposed to Lightness in picking up a very small, delicate object. Playing forte on the piano requires a Strong attitude toward the impact of body weight as opposed to playing pianissimo. The Light Weight Effort element is apparent in wiping the tears from a child's eyes as opposed to Strong Weight when spanking a child. Again, as in all the Effort elements, the contrast is between indulging, going with (Light Weight element) versus resisting, struggling against (Strong Weight element).

Weight as an Effort is not to be confused with body weight per se. There are three ways of considering body weight: 1) Neutral, in which body weight is muscularly supported; 2) Passive, in which the body weight is unsupported and gives in to gravity; and 3) Active, which occurs with overcoming the passivity of body weight by an attitude toward the body weight: A Weight Effort. Even when the Weight Effort is not dominantly strong or light, its neutral state is not passive. It has a readiness for action.

A person in a deep depression often has a quality of great heaviness resulting from an almost total — a passive — giving into body weight. When the slightest attitude toward the use of that body weight can be activated, a move that may lead out of the depression has been initiated. It doesn't matter if that attitude, the Weight Effort, is in the Strong or Light range. What is important is its indication of participation rather than passivity and the diminution of heaviness and immobility in the experience of the depressed person.

Time Effort
How does the mover exert him/herself in time? Driven by it or lingering in it? What is his/her attitude toward exertions in time?

Sudden	or	**Sustained**
urgent		taking time
hasty		leisurely

Going toward someone with immediate recognition expresses a Sudden attitude toward time (Sudden Time Effort) as opposed to the Sustained Effort action of prolonged farewells with a good friend or lingering over the photo of a pleasant experience. Response to the unexpected, such as the touch of fire, elicits the Sudden Time Effort element, while embracing a dear friend is more likely to elicit the Sustained Time Effort element. One either resists the time motion factor or indulges in it.

Time as an Effort is not to be confused with time as duration. Duration is the amount of time that a movement might take. Time as an Effort describes the attitude toward how one approaches whatever the duration of the time is. There might be, for example, one minute in which to perform an activity, but the attitude toward that minute can be leisurely (Sustained). On the other hand, there might be fifteen minutes to perform the same action, and the attitude may be one of such urgency that the actual duration of the activity will seem shorter. In both cases, it is the Effort attitude that determines the quality of the movement, the message conveyed.

Effort Observation
In general, isolated elements of Space, Weight and Time rarely, if ever, appear. In any one action, they appear in sequence and in combination. For example, in reaching for an object, one may start with a Sudden/Light reach, but, coming nearer to the object and realizing its fragility, one modifies the Lightness by extreme Sustainment and controls the easy flow of action into Bound Flow.

The skill of a mover can be recognized by the degree to which a whole activity is performed as one continuous, flowing process, each phase blending smoothly with the next. However, the flowing sequences of activity will be punctuated with many shades of exertion and recuperation, accents and fluctuations of Effort. Many small and large adjustments in Flow, Space, Weight and Time Effort elements create rhythmic fluctuations that are more or less suitable to the task.

Sometimes, the signs are barely visible. For example, a person who is anaesthetized appears to have no sign of Effort, not even Effort Flow. This is different from someone about to fall asleep, who responds to a "good night" with a slight, sleepy wave of his hand. The movement has no distinguishable Effort, except continuous flow, which might be described as Neutral Flow Effort.

Identifying distinctions requires practice. Precise observation is necessary to recognize the subtlety and range of a particular movement or movement pattern. Some of the common confusions can be avoided as perceptions are trained. For example, when Strong Weight and Sudden Time are both active Effort elements in the same movement there is sometimes confusion about the actual presence of the Weight element. When, for instance, a person is restrained by another person, he may free himself by making a Sudden Strong move. A novice observer might only see the condensed Sudden Time element and miss the added power of the Strong Weight. When carefully analyzed, it can be observed that the Sudden Time Effort actually preceded the activation of the Weight element.

A film about life in India* included a sequence in which a woman was hauling water from a well. She pulled the rope holding the vessel in short vertical pulls with extremely Free Flow and constantly renewed Sudden Time rebounding into Light Weight and Neutral Flow and Neutral Time. The Weight Effort was minimal in comparison to the dominance of Free Flow/Suddenness which gave the impression of playful ease rather than condensed Strong Weight Effort.

When Direct Space and Sudden Time are active, the movement is sometimes interpreted as including Strong Weight, which would make the action a punch or a statement: "I won't." Without the Weight, the action is actually only an alert pinpointing, as in saying, "There he is."

Bound Flow is sometimes confused with Strong Weight. However, in fact, a forward action with Bound Flow has a quality of holding back, while a forward action with Strong Weight, instead of Bound Flow, has a quality of impact, of pressing the weight forward. A person might cautiously move toward an enemy and not really want to confront him (Bound Flow), or the person might cautiously move toward the enemy with the intent to push him over (Strong Weight).

An automobile driver may seem to be trying to maintain a steady Flow in his driving but, in fact, punctuates the Flow with frequent jerks. What is happening is that his dominantly urgent attitude toward Time is interfering with the continuity of his Flow. If, on the other hand, he could appreciate these distinctions, he could activate his Flow and Time Effort elements compatibly by using Free Flow and alternate Sudden with Sustained Time.

In Labananalysis, Effort observations should always be made in relation to spatial paths, tensions, and shapes, with an awareness of the body articulations involved. It is from the combinations, their variations and relationships to each other that assessments can be made of particular functional viability or psychological and expressive messages.

Effort Combinations
Choices are continuously being made by all people in motion, consciously or unconsciously, to determine what combinations of Effort elements will best serve the purposes of their intents or modify their behavior. Whatever the action in which the Effort combinations appear — it may be a work action or a dance action or a speaking gesture in a discussion — the whole biological/psychological system is involved.

Principal Combinations to be Discussed
1.   Combinations of three Effort elements of Space, Weight and Time produce inner drives of action which Laban identified as *Basic Effort Actions*: Punch, Float, and their modifications, Glide, Slash, Dab, Wring, Flick and Press.
2.   Combinations of three Effort elements in which Flow becomes an active element at the expense of either Space, Weight or Time are identified as *Transformations* or *Drives* (of the Basic Effort Action). Spaceless is metaphorically called the Passion Drive; Weightless, the Vision Drive; and Timeless, the Spell Drive.

* *"Fifty Miles from Poona" (National Film Board of Canada).*

3. Combinations of two Effort elements are sometimes called *Incomplete* (Basic Effort Actions) or *Inner Attitudes* or, preferably, *Inner States*. Instead of drives, they produce mood-like qualities in movement that can be metaphorically described as Awake, Dreamlike; Remote, Near; Stable, Mobile.

4. Combinations of four Effort elements are called *Full Effort* or *Complete Drives*. They rarely occur because the movements they produce are so extreme.

Basic Effort Action Drive

Laban identified the Basic Effort Actions when he observed patterns of workers' movements for wartime industrial studies. By combining one element from Space, Weight and Time, the eight possible combinations emerged as follows:

<table>
<tr><td>

Float (All Indulgent elements)

Indirect (Space)
Light (Weight)
Sustained (Time)

Modifications*
  Glide
* Direct (Fighting)
  Light
  Sustained

  Wring
  Indirect
* Strong (Fighting)
  Sustained

  Flick
  Indirect
  Light
* Sudden (Fighting)

</td><td>

Punch (All Fighting elements)

Direct
Strong
Sudden

  Slash
* Indirect (Indulging)
  Strong
  Sudden

  Dab
  Direct
* Light (Indulging)
  Sudden

  Press
  Direct
  Strong
* Sustained (Indulging)

</td></tr>
</table>

* Modification indicates elements changed from most extreme contrast of Float and Punch, thus making all except Float and Punch mixtures of fighting and indulging qualities.

These Basic Effort combinations can be observed, for example, as Float when a child successfully cradles a soap bubble; Punch in an across and downward hit in boxing; Glide when using an iron to smooth out material; Slash in cracking a heavy whip; Wring in wringing out a heavy towel; Dab in applying dots of paint to a canvas; Flick in removing an insect from a dress; and Press in slowly squashing a juicy fruit or pushing a heavy piece of furniture across the floor.

These examples describe the most effective phase of the movement which may be repeated after recuperating into a two-element combination of opposite Effort elements.

In each of the pairs identified on the chart, maximal contrasts are confronted.

Float to Punch
Glide to Slash
Wring to Dab
Flick to Press

Maximal contrasts rarely appear in immediate sequence in action. The change from a series of hard-hitting, spatially precise Time-driven punches immediately into a wide open, meandering, time-indulging Light action requires more than a mechanical diminution of energy. From arousal into the Punch's high condensed "fighting" peak, it takes a number of adjusting transitions to reach a peak of Light serenity in the floating.

There will be distinctive differences in how people would make a transition or transitions to the new action. For example, in this instance of Punch to Float, the contrast is most extreme because Punch consists of all the Fighting Effort elements while Float consists of all Indulging elements.

	Punch	**Float**
Space:	Direct (Fighting)	Indirect (Indulging)
Weight:	Strong (Fighting)	Light (Indulging)
Time:	Sudden (Fighting)	Sustained (Indulging)

One may go from Punching (Strong/Direct/Sudden) to Pressing (<u>Sustained</u>/Direct/Strong) to Gliding (Sustained/ <u>Light</u>/Direct) and, finally, arrive at the full Floating (<u>Indirect</u>/Sustained/ Light). The underlinings indicate the Effort element that changed. Note that the transitions made the total change possible by changing one element at a time instead of trying to change all at once.

Or, one could make the transition from Punching via Slashing (Strong/<u>Indirect</u>/Sudden) via Wringing (Strong/ Indirect/<u>Sustained</u>) to Floating. Again, only one element at a time changed in the transition, but the changes were made in the indulging paths. There are a number of ways to change from Punch to Float. The examples above are only two possibilities. People make selections from their own preferences in Effort attitudes to express different feelings through their actions.

The transitions most often make one component change at a time, but it is possible to change two components at a time. Most difficult, as we have indicated, is to change all three components simultaneously. In the other three Basic Effort Drive pairs, the contrasts are not as total since, in each case, they are mixtures of fighting and indulging elements.

Again the changes from one to the other can be made more or less gradually according to the number of elements changed in the sequence of the process.

It is a dramatic experience to observe other three-element or two-element combinations — Transformations and Inner States — after working with only Basic Effort Action drives. Another color tone takes over and changes the quality. This can often be seen when a Basic Effort action is performed inadequately by accident or choice during the process of change, and its function — to Punch, for example — is not fulfilled. It has veered off into a Transformation drive or an Inner State. The movement has a less literal or tangible quality, not so much associated with action as with affect, or mood.

Inner States: Incomplete Effort, Inner Attitudes
A variety of inner states can be described in the movement manifestations of two Effort combinations. There are six possibilities of such combinations. Thus, Space, Weight, Time and Flow can be combined as

Space and Time Flow and Weight	1
Space and Flow Weight and Time	2
Space and Weight Time and Flow	3

59

Note that in the preceding listing, the four Effort elements each appear three times or as members of three sets. No element is shared within each set with the result that the two 2-factor combinations within each set describe contrasting moods or inner states.

For example, the combination of Space and Time in the first set, considered in terms of their characteristic qualities (see p. 53) of attention and decision create an inner state of alertness. Flow and Weight, also in the first set, have the characteristics of continuity and intention creating an inner dream-like state.

By the same analysis, Space/Flow creates an inner state that can be called remote as opposed to Weight/Time which creates an inner state of presence. And the third set, Space/Weight (stable) is in opposition to Time/Flow (mobile).

The identifying words are only approximations of the experiences that are elicited, but they can serve as guides to explorations of the expressive content of the movement. In each case, there are, of course, the variations possible in choices of either the indulging or resisting element of the Effort.

In everyday behavior, in work actions and in dance and drama, these two-element combinations often appear as fleeting transitions between major changes from one three-element combination to another. They may be the upbeat for a Basic Effort action or they may be observed as instances of failure to produce a Basic Effort action combination. For example, a person of frail body-build may attempt to "Punch" (Strong Weight/Sudden Time/Direct Space) someone in the chest, but may end only in extremely Bound Flow/Direct Space with neither Strength impact nor Time urgency.

Two-effort element combinations can also be observed as a preparative or a held attitude in the body, particularly in the face and hands, as, for example, in the Direct/Bound stare of the eyes. Observing further, one might note that stare's Direct/Boundness continues in the whole body attitude: the shoulders slightly lifted and narrowed toward the neck, the whole torso leaning slightly, rigidly forward.

Another example of two-effort combination might appear as the "nervous flutter" of Sudden/Light blinks of the eyelids, or a Sustained/Bound "rolling" of the eyes with no particular focus. These are sometimes called shadow movements that often accompany actions.

The hands are often very eloquent even when no outward movement is visible. Inner States can be strongly suggested by hands seemingly at rest. The dynamic expression is inherent in the attitude they project and may give clues to subsequent actions. For instance, when facing a row of people with their hands in their laps or on their legs, a suggestion of their inner states is revealed: Two hands resting one on top of the other in a Light/Free Flow, somewhat impulsive attitude might then initiate a Light/Free Flow gesture when the person talks to someone else.

Another person's hands might be loosely curled in his lap. No Effort is detectable, just a giving in to gravity and Neutral Flow. His total body attitude: Slumped heavily into his body weight, self-absorbed in near-total passivity.

Still another person may be holding her two hands together in a Sustained/Bound Flow attitude which, from time to time, with the addition of Weight, becomes a Basic Effort action of Pressing/Squeezing: Strong/Direct/Sustained and then returning to Sustained/Bound.

Another person sits with his forehead contracted into a Bound/Direct attitude which, all of a sudden, perhaps in response to an inner thought, is dissipated into a Free Flow/Indirectness with an accompanying smile.

Transformation Drives

By exchanging the Flow Effort for one of the Effort components of a Basic Effort Action drive, a transformation occurs that produces a profoundly different experience.

There is an intensification of the two remaining Effort elements (which can be perceived as Inner States) to which Flow adds a drive of strong sensuous quality. This is in contrast to the more tangible action quality of the Basic Effort action drives where Flow is held in reserve.

The three categories of Transformations — Spaceless, Weightless and Timeless — are identified as belonging to inner drives of Passion, Vision and Spell respectively. The identifications are developed out of the characteristic qualities of the individual Effort elements — Attention (Space), Intention (Weight), Decision (Time), Progression (Flow) — and the qualities of their combinations as Inner States (two-Effort combinations: Awake/Dream-like; Remote/Near; Stable/Mobile) and as related to Effort Action Drives (Punch/Float; Slash/Glide; Dab/Wring; Press/Flick). Again, we remind the reader that the identifying words are only approximations of the experience.

Variations within the three major categories — Spaceless, Weightless and Timeless — are possible by different combinations of indulging or resisting elements. Examples are described below:

Spaceless: If, from a Punch (Direct/Strong/Sustained), the Space Effort (Direct) is replaced by Flow (Free or Bound), the new combination of Weight, Time and Flow transforms the Punch, a Basic Effort Action Drive, into another kind of drive.

The Weight may be Strong or Light; the Time may be Sudden or Sustained. Without an attitude toward Space that can anchor Weight/Time, Flow will pulsate, intensify the Weight/Time into strong, passionate or delicate tender feelings detached from the reflection associated with the Space Effort.

Because of this effect by Flow, the Spaceless Drive is metaphorically referred to as the Passion Drive.

While Spaceless Drives with their clear, rhythmic component (Weight/Time) appear often in work and dance actions, it is not always the rhythmic aspect that dominates. When Weight is Strong, the Spaceless Drive can be detected in heated discussions. In extreme Strong, it is manifested in the violent behavior of the mentally ill; the passionate raging and yelling — perhaps a temper tantrum — of the Spaceless Drive may be a precursor of a Basic Effort action of violence such as extreme Punching or Slashing.

At the other range — when Weight is Light — a clearly defined tenderness will evolve, as in a caressing touch.

Timeless: In the Timeless Drive, Space and Weight become dominant, lending a stabilizing power to the movement. Without Time's sense of urgency or delay to loosen the stability, the steadfastness of Space/Weight becomes inescapable when Flow's "goingness" is added to it, and a spell-like intensity is created. It is comparable to "a witch's spell," or the power of an irresistible seducer. The power to break the spell is restored by a return to the active attitude toward Time instead of Flow.

Metaphorically, the Timeless Drive is referred to as the Spell Drive.

When this combination or part of it appears in a speaking gesture, it can express persuasion, seduction.

In a Russian film of *Pique Dame,* a pseudo-lover seduces an innocent girl. What made his performance only seductive and bewitching without passion could be described in Effort terms: He never used Time with Weight; he very clearly used Direct and Indirect Space, and shades of Weight with variations in Flow. In other words, Space/Weight, with Flow instead of Time.

61

Weightless:* In the Weightless Drive, Time and Space reinforce each other to mental alertness, a consciousness of precision in time and place, apart from the physical sensation of one's weight or impact. Therefore, Flow can take that awareness "where it will" into the almost disembodied state of the Vision Drive.

In speaking gestures, this Drive appears when someone outlines plans for the future without being concerned about executing a task at hand. Even more, it appears when someone describes a dream or recalls an incident from long ago. As a movement experience, the music of Gregorian chanting or other chanting monotones of the human voice evokes Weightless Inner Drives to movement.

When someone tells a fairy tale or a legend to a child or a group of children and adults, a "once-upon-a-time" story, the story teller has a characteristic tone of voice and, correspondingly, a characteristic fluency of gesture. Conspicuously present are Effort combinations of Weightless (Vision) and Timeless (Spell) Drives. However, as soon as the narrative switches to a dramatic confrontation as, for instance, when the princess or king demands a specific task of the hero, with instructions of where to go and what to do, basic Effort Drives slightly reduced or with full intensity appear in the gesturing. On the whole, the dominance of Transformation Drives defines the rhythms in such a tale. They convey to the listener the magic fascination of the fairy tale or myth, the non-real.

In ballet, the Weightless (Vision) Drive is frequently used as a theme to create the illusion of completely overcoming body weight. Some of the most ethereal adagios of a ballerina and her male partner are built around the use of this combination.

Watching charismatic leaders whip up a crowd to action reveals variations in Vision, Spell and Passion Drives that are also reflected in the symbiotic reactions of individuals in the crowd.

Shifts in Transformation Drives are facilitated or linked by the Two-Element combinations containing Flow that are embedded in them. Each Drive has one Flow/Other-Effort combination that it shares with either of the other Drives. Thus, for example, the Timeless Drive is linked to the Weightless Drive by sharing Space/Flow and to the Spaceless Drive by sharing Weight/Flow. The Weightless Drive, in addition to the above link to Timeless, is linked to the Spaceless Drive by sharing Time/Flow. This is illustrated below:

Timeless Drive–Space/Weight/Flow–contains Inner States:
  A. Space/Weight
  B. Weight/Flow
  C. Space/Flow

Weightless Drive–Space/Time/Flow–contains Inner States:
  C. Space/Flow
  D. Space/Time
  E. Time/Flow

Spaceless Drive–Weight/Time/Flow–contains Inner States:
  E. Time/Flow
  F. Weight/Time
  B. Weight/Flow

The changes from Basic Effort Action Drives to Inner States or to Transformation Drives are more or less subtle depending on the degree of change. The Inner States are particularly elusive in pure form because they become so quickly embedded in the Drives. But they are essential to the subtle transitions from Drive to another.

---

* *This does not mean without body weight. It means the absence or minimal participation of the Weight Effort: an attitude toward the use of body weight.*

However, even an untrained observer can see the principal moods and qualities of a Transformation Drive, describing them metaphorically: "He has a hypnotic (Timeless) quality," or "She was so passionately involved in her diatribe that she didn't even hear me enter" (Spaceless), or "He was drawn out of himself into the vision of the many possibilities before him" (Weightless).

Frequently a Basic Effort Action can be discerned in verbal communication — even when there may be no practical handling of materials — eliciting observations such as "He really hit it," or "He came to the point."

Changing from Transformation Drive to an Inner State or vice versa is not as dramatic as changing from a Basic Effort Action Drive to either of the other two. In fact, there is a common tendency for the former two to veer into each other.

In the course of any sequence of activity, there are many shifts from one kind of combination to another. These shifts can serve as alternate exertions and recuperations to maintain the vitality of the activity. A constantly repeated alternation between Sudden (Time)/Strong (Weight)/Free (Flow), a Transformation Drive, may bring relief from the short-lived Sudden (Time)/Strong (Weight)/Direct (Space), a Basic Effort Action Drive, perhaps as a peak in a work or a dance action.

The interpretations should be observed as possibilities, rather than absolutes. As experience and observation guides, they serve as indicators of subtle differences expressed by varying Effort element combinations. Research continues in their identifications.*

Full Effort Combinations
Combinations of all four Effort elements, Space, Weight, Time and Flow, appear in extremes of function and expression, where they seem to produce a dissolution or loss of boundaries. The simultaneous presence of all four Effort elements gives the movement a power of what appears to be self-propulsion as if the mover's volition has been usurped by the totality of the Effort involvement. At its peak, the action becomes involuntary as if the addition of Flow to the Basic Effort took the Effort beyond volition.

At one end of the range — the resisting group — the Full Effort combinations are manifested emotionally as acts of "senseless" violence, such as murderously beating up a person or tearing something apart. They can also be manifested in highly skilled athletic or dramatic performances such as those of the Peking acrobats.

At the other end of the range — the indulging group of Effort elements — the Full Effort combinations may appear fleetingly in a dancer's most delicate refinement of expression appearing to take the action beyond its form. In certain phases of skilled crafts such as fine jewel cutting, similar fleeting moments occur.

It is the addition of the fourth element, Flow, to the Basic Effort Action Drive that gives the extreme character to these movements, whether they be murderous or ethereal. There are extreme fluctuations of Free and Bound Flow in the violent acts and there are subtle fluctuations in the non-violent actions.

For example, a Punch (Strong/Direct/Sudden) becomes a senselessly extreme act of violence when repeated extreme fluctuations of Bound and Free Flow are added to it. At the opposite end of the range, a Float (Indirect/Light/Sustained) will be carried away in tender feeling when subtle fluctuations of Free/Bound Flow are added.

The Full Effort combinations involving the resisting, fighting ranges are like destructive confrontations. The Full Effort combinations involving the indulging, yielding ranges become avoidances of confrontations, escaping. Both can be interpreted as extreme survival responses.

---

* *In Chapter 11, excerpts are presented from a detailed study in the use of Transformation Drive in choreographing a specific dance.*

Examples

A Quiet Conversation

One may observe a quiet conversation between friends, over coffee. A number of times A picks up the cup in a sort of even Neutral rhythm (essentially Flow changes). B asks a question. In response, A reaches for his cup and slowly, with Sustained Time and Bound Flow, he lifts the cup, pauses before he sips. This may arouse in B a number of reactions: Is A considering my idea? Does A hesitate to accept? The changed rhythm has aroused B in a way that the previous picking up and sipping actions did not. In the same conversation, B may make a statement to which A reacts with Suddenness, lifting his right hand, pausing. Again, it will cause some feeling, thinking reaction: Is A surprised, does A want B to stop, and so on.

* * * * *

Opening a Box

In opening a spice box, for example, a Light touch will change to a Sudden yank to force off the lid; in the next moment, a Sustained, even Weight will be active in a new try to open the stubborn lid; finally, a Sudden/Strong (explosive) lift will occur as the lid comes off. This is immediately followed by a Sudden/Strong turning countermovement of the hand holding the box to prevent its contents from spilling over the floor.

Always, from one phase to another, the many small and large adjustments in Flow, in Time, in Weight, and in Space Effort elements create the constant rhythmic quality fluctuations that are more or less satisfying to the performer and the observer.

* * * * *

Assembling Ingredients for a Meal

Woman enters the kitchen in Neutral Time and Flow. She looks around, scanning drawers, refrigerator, shelves with Indirect Free Flow to Bound changes.

She opens a drawer with Sudden Directness, pauses to inspect the contents — Free Flow/Direct to slightly Bound/Indirect.

She picks up two knives separately — the first with Direct/Free Flow becoming Bound; the second with Indirect/Bound to Sudden/Direct, Free to Bound.

Closing drawer with a Strong whack Indirect to Direct/Bound to Free/Sudden, she moves to refrigerator and opens the door with Light/Bound grip and Free/Sudden motion toward herself, takes a stick of butter with Light/Bound Directness and slams the door with Free Flow/Strength.

She moves on toward a shelf, raises herself on her toes Free/Light to Direct/Bound, takes down a plastic bowl with Indirect/Free Flow becoming Sustained/Bound and sets the bowl down on the table to her left with Free Flow/Directness.

She unwraps the stick of butter with small forearm–wrist–finger movements: touching Light/Bound the fold of the paper and, with Light/Sustainment, starts to peel it off. Repeating the procedure at a place next to the starting place, she continues the peeling with shifts between Indirect/Direct, Free/Bound and Sustainment ending in a Free Flow/Suddenness.

* * * * *

Moving a Piano

Innumerable gradations in the combinations of Effort elements and their fluctuations can be observed in most action tasks. For example, a heavy piano must be moved from one end of the room to the other end. The mover will not immediately start with a Full Effort drive, or even a Basic Effort Action drive. He might not even start with a Weight Effort.

Instead, he will build himself up to it. He may first, tentatively, try Flow and Directness to pinpoint the direction in which the object is to be moved. Then, he may replace the Flow and introduce Strong Weight and, as he sets the object in motion, add Sustainment to gradually integrate the Strength and

Directness. He is now using Strong Weight, Direct Space, and Sustained Time — the Basic Effort of Pressing — arriving at it, in this case, through Attention (Space), Intention (Weight), stable combination, until Decision (Time) was added.

He may, however, slightly fluctuate in one or another of these components, or shift the sequence of them, adjusting to small impediments on his way in either Time or Space or Weight. The Basic Pressing action may, at times, because of outer impediments or his fatigue, be modified or reduced into an inherent two-element combination, such as Sustained Strength (Time/Weight), having lost the Directness (Space) and its steering potential.

*　*　*　*　*

Eating One Spoonful of Soup: a Multi-Phasic Phrase as performed by Two Different People

This illustrates distinctive characters of the activity as determined by different choices of Effort elements and Effort combinations organized in specific ways.

Subject A sits at a table, preparing to eat, and then eating the soup.

> **Phase One:** She approaches the spoon, lying to the right in front of her, with her right arm/hand. Free Flow/Directness, just before touching the spoon, becomes Bound Flow/Directness.
> **Phase Two:** She picks up the spoon with Light/Bound Flow; she lowers the spoon with Free Flow/Suddenness into the bowl.
> **Phase Three:** With Bound/Indirectness she fills the spoon and lifts it cautiously with Bound/Sustainment. Close to her mouth, the movement becomes Direct/Sustained.
> **Phase Four:** She opens her mouth Free/Indirect and, with a Sudden/Light hand gesture, she tilts the spoon into her mouth.
> **Phase Five:** She closes her mouth with Bound/Lightness as she pulls the spoon out with Free Flow/Lightness.

Subject B at the next table sits with her feet firmly planted on the floor, and veritably attacks her soup, driven to finish it "immediately."

> **Phase One:** With a Sudden/Bound Flow slight turn of her torso toward the right, she grabs the spoon with Bound Flow/Suddenness, becoming Direct.
> **Phase Two:** With another Sudden jerk, she faces the bowl and plunges the spoon into the soup with Free Flow/Directness, abruptly, Sudden/Bound, pulling it out with Direct/Boundness toward her mouth.
> **Phase Three:** She shoves it into her open mouth with a Sudden/Bound motion that includes her head (slightly backward).
> **Phase Four:** Before swallowing, she lowers the spoon in a Sudden/Direct, Free Flow motion.

Here are the two activities in Effort terms, without additional description:

Subject A:

Phase One:	Free Flow/Directness to Bound/Flow Directness.
Phase Two:	Bound Flow/Lightness to Free Flow/Suddenness.
Phase Three:	Bound Flow/Indirectness to Bound Flow/Sustained to Direct/Sustained.
Phase Four:	Free Flow/Indirect to Sudden/Light.
Phase Five:	Bound Flow/Lightness to Free Flow/Lightness.

Subject B:

Phase One: Sudden/Bound Flow to Bound Flow/Sudden to Bound Flow/Direct.

Phase Two: Sudden/Bound Flow to Free Flow/Sudden to Bound Flow/Sudden to Bound Flow/Direct.

Phase Three: Bound Flow/Strong.

Phase Four: Sudden/Free Flow/Direct.

The phases can be either clearly distinguished from each other or "slung" together. Thus, Subject A's activity consists of five phases in which the first three can be considered together as another shorter phrase. Subject B, however, has four distinguishable phases, in which the first two are slung together and the second two are almost indistinguishable because they are bound so closely to each other, with the result that the whole activity is experienced as one phrase.

By looking at just the Effort descriptions, the observer can immediately pick up the more leisurely indulgent mood of Subject A in contrast to the driven, abrupt sequence of Subject B.

In Subject A, there are frequent changes between Free and Bound Flow. This occurs in almost all of the phases. That is, the fluctuations of the Flow support the goingness of the movement. This gives the whole activity a graded, smooth progress from one phase to the next.

Subject B is loaded with Sudden/Directness throughout all phases. This is not relieved by change into the indulging range of another Effort or by a rebound into the opposite (indulging) range of its own Effort, i.e., Sustainment or Indirectness. The result is an overall impression of unrelieved high tension haste and fixed pinpointedness.

The reappearance of the same Effort components finally characterize the activity for each person, and may also, throughout different kinds of activities, eventually characterize the person. The "preferred" qualities (Effort choices) of individuals become aspects of their individuality, character attributes that are recognizable and remembered.

*   *   *   *   *

Example of Shifting Emphasis in Speaking Gestures

The subtle relationship between verbal and body movement is illustrated. The variations in Effort elements due to the change of emphasis create distinctly different rhythmic phrasing as well.

A number of people react negatively to a proposal. They say the same sentence, but emphasize different words and these differences are reflected in the accompanying head and/or arm/hand gestures.

The sentence: "I do not want it."

Version One:

I	*do*	*not*	*want*	*it.*
Free Flow	Free Flow	Bound Flow	Direct/Sudden	Bound Flow
to Strong/Bound				
to Strong				

Version Two:

I	*do*	*not*	*want*	*it.*
Light	Strong	Bound Flow	Light	Bound Flow
Free Flow	Direct		Sudden	
	to Bound Flow		Bound Flow	

66

Version Three:

I	*do*	<u>*not*</u>	*want*	*it.*
Light Bound Flow	Bound Flow	Strong Sudden Bound Flow	Sudden Free Flow	Bound Flow

Version Four:

I	*do*	*not*	<u>*want*</u>	*it.*
Free Flow	Bound Flow	Free Flow Sudden	Indirect Sustained Free Flow to Strong Direct Sudden	Bound Flow

Version Five:

I	*do*	*not*	*want*	<u>*it.*</u>
Free Flow	Bound Flow	Bound Flow	Sudden Bound Flow	Direct Sudden Strong

*　*　*　*　*

Two People Performing the Same Activity

A woman opens the door, with Sustained/Slightly Bound Flow and walks with Free Flow/Lightness becoming increasingly Direct/Free, toward the table where there is a bowl of fruit. As she passes the table, she snatches a peach from the bowl with Sudden/Light/Free Flow becoming slightly Bound as she seizes the fruit. She continues to walk in Free Flow/Lightness. As she almost reaches the door, she hears the man enter at the other end of the room and stops with Sudden/Bound Flow, then turns around with Indirect/Free Flow, inclining her head toward the man with Indirect/Bound Flow. She pauses.

The man enters with Free Flow/Strength which becomes Direct/Bound as he reaches the bowl and takes an orange with Indirect/Free Flow becoming Direct/Bound. Then, he turns the fruit from side to side, examining it with Light/Bound and Light/Free Flow and, with Sudden/Bound to Direct/Free Flow, drops it back into the bowl.

For both, from one phase to another, there were many small and large adjustments whose fluctuations created particular rhythmic qualities and movements as telling as melodies of songs or speech patterns. Whereas her organization was generally in one sequence, he had several phases in his sequence. Her melody had a Light Direct quality with Sudden accents, while his had a more hesitant quality, a Strong accent, then a deliberative ritard ending with abrupt Suddenness.

Dominant Qualities

Effort	**Woman**	**Man**
Flow	Free	Balanced Free/Bound
Space	Slightly more Direct	Balanced Indirect/Direct
Weight	Light	Strong
Time	Sudden	Sudden
	Casual, easy-going, flowing	Thoughtful, deliberative

*　*　*　*　*

Shepherd's Dance: Effort Exertion/Recuperation

Another example of maintaining continuity, illustrating how Effort elements need to be recreated in the process of repetition by recuperative transitions between each repetition, can be observed in various folk ballets of Central Europe — Poland, Yugoslavia, Ukraine, Romania, Hungary. They have richly developed their indigenous folk material in rhythmical variations and extraordinary feats of jumping, acrobatic thrusts of the body, whirling turns at all levels. These "natural" feats have been the source of highly polished performances in the professional folk ballet. The original folk dances and the professional performances of them are "the same — but not the same;" the difference in the continuity of their mobility and intent can be described in Effort terms.

To do this, we observed one of these professional groups of young, highly-trained dancers in a Romanian film. We also observed some village dancing (Kalusha) of Romanian shepherds. We analyzed a piece of the professional folk ballet film when the dancers were turning at high speed with fast footwork and we saw, on the frame-by-frame analysis, six or seven or more frames blurred, indicating that fast tempo was maintained without fluctuation.

The shepherd's performance also gave the impression of high intensity speed action. However, in this case, there were alternations between Effort elements as peak accentuations: Sudden (Time)/Strong (Weight)/Free Flow alternated with Sudden (Time)/Strong (Weight)/Direct (Space). In the frame-by-frame analysis, one or two frames would be blurred by high speed, followed by one or two recuperative frames not blurred and followed by another one or two frames again high speed blurred, followed by another recuperative transition.

Thus, the shepherds stayed within the quick tempo by a constant re-creation of the Sudden Effort element in various combinations with other Effort elements. The professionals' fast tempo, lacking the Sudden Effort element, and lacking the combination changes that continuously renewed it, had a static rather than a mobile quality. It was the constant re-creation that gave the shepherd's dance more excitement and gusto, while the professionals' training for high-speed tempo produced a "conditioned," overpolished performance.

In the examples of repetitive work action and of the shepherd's dance, spontaneous recuperative Effort involvement sprang from the rhythmical alternation of work and leisure. However, in the professional performance of a folk ballet this inherent recuperation necessity was negated by over-trained, mechanical skill. The vitality of continuity and of authentic spontaneity was lost in the process.

*　　*　　*　　*　　*

Rehabilitation: Learning a New Task

A child of eight, sitting on a low bench, tries to pull her paralyzed legs up the next higher bench. The benches are arranged in threes like steps of some staircases. Her natural Effort tendency is to linger, in Time Sustainment, with Flow and Neutral Weight. She has to be reminded to "do it all at once in the fastest, strongest way." Then she succeeds by following instructions that incorporate her Flow and Weight changes with Time.

A tall, slim dancer solved the same problem through her fluent mobility: She learned to wriggle herself up by serpentine-like convolutions, constantly changing from right to left weight shifts, Free Flow, interspersed with occasional Suddenness.

The child solved the problem with essentially Effort changes; the dancer with essentially Shape changes and their accompanying Effort changes.

CHAPTER 5

Rhythm and Phrasing

Work and festivities have their rhythms, their laws, and they must be organized according to the sense of these rhythms. People cry for rhythmic power waves — work and festive — to revive and enliven into meaningfulness their suppressed sense of life.

— Rudolf Laban

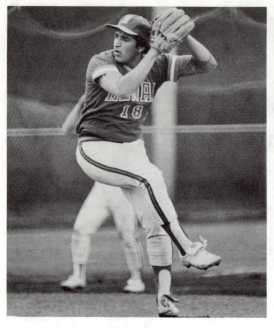

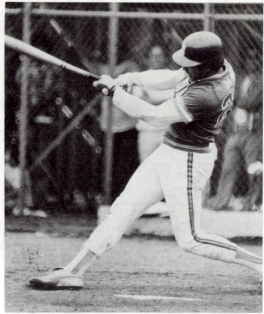

Pitcher and Batter © Leonard Nakahashi
Total shaping. All three dimensions are involved and clear diagonals connect the whole body, from head through center to tips of fingers and toes.
Pitcher: Free to Bound, Suddenness to moment of Sustainment and Strength.
Batter: maximal Flow, Strength and Directness on swing; maximal Flow, Suddenness and Strength in follow-through.

Top left: Pitcher at beginning of phrase. Both shaping and Effort rhythmical accents of condensations and explosive swings color the phrases in the whole sequence of the three photos.

Top right: Batter in middle of phrase.

Right: Batter at end of phrase.

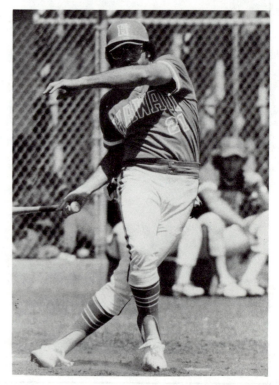

Rhythm and Phrasing

Rhythm can be perceived in many ways. It can be visible and/or audible, and can be observed in the accents of changing body tensions — all of which are interrelated.

Visible and audible rhythms can be transposed into body tensions, or, in some cases, can be identified by the neutrality of the body tensions. Moreover, the deep association (conscious or unconscious) with body movement is reflected in the emotional content elicited by various rhythmic patterns. The sensitivity to body, space and Effort rhythmic sequences is essential to the movement observer.

Judith Kestenberg's studies of newborn babies observed fluctuations in their tension flow changes while they made drinking and biting attempts. Diagrams of their patterns were recorded as in Figure 28.

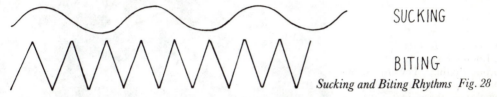

SUCKING

BITING

Sucking and Biting Rhythms Fig. 28

Note that sucking produces a wave-like rhythm and biting an angular rhythm. Other biological functions were also recorded and studies were made of the relationships of all these rhythms to total body activity rhythms.*

Laban encouraged dancing without music to increase sensitivity to the rhythms of body tensions and to free performers from rigid, symmetrical rhythmical patterns with metrical emphases. Delineations of character and mood are evoked by their rhythmical associations with the body tensions they reflect.

One's whole organism is organized into rhythmic patterns. Heart beat, breath, intestinal rhythms are only examples of the most vital functions. The continuity of the patterns is protected by regulatory mechanisms that maintain the balanced alternations of their essentially two-phasic activities through many forms of stress. Syncopated rhythms always arouse excited body involvement; they might be related to the primary startle reflex of infants.**

We will confine our attention to the immediate experience of rhythm in body movement as it is determined by shifting tensions in the body relating to space and to Effort. In other words, by reviewing the Body/Effort/Space perceptions previously discussed, but with the focus on rhythms intrinsic to that analysis.

Laban considered elemental rhythms as those based on polarities of exertion and recuperation, such as Awake/Asleep, Work/Rest, Condensation of Tension/Dissipation of Tension — all expressed in spatial and Effort patterns and in the use of body parts. Changes within movement — contrasts and near-contrasts — produce rhythmic patterns of stresses and phrasing, which can be experienced in the spatial scales. A phrase is that organization of movement process that consists of a beginning, middle and end of a statement. Each section may have one or more phases and each activity may have one or more phrases.

The sequences of direction changes in the spatial scales are ordered so that each exertion is followed by a recuperation before the next exertion in another dimension. There are inherent accents in these changes which create the dynamics of the rhythm. This is analogous to a musical conductor's movement eliciting music that is also dependent on his/her active Effort involvement.

---

*   *See Bibliography: Kestenberg.*   * * *See Fries and Kestenberg references in Bibliography.*

Right: *Girl Jumping Rope*
© Morris H. Jaffe
Light Weight and Sudden Time,
accelerating and diminishing
rhythmically, accent the Free
Flow in cyclical sagittal
movement. Phrases could be
identified as two-phasic (back and
over) or could be extended until
the jumper makes another
variation. Body shaping convex in
countertension to pull of swinging
rope.

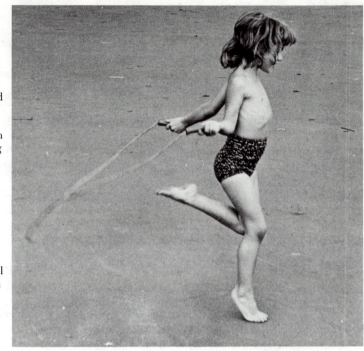

Below: *Whaleboat Race*
© Bonnie Freer
Group rhythms. Toward end of
exertion phase. They are not in full
synchrony: there are variations in
body shaping and in Weight and
Effort combinations. Coxswain
clearly sagittal, concave in
countertension to forward
movement of boat.

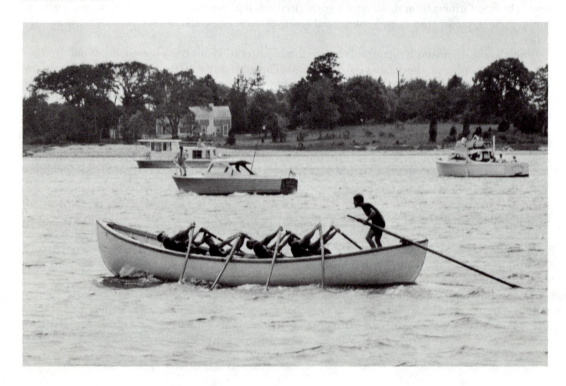

72

In a sequence from a prison work camp film, the exertion/recuperation spatial Effort rhythms of a work action were observed: Three men fell a tree with an axe. They strike with power, one after the other, leaving each man a time of recuperative and preparatory action. Thus, a particular triadic rhythmical sequence is established which allows each to contribute his Strength Effort maximally at the right moment. The action is accompanied by singing which reinforces the rhythm and keeps it going. The main Effort element of the striking action is Free Flow and the action adds Sudden (Time) and Strong (Weight) in a wide scooping arc.

Exertion/recuperation rhythms are inherent in preparatory action/main action sequences. The simplest example is an in-out limb swing toward the body and away from the body. Toward the body represents the preparatory phase. It is a condensed movement close to the body that, in the main action, swings out towards space. It is like the up-beat or anacrusis in music.

In Effort/Shape terminology, the preparatory movement sometimes consists of Effort elements that are opposite to those of the main statement. For example, a Light (Weight) up-beat will prepare for a Strong statement.

Repeating a series of such in-out swings in different directions produces different rhythms according to the direction or combinations of directions of the swings. A forward/upward/sideward swing results in a slightly asymmetrical shape and rhythm, while a swing that is only forward/backward has a symmetrical shape and basic beat.

The rhythms built on this in-preparation that swings out into space can be seen in many familiar movements, such as gestures in dance, thrusts in playing ball (where the sequence is reversed). When preparing a horse for a fence jump, the rider starts the pre-jump run with a slight body and/or spatial retreating. That provides the rhythmic up-beat for the forward run and jump.

The characteristic rhythm of any given activity evolves out of the spatial/Effort sequence and phrasing of its components.

Phrasing of body movement, again as in music, requires an intimate connection to the intent of the performer and to the breathing patterns that support the intent. The subtlest change in phrasing can color the quality of the function and expressiveness of the movement. In music, the phrasing is experienced without reference to the measures; phrases often cross the bar lines in order to place emphases, usually followed by a breath, at appropriate points. This is also true of movement phrasing.

The sequence in which the movements of an activity occur and the emphasis within the sequence define the phrasing on the simplest level. On a more complex level, the sequence of constellations of movements in the activity and the emphases among them define the larger structure of the whole behavior pattern. Thus, it is not just the activity that identifies the behavior but it is the sequence and phrasing with their distinctive rhythms that express and reinforce verbal and emotional content. All are related to the spatial intents of the movements.

What is generally recognized as an "action" in movement terms can actually be perceived, as we have indicated throughout the book, on several levels — as a body action, a spatial action, and/or an action with varying degrees of Effort qualities. In each case, the action can be simple, i.e., moving one body part in one direction with one Effort dominant, or, complex, involving more body parts in more directions with more Effort elements. The complexity of the phrasing is increased as the body, space, Effort factors of the actions include more variations.

A combination of actions produces an activity such as writing a letter, turning on a radio, picking flowers. Each activity contains a number of actions ordered in a sequence and phrased by particular spatial and/or Effort emphases that will best fulfill the intent.

The phrasing can be two-phasic or multi-phasic, short or long, explosive or gradual in development.

The simplest form of activity is two-phasic: one phase is the exertion and the second phase is recuperation. Spatially, this could be, for example, bending/stretching, or pushing/pulling. Two-phasic Effort sequences are found in, for example, an action of Strength followed by a rebound into Lightness or one major Effort combination and a recuperation on the same path with just Flow.

When performed in exact repetitions, these two-phasic phrasings produce rather monotone rhythms that can be dulling or soothing. With hardly any stress from Effort or spatial path, young children use such rhythms in rocking back and forth; mothers use them to rock their children to sleep or console them when they are upset. Therapists use them with disturbed patients. They also appear as expressions of deep grief. The monotone consisting mainly of flow that has not yet crystallized into specific Effort elements and shapes produces a basic rhythm of evenness.

As activities become more complex, canoeing, for example, or threshing or hoeing, simple two-phasic forms are still central, but there are more of them — repetitions of the same two-phasic forms or several different two-phasic forms in series. Therefore, more space and Effort variations and more complicated phrasing appear within the sequences but the underlying quality of two-phasic stability remains. Examples at the end of this chapter illustrate other two-phasic activities. Both space and Effort are considered in repetitive, non-repetitive, symmetrical, non-symmetrical, and continuous actions. The stability of the two-phasic monotone quality lends itself to easy sharing in a group. Continuous repetition of two-phasic phrases, without space or Effort variation, can lead away from alertness into wandering states of consciousness. When this is interrupted by adding phases increasingly asymmetrical (either in Effort or space), new rhythms result that restore alertness and change the communication.

Spatial intent, initiation, transitions, recuperations, continuity of breathing patterns — all temper the phrasing within and between the continuity of sequences and, therefore, the functional and expressive meaning.

The dimensional scale has a basic rhythm that is different from the rhythm of, for example, a diagonally inclined "A" scale. The dynamic quality of the metrical rhythm is determined by the order of the sequences. In the move from an opening shape to a closing one, the dynamics of the rhythm are different than when that sequence is reversed. Illustrations of the rhythmic structure of sequences derived from the icosahedron are described in Effort/space terms in examples at end of this chapter.

Symmetrical movement has a symmetrical rhythm count. Asymmetrical movement has an asymmetrical rhythm count. A step in any direction causes countertensions in the body that influence the rhythms. A simple alternation of forward/backward steps or side/close supported by a vertical body attitude produces a simple 2/4 or other binary rhythm. But as soon as the side steps include crossing and uncrossing, that is, a slight forward/backward tension, the rhythm tends toward a ternary (3/4) model. This may be additionally influenced by progressing on a circular floor pattern which reinforces countertensions of twisting. Balkan dances have many examples of crossing/uncrossing steps on a circular line which may frequently alternate from clockwise to counterclockwise progressions. When these are also interspersed with forward/backward sequences in place, the rhythm has great variation between binary, ternary and more complex combinations.

The "simple" act of walking is an excellent illustration of the different relationships between shapes and rhythms. Walking to rhythms, perhaps accompanied by a musical instrument, can be repeated with definite Time/Weight changes that will either enliven or dull the movement with rhythmical tensing and detensing consistent with body usage. In western culture, walking emphasizes the regular alternation of right and left progression with minimal contralaterality between the upper and lower body. This results in a symmetrical, binary (2/4 or 4/4) beat.

However, in other cultures, walking emphasizes an ornamented alternation of right and left progression which reinforces the contralaterality between upper and lower body. This results in a less symmetrical beat that is closer to a 5/4. In some cases, arm gestures add complexity to the rhythm to such an extent that steps become accompaniment to their basic beat. (See Walking details, p. 205 ff.)

Some audible and body rhythms reinforce internal moods, and others, group moods. A single flute spinning out a long drawn-out melody with minimal rhythmic variation puts the listener into a mood of quiet meditation or may stir intensive feelings of longing and body movements with Flow and Sustainment. The noise that workers produce in a regular repetitive activity, such as old-fashioned threshing with flails, makes a rhythm that keeps the activity going in either a maintained synchrony or a successive alternation. This will depend on how the group arranges itself spatially — in a straight line, for example, or in a half circle, or in a square of four workers. It must feel comfortable to join and to maintain the activity. The territorial arrangement makes the difference between a shared, massive input or a contributory successive input, that is, either sharing or rhythmically distributing main exertion and recuperation. All of this may be further reinforced by the workers making vocal sounds accompanying the action. Both the audible rhythm and the rhythm felt as body tension supports the mood and flow of work. In all cases, the moods can be identified also in terms of the combinations of Effort elements, particularly Incomplete Effort combinations and Transformation Drives.

To summarize, rhythm is not just a duration of time, accentuated by stresses. It is also the result of the interaction of Effort combinations with variations in spatial patterns.

Since time relationships and all divisions of time are actually perceived in space, the movements of the body in space, the movements of sound in space and the movements of lines and colors in space can be related to the time divisions to produce visible and audible forms of time in dance, music and art as well as in functional activities.

The move away from fixed metricality is toward a greater sense of relativity in both dance and music. In executing the Laban movement scales, the givens — body limitations, intent and spatial goals — are modified or stretched by their intrinsic relationship to each other, their affinities for particular Effort elements or combinations of Effort elements and their resulting tensions and rhythms. Choices can be made to move in opposition to those affinities. This is also true of musical scales.

All live movement has a fluctuating exchange between a structured framework and the enlivening Space/Weight/Time/Flow tensions and their particular rhythms. Individual preferences support tendencies to variations as can be seen when observing different people perform the same actions in dance, music, work and play. The contribution of the individual preferences is weakened when a performance is accompanied by taped music because the flexibility of mutual rhythmical adaptions is reduced. Observe the difference between a dance performance with live musicians as opposed to one given with taped music. In the latter, the subtle flexibility and spontaneity which give vitality to rhythm is destroyed and the rhythm itself becomes pallid.

Industrialized society often has a devitalizing effect on organic rhythms. Its pressures reduce the flow of exertion/recuperation rhythms necessary to the continuity of vitality in activity. New technologies may introduce new rhythm possibilities, but when they confine themselves to actions without recuperations or attempt to fit the actions totally to the machine, the human element on which the next levels of creativity depend is abandoned.

It is not Effort alone, nor spatial shifts alone, but the combinations of their many variations in relationship to the body parameters that create the shifting tensions underlying rhythm. And the continuous environmental changes require continuous adaptations at every level.

Music and the other arts relate to those rhythmic tensions and additional instruments can extend them in particular ways. For this reason, it is of great value to movement observers to include the subject's music and art activity in the overall observation. It is the experience of the body tensions that provides points of reference for rhythms. The vocabulary which heightens the clarity of those rhythmic keys can also be invaluable in relating the arts to each other and extending the ranges of performers into the work and play activities of their communities.

Examples

Two-Phasic Activities: Three Examples

1. Polishing a smooth surface going horizontally over the surface. A repetitive action.
   Phase One: going to the right
   An up-beat, Free Flow/Light, initiates the action's Neutral Flow/Direct/Sustained/Light.
   Phase Two: return
   Free Flow/Slightly diminishing Directness and Sustainment/Light.

2. Squashing some leaves, for a primitive dyeing process, with a stone forward/back over the surface in two uneven repetitive actions, slightly asymmetrical.
   Phase One (main phase): forward contact with stone
   An up-beat, Free Flow/Light, precedes the action's Sudden/Light/Bound to Bound/Strength.
   Phase Two (return): backward taking hand off stone slightly
   Free Flow/Light. In the repetition, the return functions as up-beat.

3. Pulling tape off a package and letting the arm drop. Non-repetitive and asymmetrical.
   Phase One (main phase): the pull
   An up-beat of Sudden/Free Flow precedes the action's Exaggerated Sudden/Strong/Bound.
   Phase Two: arm drop into collapse
   Force and Time are given up completely and Free Flow diminished to zero, and the arm gives in to gravity with passive weight.

The first two examples illustrate repetitive actions; the first is evenly repetitive, the second is unevenly repetitive, therefore slightly asymmetrical. The third is not repetitive; it is asymmetrical. Because of the repetitive intents in the short examples, phrasing is less significant than when the ranges of intent are expanded.

$$* \quad * \quad * \quad * \quad *$$

Picking Flowers — Phrasing

Picking flowers involves bending down or squatting, reaching for and grasping the stem of the flower, tearing it off its stem, collecting it into the other hand in a complex of shaping actions.

One could pick the flower with one of several possible intents, which would determine Effort choices and emphases. If the intent is to tear the flower off rather than to pick it, the phrasing is likely to be shorter, two-phasic (out and back), the spatial and Effort fluctuations would be more limited, and the shaping of the phrase would be simpler and less rounded.

If the intent is to pick the flower in order to enjoy it, the phrasing is likely to be longer, with more internal divisions. The fluctuations in spatial path and Effort would be more varied and the shaping of the phrase would be more rounded and two- or three-dimensional.

Phrasing is not to be confused with phases of activities. For example, when picking flowers by bending over with a straight back or curling up into a squat, there may be a spatial pause before reaching out with the arm. That pause would end the first phase of the activity, but the phrase could actually end when the arm has reached the flower, or if there is no interruption, the phrase may not end until the flower is brought to the nose. Phrasing could also be determined by Effort variations. For example, the Time Effort might be active as Sustainment going down to the pause in the squat, marking the first phase, and then suddenly accelerating to reach out and touch the flower, thus ending the second phase and the phrase with the touch of the flower.

$$* \quad * \quad * \quad * \quad *$$

Effort and Spatial Phrasing — Verbal

The following verbal example illustrates the Effort phrasing in a multi-phasic phrase of several short actions that are repeated and lead to a climax of high intensity: "I warned you again and again, but this is the end." There are at least two possible perspectives — main stresses only or main stresses plus transitions between them. The first chart shows Effort stresses; the second spatial stresses.

A. Main Stresses Only		B. Capturing the Subtleties (Transitions)
	I	Light/Bound
	warned	Diminished Strong/Bound
	you	Neutral Flow
Direct/Bound/Sustained	again	Sudden
		Direct/Bound/Sustained
Sudden	and	Sudden
Direct/Bound/Sustained	again	Direct/Bound/Sustained
Pause		Pause
	but	Bound/Sudden
Strong/Bound Flow	this	Diminished Strong/Direct Bound
	is	Direct/Bound
	the	Neutral Flow
Direct/Strong/Bound	end	Sudden Up-beat
Indirect		Sustained/Strong/Bound
		Indirect

In Column A clearly-observable Effort stresses are identified as they appear in the sequence, while Column B adds identification of transitions between the major stresses. This means particular attention to Flow changes. When the subtle Flow changes have been excluded, as in the first (A) perspective, the melody of the phrase is lost, and with it, the subtle fluctuations of mood.

The Spatial Pattern of right forearm/hand in the gesture accompanying the sentence shows the three phases of the one-phrase sentence.

I	raising right forearm/hand up
warned	to forward
you	pause — phase 1
again	slight lift forearm/hand to forward pointing
and	slight lift of forearm/hand
again	to forward pointing
	pause — phase 2
but	lifting forearm high, slight pause
this	spreading hand and right forearm
	toward right/forward
is	slight lifting of hand/forearm
the	spreading palm, forearm
end.	to the side
	pause — phase 3
	Turns head away — end of phrase
	and sentence.

*   *   *   *   *

Rhythm in Work: Two examples

Observing a Cleaner in an Office Building

The man had just finished cleaning the floor with a vacuum cleaner. He was winding the long electrical cord around the two prongs, designed to hold it in place. After a first haphazard attempt, this developed into a clearly organized two phasic phrase, a repeatable Effort/Shape rhythm.

First Phase: Pulling the long cord along the floor toward himself in a wide spiral-like shape up and slightly outward with an upbeat of Free Flow/Strength/Suddenness.

Phase Two: Starting at the lower prong of the upright vacuum cleaner, he wound the cord with even Flow, fluctuating into slightly Bound Flow/Directness, "channeling" it between his fingers of one hand and becoming Bound Flow/Sustained when he fastened it around the upper prong.

Then he started again: Sudden/Free Flow and Strong spiral-like arc and so on. It took only one or two repetitions to establish the rhythmical structure. The contrasting Effort combinations of phases one and two obviously gave pleasure to the man as they accompanied contrast in shaping from the dramatic wide pull of the start to the linear precise fastening of the cord on the vertical prongs of the upright machine.

Group of Workers in Synchronized Rhythm

In a film made by the American folksinger and folklorist Pete Seeger, a group of workers, working side by side in a row, are hoeing in a synchronized rhythm. In a wide swingy arc forward/down they hit the ground simultaneously.

Frame-by-frame analysis of their movement revealed that it started with diminished Suddenness/ Free Flow which developed to full Suddenness and Strength in the last fourth of the arc. If the Strength came in sooner or later, it would change the rhythm and the nature of the impact.

The rhythm that evolved from the whole activity was a composite of sequencing spatial direction, Sudden Time and Weight. The main exertion of the downward/forward strike done in succession established the beat with precision.

The recuperative phase was essentially a graded Indirect stretching-lifting on a serpentine curve in space with Sustainment and Free/Bound/Free/Bound Flow changes. The recuperative phase allowed for rhythmic dynamics for individual expression as some workers made more of the shaping trace form while some accentuated the Effort elements. They may have reduced the path and Flow/Strength variations, or enlarged the path by spiral pathways and Indirect/Flow/Strength accents, or by throwing the hoe up into the air, catching it and, with Sudden/Bound/Lightness, becoming ready for the impact.

*   *   *   *   *

Dance Examples of Rhythm

The "Water Study" of the dancer and choreographer Doris Humphrey is a pure example of returning to the body rhythm of breath. The extremes of high body tensions in Martha Graham's vocabulary — her contractions — often reflect body rhythms communicating neuroses because the tensions are extended to distortion. Today, both ballet and modern dance choreographers are increasingly tuned in to body rhythms as observed in ordinary life, which can be transformed into dance rhythms. These appear particularly in the American genre of Broadway musicals, such as Charles Weidman's "Lynchtown," Jerome Robbins' "West Side Story" and Agnes de Mille's "Oklahoma."

The basic patterns of ballet, although shaping with all the limbs, actually accentuate the step movements. Until the early part of the 20th century western choreographers adhered strictly to such patterns. Modern dance has modified these patterns by involving the movements more totally throughout the total body. In other cultures, this more total activation of all parts has been done in different ways throughout history. Dancers often connected sound-producing props such as bells around ankles, finger cymbals, tambourines, hand drums, castanets to reinforce their body rhythms.

The combination of symmetrical and asymmetrical rhythm in a Yugoslavian folk dance was the subject of a painstaking study by the folklorist Ljubica Jankovic of what she called "arrythmie" in Yugoslav dance. Using as an example a dance where the steps are in 2/4 and the accompanying score is in 3/4, she found that dancers and musicians start together and end together at either a sixth or twelfth measure. But, in between these points, the pulls of each other's rhythms produce small stretchings and shrinkings in the step patterns that affect the spatial shapes and Effort stresses adding extra vitality to the dance that could not be explained in explicit metrical terms.

Alphons Dauer, an ethnomusicologist at the Institut für Wissenschaftlichen Film, Goettingen, Germany, now Professor of African Music, University of Graz, Austria, has done a detailed analysis from a synchronized film of two drummers, each with two motifs in 3/4 and 2/4, accompanied by a group of girls, singing and clapping an even 4/4. The drummers were always in opposite rhythms, varying them, so that actually the whole group was never all together at one beat. This gave the whole sequence a continuous, powerful, varied drive ascending to peaks of excitement.

This dynamic development can also be observed in Effort terms by watching the movements of the participants. As the rhythms shifted, there were changes in the spatial shapes and Effort configurations. Space and Effort matched the aural drive to the peaks of excitement.

In the production of tone, the spatial build-up is an indivisible part of the production of a particular quality of tone. That quality also affects the rhythm. For example, to hit the center of a hanging large gong takes a spiral right/left/up *preparation* for a down Direct/Light/Free Flow straight touch. Just touching without that spatial preparation would produce only a weak tone without the appropriate reverberations. This preparatory sequence also represents a rhythmical phrase leading to the accent of the touch. Without it, there would be a dull, flat, arhythmical sound, without vibration.

*   *   *   *   *

Illustrations of the Rhythmic Structure of Sequence in the Scales Derived from the Icosahedron

The Three-Ring: The Rhythmic Structure of a Spatial Shape Developed from Transversals of the Icosahedron

The three-ring is defined as follows: Two transverse inclinations of the "A" or "B" scale that form a volute closed by a third inclination to form a rounded triangular shape. Now we re-examine the three-ring, introduced as a spatial form on page 43, to illustrate its spatial and Effort rhythmic pattern.

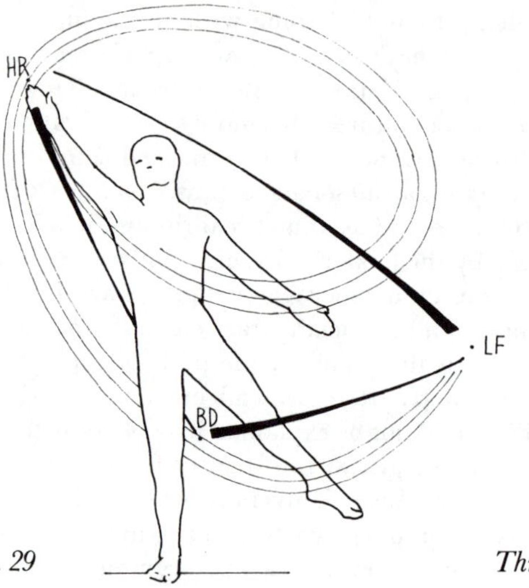

Fig. 29   *Three-Ring*

Spatial Sequence

left/forward	to	high/right	to	back/deep
(horizontal)		(vertical)		(sagittal)

Effort Affinity Emphasis

direct/sustained	to	light/indirect	to	sudden/strong
(across reach)		(wide lift)		(steep fall)

Rhythm

If, for example, you start as indicated above, there is a crescendo-like "grand" opening, which moves through the next points toward a fall as a closing. This almost necessitates a pause at the peak, marking the close of the first phase, followed by a quick drop, immediately recuperating into a slow closing of the phrase. This could be counted in 5/4 metrical time as 1–2–3 — 1–2.

If, however, you start high/right, there is a quite different rhythmical sequence: You drop back dramatically with Suddenness and Strong Weight. Gradually you recuperate by closing in front of yourself with Directness and Sustainment. You then rise and open with Lightness and Indirectness to return to the beginning. The metrical count would still be 1 2 3 4 5 (5/4), but divided as 1–2 — 1–2–3.

Wherever you start, you are in a triangular shape, but the moves from one corner of a plane to another create different stresses. Thus, a complete ring around the triangle will include shifting rhythms.

Two-Ring: Another Spatial Shape Developed from the Icosahedron

It is defined as follows: Two parallel transversals of the same category (either flat or steep or suspended) linked in a cycle by two parallel peripheral inclinations. Together they form a rectangular shape within the icosahedron.

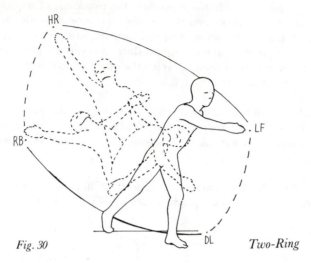

Fig. 30   *Two-Ring*

Flat Transversal			**Peripheral**	
left/forward (horizontal)	to	high/right (vertical)	to	right/back (horizontal)
Flat Transversal			**Peripheral**	
	to	deep/left (vertical)	to	left/forward (Return) (horizontal)

Effort Emphasis

Flat Transversal
Light/Indirect
Rising and widening with slight retreating

Peripheral
Diminished Indirect/Diminished Free Flow
This peripheral sinks slightly and retreats slightly which extends the retreating component of the transversal

Flat Transversal
Strong/Direct
Sinking and narrowing with slight advancing

Peripheral
Diminished Direct/Diminished Bound Flow
This peripheral rises slightly and advances slightly which extends the advancing component of the transversal

N.B. The peripheral inclinations extend the third — but minor — quality of the transversal in the creation of the two-ring. In this case, for example, the third quality of the two-ring is the advancing/retreating (sagittal) component which extends the major components of rising/falling (vertical) and widening/narrowing (horizontal).

Rhythm

Two-phasic. The first phase is a rising and widening with slight retreating; the second phase is a sinking and narrowing with slight advancing. This lends itself easily to a 6/8 metrical count as 1–2–3–4–5–6, or two phases of 1–2–3.

There is a distinct rhythmical difference between the two kinds of sequences because one (the three-ring) includes three transversals on three different diagonals while the other (the two-ring) includes two parallel transversals on one diagonal. Moving in the first shape produces more of a dynamic stir, while moving in the second shape produces an even, calmer rhythm.

Moving in vertical, horizontal, or sagittal cycles, the time divisions will be influenced by the main spatial stress of each cycle approximately as follows:

Vertical cycle tends toward binary symmetrical beat, as in cranking a vertical wheel.
Horizontal cycle tends toward ternary asymmetrical beat, as in stirring a soup.
Sagittal cycle, which is asymmetrical, tends toward a combination of binary and ternary (such as 5/4), as in performing a somersault.

These affinities explain the dramatic quality differences in performance of the two shapes illustrated in Figures 29 and 30, which have produced such different rhythms.

*   *   *   *   *

CHAPTER 6

Affinities of Body, Space and Effort

In observing a movement we must visualize all the intermediary stages of its unfolding. In describing movement, we must make a mental note of the most important intermediary positions.

Rudolf Laban

Right: *Two Men at Poor People's Campaign* © Bonnie Freer
Active repose. Man in chair is the more active: shows more differentiation in Effort and shape. There is asymmetry between his upper and lower body and between his right and left sides. Differentiated shaping in hands. Relaxed twist in body. Free Flow. Fluctuations in Effort. The other man is more symmetrical, shows less differentiation.

Below: *Two Women in Store* © Bonnie Freer
Woman on right is active, shows Postural Effort, fluctuations in Sudden/Sustained and Free/Bound. Clear Lightness/Direct. Indulging rather than Fighting range. Other woman shows Neutral Flow/Diminished Directness/Bound.

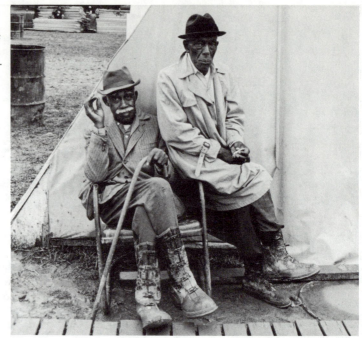

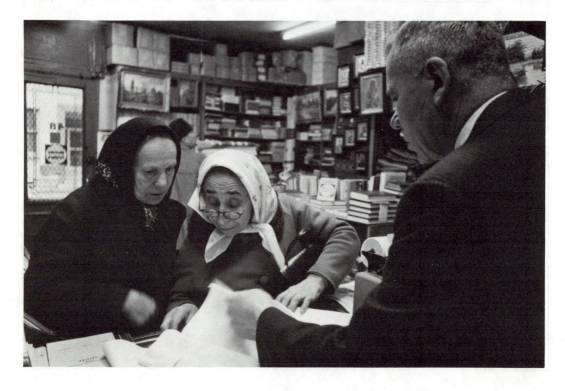

Affinities of Body, Space and Effort

Although it is reiterated throughout this book that body, space and Effort are inextricably interrelated, they have thus far been described as individual components of Labananalysis.

If, however, one examines them developmentally, their interrelationship becomes more clear.

Primary body movement shapes, supported by the process of breathing, foreshadow later spatial shapes. The earliest identification of the primary shapes can be seen in the baby's amoeba-like movements that go toward or away from the body center. The continuity, flux or flow in the movements, already has a shape quality, Shape Flow, as the body hollows and bulges, shrinks and grows with breathing. Such movements also have a quality of Effort Flow — either Free or Bound. These Effort Flow fluctuations between Free and Bound and the shaping flow fluctuations between shrinking and growing initiate all later spatial actions. They are still body focused; they do not yet go toward a goal in space or carve up the space around them.

In semi-conscious states, the Effort Flow and Shape Flow are barely distinguishable, but close analysis can identify them and their potential for more crystallized Effort and shaping activity. For example, when a tired child sleepily waves his hand in the air, just barely flexing and extending the wrist, we observe Flow, the "goingness," the continuity of movement, without distinguishable Space, Weight, Time Effort elements, or shaping of form. There appears to be only fluency, which, in a more conscious state, could start and sustain the kinetic drive of a movement with more form.

Even in this semi-conscious state, the flexion/extension of the wrist which shortens and lengthens the arm is a Shape Flow — shrinking/growing — process. And it is possible, on close analysis, to distinguish some fluctuations between Bound and Free Flow Effort elements. Without the continuity of Effort Flow fluctuations, there would be an arrest in either the flexion or the extension.

This dependency between Effort Flow and Shape Flow develops into the spatial shapes and Effort interrelationships that can be observed in all movement behavior. What may, at the simplest level, appear as Shape Flow and Effort Flow, as in the flexion/extension of the wrist, can, in another situation, with spatial intent, crystallize into spatial shapes with clearly defined Effort elements.

Judith Kestenberg, at her Child Development Research Center for Parents and Children, studied, for many years, the fluctuations in Shape Flow and what she called Tension Flow, a precursor of Effort Flow, in newborn babies. Her observations showed how the fluctuations in early Tension Flow have rhythmical patterns that foreshadow the later Space, Weight, Time Effort elements. She traced the development from Shape Flow to more clearly defined, more complex, spatial shaping.

The shrinking of the body, for example, especially in extreme form, can be clearly perceived in space as a spatial retreating in the sagittal plane, or, sinking in the vertical plane, or, narrowing in the horizontal plane. The form can be said to have a relationship to space rather than just an involvement with body. In the opposite range, the opening or unfolding of the growing phase of the body Shape Flow process might be perceived as a spatial advancing in the sagittal plane or, rising in the vertical plane, or, widening in the horizontal plane — again, relating to space.

As the spatial shapes emerge from the Shape Flow, more clearly defined Effort elements will also emerge, such as Sudden Time with retreating, Strong Weight with sinking, Direct Space with narrowing or Sustained Time with Advancing, Light Weight with rising and Indirect Space with widening. Laban observed that these Effort qualities and spatial shapes so frequently appeared together that he identified them as affinities.

Many possible paths creating many possible spatial forms can fulfill spatial intent. When a baby is merely playing with the movements of his arms, some Effort Flow and Shape Flow can be observed. When, however, a baby reaches for his mother, he creates a simple spatial form — a line, with some Effort elements activated, especially Sudden Time and Strong Weight. When the mother cradles a baby's head, she creates a more complex three-dimensional, rounded spatial form, with more

85

Right: *Boy in Wheelchair Reaching to Catch Ball* © Morris H. Jaffe His Direct Space Effort is increased because it can have so little support from total body shaping.

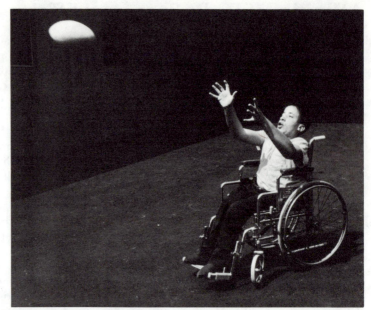

Man Splitting Sticks © Kim Bailey Basically linear activity toward body rather than three-dimensional movement. Some two-dimensional shaping indicated by scapular involvement. Right arm Sudden with Free-Bound Flow and some Direct Space. Counterhold of left arm away from body with Strong, Free/Bound Flow fluctuations to maintain stability.

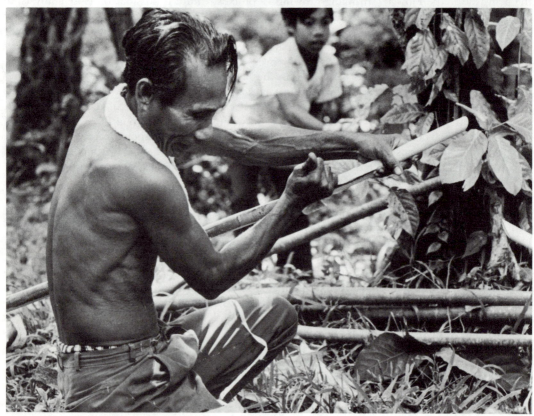

fluctuations in all the Effort ranges. To identify subtle changes in movement behavior, either functional or expressive, the observer's ability to distinguish subtle component changes is critical.

Kestenberg's studies have identified latent or reduced Effort tendencies in late childhood and among adults. In those studies, the dominant presence, in the newborn and infants, of primary Effort (or Tension) Flow fluctuation patterns served as clues to existing or potential pathological states. Treatment can be aided by insight into the body/space/Effort components of the movement patterns which accompany the pathology and by exploration of variations of those components.

Observations of patterns can also help to define basic cultural patterns and to distinguish individual or group preferences that emerge as clear shapes and Effort combinations. It is hoped that such observations will be incorporated more into research studies.

In ordinary conversation, Effort Flow and Shape Flow predilections of the participants can be perceived as baselines for the observable Effort elements and shapes that become clearly defined in the conversation. Different degrees of spatial activity, dependent on the spatial intents of the participants, can be seen. The changes can occur in one concerted use of the whole body and limbs or in one or more limbs accompanied by just Shape Flow changes in the trunk. Or there could be just trunk movement without use of any limbs, as when someone sits with folded hands and leans forward. In any case, it is not just the physical movement of the body that gives the statement communicating power. The communication of the move is expressed by combined spatial and Effort patterns.

One participant in a conversation may tend to shape the space into piercing lines moving forward/backward. Another may take in more space as he shapes his reply by curving forward/upward as well as left/backward. A third carves spirals in the space, encompassing forward/backward, upward/downward and side-to-side. Different Effort combinations will appear with each spatial choice. Slight variations in the combinations will change the meaning of the move. If the piercing gesture is done with Sustained (Time) and Free (Flow), the partner experiences a gentle two-way exchange. If, however, the gesture is performed with Sudden (Time) and Strong (Weight), the partner will be threatened.

In different situations, one of the three components — body, space or Effort — will be dominant over the other two. In many floor exercises, for example, the body aspect is dominant. The emphasis is on relationship of body parts, awareness of the center of weight and how it relates to initiation of action. Later, in the upright position, when less of the body surface is getting support from the floor, space and Effort become more dominant for different movements. The Bartenieff Fundamentals, which were discussed in Chapter 2 from primarily a body perspective, also point out the developmental process of space and Effort relationships in increasingly complex body movements.

The first exercises are close to the "pre-space" period and then progress to other levels although the progression is not necessarily the same for each person. Some have earlier body development, some earlier spatial development and others may have stronger Effort predilections.

As the mover gets up from the floor, the "pre-space" period with its predominance of Effort Flow and Shape Flow gradually assumes a more interrelated body/space/Effort quality. For instance, as soon as both hips are raised — while still lying on the floor — the mover is beginning to establish "where" he/she is going, dealing with another aspect of space and shape. When the mover rolls from backlying into a crawling position, Sudden Time and Strong Weight come into play.

There is always the potentiality for activated Effort involvement, but either the challenge of the environment or the intensity of the mover's liveliness elicits certain constellations of particular elements and their particular qualities.

As soon as the mover sits up, establishing the vertical axis through body/limb reach, space all around opens up. Direction is differentiated: where the arms aim, how the weight is shifted to get from place to place, what different degrees of Effort combinations will work. The body/space/Effort

Right: *Broad Jumper*
© Morris H. Jaffe
Shaping forward and up in sagittal plane is crucial, with initiation from pelvic center and Sudden Time, Strong Weight, Free Flow.

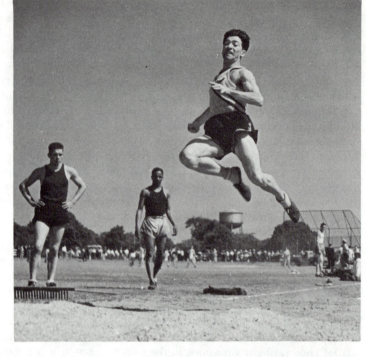

Below: *Two Boys and Girl on Twig Bridge* © Morris H. Jaffe
Boy on left is trying to guide girl's mobile sagittal progression by emphasising his vertical support from below with some complementary sagittal shaping from above. Her Light Weight Effort with Free Flow balances his Strong Weight Effort going toward Bound Flow.

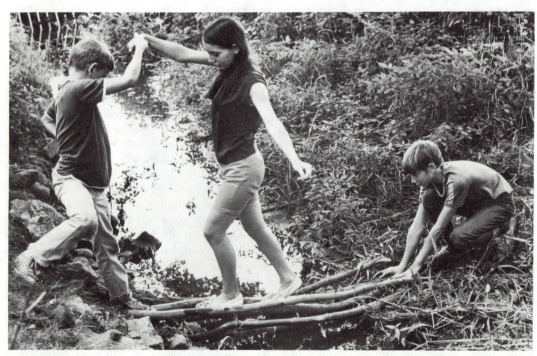

triad reaches a greater degree of balance or cohesiveness, with none of the elements taking a lop-sided constant overdominance.

This is further developed as the mover stands upright. Now, the whole range of the four Effort elements — Space, Weight, Time and Flow — and the full potential of space — rising, widening, advancing and sinking, narrowing, retreating — can be differentiated.

One- , Two- , Three-Dimensional Movement and Effort

When a mover tries to lift his/her arms to a vertical-up direction, he/she automatically veers forward on the way up. Such one-dimensional movements are always about to slip into two- or three-dimensional movements because of the three-dimensional potential of the ball and socket joints of the shoulder. The global structure of those joints causes subtle rotary adaptations to every change of direction and the torso will slightly shape itself for support. Only a "poke," a clear forward or upward or sideward movement from a *flexed* arm or leg, as in fencing, is possible as a near-perfect one-dimensional movement. Such one-dimensional movements can also appear in small gestures, such as pointing. The constant fluctuations fighting the intent to stay purely in one dimension create a quality of high intensity in such movements. The execution of the defense scale, for example, produces a characteristic intensity reinforcing the impact of its movements. It requires strong, central, vertical control to support the scale's struggle to stay within one dimension.

In pursuing the directional goals of up–down, side–across and out, and forward–backward, the total body, including its center, becomes involved in spatial shaping or rising–sinking, narrowing–widening, and advancing–retreating. The body shape becomes convex in rising, widening and advancing and it becomes concave in sinking, narrowing and retreating. At the same time, the Effort elements are crystallized and shifting with each change.

For example, the changes in the Flow Effort in each of the moves can be observed as an increase in Bound Flow in moves toward the body center while moves away from body center ease into more Free Flow.

Similar affinities between all directions and Effort elements can be observed as follows:

Dimension	Direction	Shape	Effort Factor	Effort Range
vertical	up	rising	Weight	Light
vertical	down	sinking	Weight	Strong
lateral	across	enclosing narrowing	Space	Direct
lateral	out	spreading widening	Space	Indirect
sagittal	backward	withdrawing	Time	Sudden
sagittal	forward	advancing	Time	Sustained

Note the vertical affinity for Weight Effort; the horizontal affinity for Space Effort and the sagittal affinity for Time Effort. This does not mean exclusive involvement; it means that the "affined" Effort is dominant over the other two although the mover might consciously or unconsciously fight it.

The affinities can be differentiated in observations of movements that support them as compared to observations of the same movements performed with oppositions to the stated affinity. For example, Strong Weight is most naturally dominant in smashing an object with a fist, performing the blow in a downward direction. When an attempt is made to perform the task by going in an upward direction, additional energy must be exerted to maintain the necessary impact because the natural affinity of upward with Light Weight has to be overcome.

One might initially feel this to be synonymous with going with or against gravity. But just to go with gravity is not the same as using the Strong Weight Effort element. The former is a passive giving in to the weight of the body. The latter (Effort) requires an attitude of using the impact of body weight for a particular purpose. The greater impact results from an attitude that reinforces the natural gravity pull, that is, a Strong Effort with its affined downward direction. Additional examples appear at the end of the chapter.

These spatial/Effort affinities are a central aspect of Labananalysis whether they occur as affinities or whether they occur as deviations from affinities. In each case, an expressive statement or level of functional adequacy is identified. In all cases, the spatial/Effort affinities are interdependent with the body's potential and limitations.

In any sequence, there are built-in gradations in spatial and Effort tensions that allow for a certain amount of recuperation from the opposite range possibilities. For example, in the defense scale, the exertion down is followed by a recuperative going up and vice versa. In shaping and Effort terms, exertions and recuperations in the whole scale can be charted as follows:

Exertion: Spatial and Effort	Recuperation: Spatial and Effort
down (sinking)/Strong Weight	up (rising)/Light Weight
across (enclosing)/Direct Space	out (spreading)/Indirect Space
backward (retreating)/Sudden Time	forward (advancing)/Sustained Time

The same principle of exertion and recuperation can be applied to all movement sequences and scales. Survival endurance is dependent upon the continuity of such patterns. This physical reality has, of course, an inherent emotional concomitant which is equally significant for survival.

Two-Dimensional Movement

The planes and cycles of two-dimensional movement offer distinctly different functional and expressive possibilities from those of the defense scale model because more complex space-Effort ranges are added with the additional dimension involvement.

In moving in each plane, as noted earlier, the pull of one of the dimensions of the plane is dominant over the other. The continuous change of dominance between the two spatial tensions involved appears also in the shifting dominances of the Effort elements affined with the active plane. Thus,

Plane	Dimension Dominance	Effort Dominance
door	vertical (horizontal secondary)	Weight (Space secondary)
table	horizontal (sagittal secondary)	Space (Time secondary)
wheel	sagittal (vertical secondary)	Time (Weight secondary)

Various speakers can project different images — each moving primarily in one of the three planes. The observer can identify the corresponding Effort elements or might first recognize the Effort elements and then identify the planes. Such observations communicate additional meaning to the words of the speaker. When, for example, the Weight Effort/door plane is dominant, a vertical stability and assertiveness is communicated. When the Space Effort/table plane is dominant, the horizontal movements of including and sharing are communicated. When the sagittal movements of Time Effort/wheel plane are dominant, a reaching toward or withdrawing from are communicated. Observations of these interrelationships can be made of partial or full cycling movements.

Differences in degrees of stability and mobility are also reflected in the affined Effort elements. Moving around in the vertical (door) plane in a cycle, the dominance of the vertical axis produces gradations of Light Weight to Strong Weight to Light Weight (depending on where the movement originates), with slight changes in Indirect to Direct to Indirect Space.

Moving around the wheel plane, the driving Time Effort goes from Sustainment to Suddenness to Sustainment (again, depending on where the movement originates) with secondary changes in Strong to Light to Strong Weight.

Moving in cycles around the table plane has predominantly Space Effort going from Indirect to Direct to Indirect, with secondary changes in Sustained to Sudden to Sustained Time.

These movements rarely appear in pure form. But they can be observed constantly in smaller movements and gestures and in attempts at total pure forms.

Three-Dimensional Movement

Each diagonal has distinctive body/space/Effort tensions associated with the dimensions involved. The impact of the combined three tensions is diminished if any one is weakened; in the natural veering toward stability, the mover frequently allows this weakening to occur. Only in extraordinary circumstances does a mover come close to the peaks of kinetic power, but even attempts toward movement along a pure diagonal will have some of the dramatic power of its extremes of flight and fall.

Cube Diagonals and Basic Effort Affinities

The high driving tensions of the pure space diagonal are accompanied by the affined use of Weight/Space/Time Effort elements, with some Flow in moving between diagonals. There are some actions in which one or more of the Effort elements dominate, but in the pure diagonal all three are equally important. This is comparable to the spatial stress balance between the diagonal's three pulls: vertical, horizontal and sagittal.

Performance of the diagonal scale illustrates the affinities between specific sequences of paths (shaping) and Effort elements combined as Basic Effort Action Drives.

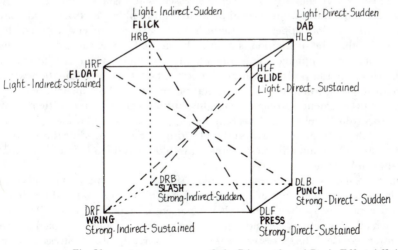

Fig. 31   Cube Diagonals and Basic Effort Affinities

91

As can be seen in Figure 31, performance of the diagonal scale could be described in Effort terms as Float to Punch to Glide to Slash to Dab to Wring to Flick to Press. Note that the two Basic Effort Action Drives on the same diagonal are opposites in their Space/Weight/Time elements. Just as the three spatial tendencies are evenly stressed at each corner, so are the three Effort elements evenly stressed at each corner.

If there were no body limitations, the diagonal scale would utilize all four Effort elements evenly with full use of space as Full Effort Action Drives. That is like a goal of pure physical/emotional aspiration. In some extraordinary performances, such as the acrobatics of the Peking Opera, it sometimes appears that the impossible has been accomplished and that the maximum mobility required by the diagonal has been realized.

Effort Affinities with "A" and "B" Scales

When these scales or spatial pathways related to diagonal axes are affined with Effort they reveal infinite varieties of behavioral possibilities, incorporating curves and interweaving play, nurturing and aggression. Other ranges are added to the fight defense behavior of the dimensional scale with its single vertical axis and to the more complex character of two-dimensional movements.

"A" scales suggest actions that predominantly move on diagonals that rise forward and fall backward. They are gentle and retiring, as, for example, in the receptive gesture of a beggar, or, on a larger scale, an open pleading gesture to the gods. "B" scales suggest actions that predominantly move on diagonals that fall forward or rise backward. They are harsh and aggressive, as, for example, in the working action of using a scythe for cutting wheat or in the fencing action of lifting the opponent's sword in a turn.

These affinities to Effort are much more subtle than the affinities found in the dimensional scale where one spatial direction affines with one Effort element as, for instance, up/down affines with Light/Strong (Weight). They are also more subtle than those of the diagonals, emerging from the cube. Each cube diagonal has three equally stressed spatial tensions, each of which is affined to an Effort element. Thus, the diagonal scale affines to a series of Basic Effort Actions; for instance, going down in the diagonal high/right/back — deep/left/forward is affined to the Basic Effort Punch.

The greater subtlety of the "A" and "B" scale Effort affinities is due to the unevenly stressed tensions. Each of the modified diagonals — transversal inclinations — of the icosahedron scales has three spatial tensions but they are not evenly stressed. For instance, in the "B" scale, a steep inclination occurs in the move from vertical plane to sagittal plane: high/left to forward/deep. It is because the vertical directions appear in both the beginning (high) and end (deep) of this inclination between the planes that the inclination is steep. The sagittal plane, toward which the inclination moves with its forward component, is secondary in dominance, while the horizontal plane, the weakest of the three spatial pulls, is still an important factor in the inclination which must veer toward the right in going from vertical to sagittal planes. The whole inclination would invite the affinity of the Effort elements Strength (Weight)/Sustainment (Time), with minimal stress on Indirectness. Proceeding from forward/deep to right/back, a suspended transversal, accentuates the spatial tensions of depth (sagittal, retreating) and width (horizontal), while there is only little stress on height (vertical). The main affinities, therefore, would be Sudden (Time) and Indirect (Space) with little change in Weight.

The two transversals described here form a volute that appears somewhat modified in both sword fighting and in the greeting gesture of a cavalier lifting off his large hat and bowing to a lady. In fighting, it is sweeping away the adversary's weapon in an expansive move. The specific spatial character in each of these actions depends on how the two inclinations are linked together, and how that linkage influences the Effort stresses. In the fight gesture, the spatial stress may be the forward component with going down secondary, inviting emphasis on Sustainment and increasing Strength.

This is immediately followed by opening into a wide sweeping retreat supported by Indirectness and Suddenness which prepares for the next attacking move.

In the bowing to the lady, the Effort affinities may not be played up to their fullest. They may accentuate a Sustained bending down and opening into an Indirect, slight diminished Suddenness. Thus, in these transversal shapes that are built on the same volute, there is a greater fluctuation of affinities. This, as noted above, is because the modified diagonals in the transversal shapes, unlike the pure diagonals, do not have evenly stressed spatial tensions, but instead have primary, secondary, tertiary spatial tendencies. The affined Effort elements vary accordingly.

In Effort combinations other than Basic Effort Actions, the affinities between the Effort and spatial elements may be less apparent because the Effort elements are frequently less stable. The fluctuations of the Effort elements are more numerous, but more subtle; the spatial tension varies accordingly and the shapes reflect the variations. But the subtle differences make profound distinctions in communication.

The understanding of affinities opens new possibilities in learning and changing movement for different purposes: To switch moods according to the demands of a task, a role or a rhythm; to modify behavior, such as hyper-excitement toward calmness, through a movement experience; to add subtleties to communication.

For specific tasks, performance can be evaluated in terms of the extent to which body/space/Effort components are appropriately combined, that is, what deviations from pure affinities are necessary for the task. Expressive communication can also be perceived or created by incorporating affinities or by deciding to make another statement that would result from other combinations.

Examples

Removing a Book from a Mail Envelope for Single Books
Example for affinities of:
   a)   side-across/side-open with Space Effort Direct/Indirect.
   b)   up/down with Weight Effort Light/Strong.

The unpacking of these usually tight-fitting envelopes for mailing books sometimes offers spatial and Effort challenges. After removing some of the tightly fitting and firmly glued tape, one may try to pull the book out laterally, constantly changing the accompanying Space Effort elements Direct and Indirect, as one tries to anchor the package at the opposite end. If there is resistance due to the material of the envelope or the too-tight fit of the book and envelope, non-affined Weight Effort may also come into play. If Strong Weight becomes more dominant, the performer might try to upend the whole package into the vertical which is affined to Strength/Lightness.

*   *   *   *   *

Advancing Retreating
Trying to straighten out a crumpled piece of paper lying in front of oneself on a table.
   The tendency is to accompany the forward stroke of smoothing out with Sustainment, then as the job is almost done, one hand holds one corner of the paper while the operating hand finishes with some Sudden superficial strokes toward oneself (retreating) and a series of Direct Suddennesses.

*   *   *   *   *

Cyclic Movements in Functional Gestures
Cyclic motions in the planes occur in many functional activities. Some are constantly repeated, some are interspersed with other spatial shapes. The following are examples of activities in which one plane is dominant.

Vertical (Door Plane) Cycle
The act of polishing a vertical surface, a window or a door, with a piece of cloth is frequently a cyclical motion. One goes over the surface evenly with clockwise vertical cycles that start deep/left progressing to high/left, to high/right to deep/right. This allows for a smooth covering of the vertical surface, the smoothness resulting from the emphasis on the high/right which invites the Effort affinities of Light/Indirect. Wherever one finds resistance to this cycle of wiping, one may want to apply greater pressure and therefore may reverse the cycle to counterclockwise (high/left to deep/left to deep/right to high/right). This, particularly high/left to deep/left, allows one to bear down with increased Strength and some pinpointing Directness. As the stubborn resistance diminishes, one might smooth the whole surface with the upward-aimed (clockwise) cycle which emphasizes the action of widening with Indirectness in contrast to the downward cycle that is reinforcing the narrowing component with its affinity for Directness.

Sagittal (Wheel Plane) Cycle
Winding up knitting yarn into a ball from a horizontally spread skein of yarn can be done as a cyclical action in the sagittal plane. The operator may first lift a few yards of yarn from the horizontally fixed skein with Free Flow to slight Bound Indirectness. The actual winding will be performed in a sagittal cycle where one can observe tendencies toward single Effort elements of Sustainment in the rising (forward/high) phase and Suddenness in the sinking (back/deep) phase. Also, secondary components of Effort, Strong and Light, may come into play. When the latter assume dominance, the thread

may break from overuse of Strength on the sinking phase or, when too much Lightness is used on the rising phase, the ball may become a tangled mess or even fall apart. It is the four spatial ingredients, high, deep, forward, backward, with the affined four Effort elements, Lightness, Strength, Sustainment, Suddenness contributing together and successively in variation that make for a perfect job.

Horizontal (Table Plane) Cycle
An example of a cyclic movement in the horizontal plane is stirring a thick soup in a round pot. It requires a meticulous blending of the forward and right-side with the backward and left-across, along with the additional subtle changes in Space and Time Effort elements.

*   *   *   *   *

Conversation
In a conversation between Mr. A and Mr. B, Mr. B leads the conversation; Mr. A is a quiet listener. Mr. B underlines his verbal statements with varous gestures of forearm/hand/fingers. Though not hearing the words they exchange, one gains impressions of their mutual relationships and the changes in mood between them are observed as Effort changes and variations in their spatial shapes. Mr. B uses a recurring back and forth, a slight fluctuation in Effort and Shape flow: growing and shrinking with increased Free Flow on the Growing and Boundness on the shrinking. At one point, this changes to a sudden pointing toward Mr. A with an almost limp return toward himself. In the next minute, the pointing becomes Sudden, Strong, Free Flow and the return to himself a Sustained/Boundness. Mr. A had so far responded only with a Light/Boundness or Indirect/Sustainment. He stays calm as Mr. B gets more and more aroused. Mr. B changes his spatial pattern: a whole series of up-down gestures with Strong/Sudden/Boundness on the down and slight rebound into Free Flow on the up, ending with a final broad sweep to the side that is Direct/Strong going from Sudden into Sustained/Bound/Strength. Mr. A bends forward with Light/Sustained/Boundness.

*   *   *   *   *

Preparing Pizza – A Labananalysis
The chief pizza baker in a restaurant, preparing the dough and its fillings for the oven, was observed. The dough, a pale yellow ball of slightly moist consistency, was forcefully dumped with Sudden/Free Flow on a large wooden plank, ready for the truly spectacular ritual of transforming it into that elastic circular shape, the pizza. The baker was a young man, muscular and swarthy of complexion, with almost overdeveloped upper trunk, shoulders, arms and hands. The reason was clear: the operation was a three dimensional feat, a treat for the movement analyst.

First, the ball was assaulted with a few Strong Weight, Free Flow downward slaps, followed by a series of wormlike kneadings with Free Flow, Strength, sagittal kneadings. Each time the dough was slightly lifted off the table and slapped down again, the ball began to look like a thick slab. He continued the sagittal kneadings and lifting the dough off (up) in the air, continuing the right and left slappings in gathering/scattering shaping: the slab began to expand.

At a certain point, he got his powerful hands–fingers underneath the dough with palms and fingers widely spreading in the horizontal plane. The dough was lifted to chest height, essentially balanced over the palm on the right hand fingertips but at the same time the left hand was turning the whole dough shape like a carousel, continuing widening rounding shape tensions multidirectionally. It became a hollow tentlike shape, constantly expanding in all directions, exposed to rapid fluctuations of Weight/Flow with renewed Suddennesses. Then, slowing up, came the last phase: he stretched the tent in an even right/left countertension. When the dough reached the desired thinness of about half an inch, he gently — with Even Flow, Decreased Time — let it slide on the board and, in a few seconds, sprinkled the various ingredients of the filling onto it, transported it in a few quick steps to the oven when he let it slip into the oven in a steep forward/down diagonal with a controlled even Effort Flow. With Sudden/Free Flow and with serpentine shaping, he whisked away the board from the oven and returned to his working table, where he immediately reached for the next ball of dough at his left side.

The whole operation was a matter of a few minutes, an exquisite demonstration of multidirectional shaping accompanied by a constantly varied performance of Flow/Time/Force combinations. Flow was dominant in all phases. Within a few minutes an Effort/Shape "packed" action spectacle had been performed. It was on the continuity of the Flow that the elastic consistency of the dough depended, while its rounded shape and thickness was the result of the multidirectional assault to which the dough was subjected, guaranteeing its final even shape and thickness. And it was the constant practice of interaction of the two that created the structure for the most efficient method of making pizza.

In looking at this spectacle, one was reminded also of the flourish of the Italian speaking gesture, the "style" of the commedia dell'arte gestures of Italian street theater. It is the characteristic interrelation of Effort and spatial shapes, the characteristic shapes and characteristic Effort combinations that recur and would be found in any structured activity from food preparation to architecture and painting that identify cultural style and identity.

*   *   *   *   *

Two Political Candidates

In observing a confrontation of two politicians, candidates for U.S.A. president, in a TV presentation, we noted interesting interrelationships between body, spatial shaping and Effort expression. The intensity of such a confrontation was heightened by the competition between the two speakers in their attempts to persuade the audience to their individual points of view. There was also a restricting factor of concern with civility; they wanted to avoid an open fight. Thus, gestures were relatively small in amplitude and most of the Effort elements somewhat reduced in intensity. The spatial forms of these gestures additionally reinforced the nature of each speaker's contact with the audience. Even within the limitations of a TV format, their movements were expressive and explicit.

Speaker A: He was verbally loaded with facts and figures of past achievements, reiterating many items. His body attitude was essentially vertical but with somewhat hunched up shoulders and solid support from the floor. He was "grounded." His action space was either right in front of him or changing toward slight increases in verticality with the hunched shoulders maintained throughout. Hand–forearm gestures stressed up/down linearity or reaching forward and back to himself, slightly leaning toward the audience. The Effort combinations in the repeated up/down gestures were Bound Flow/Directness changing to Bound Flow with occasional Strength accents and giving in to gravity. The Effort combinations were essentially reduced punches and presses, with variations in either spatial pattern or in Effort and Neutral Flow transitions. The Effort combinations rarely became postural (that is, involving the total body). With a monotone repetitiveness, he seemed to hit the same place. There was a preponderance of two-Effort element combinations; no use of three-Effort element combinations of the Transformation Drives occurred.

Speaker B: He verbally conveyed ideas and described how he was going to operate. His body attitude was a clear verticality, presenting an open chest. His action space, though small, extended into width and depth and some height and he used this space in various ways emphasizing the width and depth. In contrast to Speaker A, he used subtle variations of the Weightless (Vision), Timeless (Spell) Drives, emphasizing the indulging rather than the fighting qualities of the combinations. Thus, there was more Lightness than Strength, more Indirectness than Directness and a great subtlety in varying Effort and action space. He was not storming the audience with Passion (Spaceless) Drives emphasizing resisting rather than indulging qualities. Rather he invited them to see new vistas and suggested the ability to change.

Thus, the overall impression of this low-keyed discussion left the viewer with the impression that Speaker A was thinking in terms of preserving and holding on to established patterns while Speaker B came off as a man of ideas.

There are open questions about both. Would Speaker A be able to find new solutions for new problems in new situations? Would Speaker B be able to condense his Drives into Basic Effort Actions when it came to carrying out his ideas?

The movement behavior communicated these questions, whether or not the viewer could consciously analyze it in Body/Effort/Space terms.

*　*　*　*　*

Tetrahedral Tensions Example

Two photos of dancers capture the peak moment of a leap, especially the intensity of the lift and the transport of the body sagittally. Spatially, there is a juxtaposition of two one-dimensional spatial tensions: a horizontal side/high tension in the arms/upper body against a forward/backward (sagittal) in the legs, causing a twist of the upper against lower body. The power of that spatial twist together with the centrally initiated Effort (Strong/Sudden) sends the body flying through space: the twisting initiated at the center of the body transforms the vertical downward pull of the body weight into lifting/twisting power. This partial overcoming of the gravitational pull makes the performer extremely airborne to play with Weight and Time and Flow Effort elements. It all happens simultaneously — a concerted exertion defining the height and the impactiveness of the progression in space.

Woman Dancer Leaping
© Steve Turi.
Courtesy Robert Shuster and
Downtown Ballet Company.

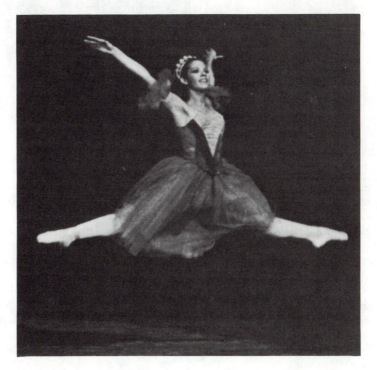

97

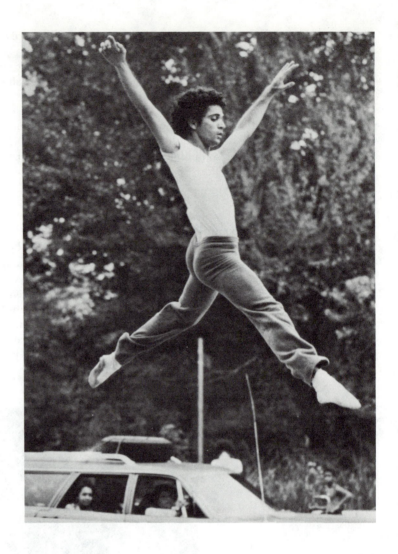

Differences can be observed between the male and female dancer not only in the timing of spatial and Effort elements, but also in the attitude toward space and mood: Paschal has shot vertically up in space and spread himself laterally and sagittally from an attitude predominantly of rising, losing the sense of weightedness. The woman explodes high into sagittal space, the sagittal component becoming dominant to the degree that her lateral spread of the arms has a slight backward–up component reinforcing the flight forward, adding acceleration in the upper body and intensity, Strength/Suddenness, in the lower. She seems to attack space while Paschal overcomes body weight essentially with Flow and Weight.

Tetrahedral tension in leaping is not just the prerogative of the dancer. One has only to open the sports section of a daily newspaper during the baseball season to find such leaps in the reach for the balls. Here the spatial intent to reach the ball seems to transform spatial energy into tetrahedral crystallization. In fact, tetrahedral tensions can be particularly well observed in spontaneous situations in contrast to the formal practice leaps and jumps of ballet technique where the dancer is required constantly to correct spatial placement of arms and legs, thus structuring the spontaneous timing that originated from the desire or necessity to leap. In the athlete, the excitement of the competitive game arouses the fighting Effort elements of Strong, Sudden, Direct, together with the spatial intent to get places. Both dancer and athlete, through stimuli of music or other rhythmic accompaniment, can be steered into explosive outpourings of Effort with Flow from an inner motivation of wanting to leap. The freedom of action on a stage might restore to the dancer the original quality of spontaneity.

*   *   *   *   *

Mathematics Offers Key to Choreutics

Excerpts from a report* on a workshop conducted by Valerie Preston-Dunlop in her continuing exploration of the logical forms of choreutics and their aesthetic implications. (See Bibliography for Preston-Dunlop publications.)

Ms. Preston-Dunlop began by having the participants perform the zig-zagging axis scale which rises and falls along the diagonal high/left/forward to deep/right/back. Peripheral transitions were substituted for the transversals of the axis scale forming a primary scale:

high/left to	left/back to	back/deep to	deep/left to
1	2	3	4
left/forward to	forward/deep to	deep/right to	right/forward to
5	6	7	8
forward/high to	high/right to	right/back to	back/high
9	10	11	12

These locations were then numbered as shown above. (See Footnote** for an example of the same sequence in Labanotation.)

The 27 participants were divided into smaller groups and assigned "number game" tasks to find different choreutic forms within the primary scale.

"If you identify the spatial locations by number, you can find through numerical relationships the basic harmonic forms," Ms. Preston-Dunlop explained.

For instance, if you start with 1 and add 3 to each subsequent number, you create the series 1, 4, 7, 10, which gives you the vertices of the vertical plane. The series beginning with 2 and adding 3 to each subsequent number (2, 5, 8, 11) produces the horizontal plane. A similar series beginning with 3 (3, 6, 9, 12) produces the sagittal plane.

Every even number yields a peripheral six-ring or girdle. Every other even number starting with 2 (2, 6, 10) and with 4 (4, 8, 12) produces transverse three rings.

Every other odd number starting with 1, (1, 5, 9) or 3 (3, 7, 11) yields polar triangles or peripheral three-rings. The series beginning with 1 and adding 5 to each subsequent number (1, 6, 11, 4, 9, 2, 7, 12, 5, 10, 3, 8, 1) produces the right B-scale.

---

* Carol-Lynne Rose, Editor, *Laban Institute of Movement Studies Newsletter, January 1979.*

**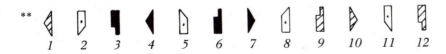

"You can find many regular forms this way," Ms. Preston-Dunlop stressed. "Transposition has to be made to find the forms on the other three diagonal axes. By taking a primary scale, transposing it vertically and horizontally (both laterally and sagittally) three further primaries emerge. (They should be numbered 1 through 12, grouped into four sets.)

"The numerical relationships within these three new primaries produce a further component of regular forms. But the problem is what should be done with them. These forms exist outside the body. One must take the leap into aesthetic embodiment by taking the original performance style of the forms apart and synthesizing the bits again in a new way."

To experience this leap, the group first took the sequence deep/left to right/forward to back/high (4/8/12) and performed it in Laban's original style, through body congruency, leading with one side of the body, counterbalancing the other side with opposing spatial tension, emphasizing mobility and the flow of the phrase.

The same form was then performed with different body organization — stepping left/deep while the hands moved towards right/forward and the left leg gestured backward and upward. These actions were danced sequentially, as a phrase, and simultaneously as a spatial chord. The sequentiality was seen in one dancer's body and then in three dancers, each taking one part. Similarly, the chord was danced by one dancer and by the three simultaneously, each taking one part.

The form was danced with both the standard cross of axis reference (according to the dancer's front) and with the constant cross reference (according to the front of the room or stage).

"Laban had the vision that this work could lead to new choreographic methods. This requires imagination, the taking apart of things formerly thought to be inextricably related. That is what I think contemporary choreutic study is all about," Ms. Preston-Dunlop concluded.

*   *   *   *   *

CHAPTER 7

Tensions and Countertensions

. . . The law of counterbalance (tension) demands that any limb moving in one direction be given a counterweight which would be led in approximately the opposite direction, in certain definite measures and angles . . . These basic laws (degree of flux and counterbalance) are variable in the most manifold ways . . . A whole accord of spatial direction may occur and these spatial directions have their definite proportion of angles in relation to each other. The control — that is, the central control of a limb leading into a certain direction — can happen in more than one way: on this fact a whole series of movement sequences can be built.

Rudolf Laban

Dynamic space, with its terrific dance of tensions and discharges is the fertile ground in which movement flourishes. Movement is the life of space. Dead space does not exist, for there is neither space without movement nor movement without space. All movement is an eternal change between binding and loosening, between the creation of knots with the concentrating and uniting power of binding, and the creation of twisted lines in the process of untying and untwisting. Stability and mobility alternate endlessly.

Rudolf Laban

Right: *Boy Receiving Bowl*
© Kim Bailey.
Three-dimensional shaping with hand and forearm provides synchronous link between the two people. The adult shapes around and down with even Flow/Light/Sustained Effort. Adult shaping and Effort are more crystallized.

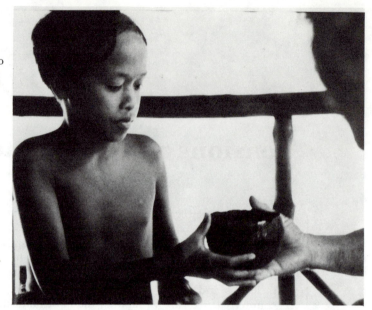

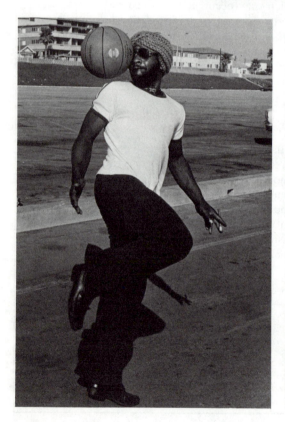

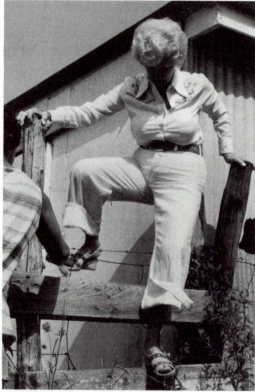

Tensions and Countertensions

Laban perceived the skeleton as a crystalline structure created by the numerous (one- and multi-dimensional) pulls of active muscles on individual bones, spreading muscular tensions through larger or smaller segments of the skeleton in ordered tension sequences.

It is an established anatomical fact that bone deteriorates when the musculature attached to it is not used, and that bone can be built up anew when exposed to the demands of activated muscle pulls. Function, therefore, affects structure.

The muscle pull on the bones is a process which shapes the structure of the skeleton. This can be called an *inner* shaping process. Spatial intent exerts a pull of the body-reach possibilities to create an *outer* process of shaping space. Each affects the other in both functional and structural adaptations to movement tasks.

In the spatial shaping process, the muscle pulls of limb-trunk or limbs-trunk or several limbs or parts of limbs create lines of different spatial designs which reflect the condensations and expansions of body-spatial tensions.

Spatial tensions are the springboards for mobility. A state of two opposing pulls as, for instance, the dominant up/down tension of vertical standing can be rescued from stasis by continuous — often infinitesimal — shifts to other directions: forward/backward and right/left. These shifts are exertions and releases, which can also be described as recuperative transitions to maintain the continuity of mobility. A continuous shifting between these sets of spatial tensions guarantees upright stability as well as continuous readiness to move in space, creating new adaptations to the environment.

The geometric, architectonic principles illustrated in the Laban spatial models (Choreutics) are not artifices imposed on flexings, bendings and rotations; they are biologically valid sequences of movements of limbs and spine. The principles correct misconceptions of movement process which emphasize only muscle tensions and changing joint angles in movement as predominantly muscular/articular tensions without reference to *spatial* tensions. In highly dynamic, centrally initiated sequences in the air, such as a "run, run, leap" sequence, for example, a spatially peripheral groping upward/sideward in the arm-upper body creates a countertension in the forward/backward striving of the legs. This spontaneously created countertension helps lift the body weight and prolong the forward progression in the air. This is in sharp contrast to just jumping with the arms hanging limply at the side, without creating countertension.

The Developmental Experience of Countertension

When there is minimal countertension, an initiating folding movement will be followed by the rest of the body into one total folded, passive, concave shape. One of the simplest experiences of countertension is to unfold from such a rounded shape on the floor downward from the feet and upward from the head into an open convex shape. Countertensions must be strengthened to further activate the shape.

Far left: *Man with Soccer Ball* © Elizabeth L. Stopol.
Countershaping in arms and head supports his total shaping in full spiral. Effort fluctuations: *Free*/Bound, Sudden/*Sustained*, *Light*/Strong, *Indirect*/Direct.

Facing page, left: *Woman Descending from Fence* © Carol Fenner Williams.
Countertensions provide support in precarious position. Total shaping, slightly concave to balance forward-downward progression. Left and right diagonal countertension: left arm down, right leg up; right arm lateral, slightly forward, down as left leg is down.

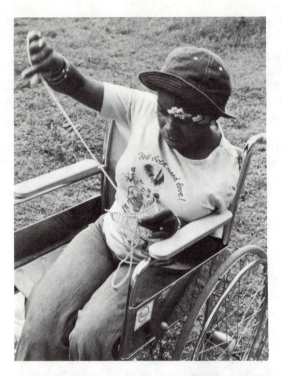

Left: *Girl in Wheelchair Sewing*
© Morris H. Jaffe.
The clear Effort and shaping of the
right side compensates for the
handicapped left side.

Right: *Man with Outstretched Arm*
© Bonnie Freer.
Gestural movement. Only the
forearm is active with shaping in
the hand. Everything else goes
toward giving in to weight. Head
in back diagonal with side tilt
underlines sinking stance.

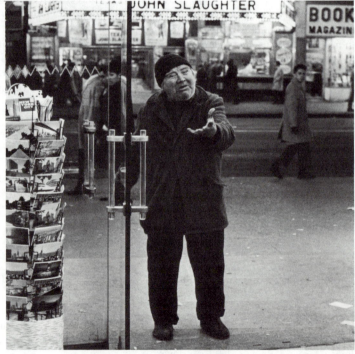

When a baby lifts his head up for the first time he will soon try to support himself further by pushing down on his arms or elbows and forearms. He creates the vertical countertension which leads to uprightness. Gradually, the many possibilities of counteraction and its spatial form, countershaping, develop and full uprightness becomes possible as a result.

As the tensions and countertensions of shapes increase in complexity, they reflect the constant primary stability versus mobility contest that starts as soon as the limbs and body reach into space. The most subtle tension changes of paths, Effort and resultant shapes, will affect the function and expression. As in music, the nature of the progression, not just the particular tones struck, determines the distinctive quality of the key or mode of a melody.

Moving in the kinesphere away from the body into even one direction causes a tension between the body and the point reached. Spatial tensions develop in constantly changing degrees throughout the whole path, not just between the beginning and end of it. They are not isolated tensions, but are interdependent with other systems of tensions within other body-space configurations.

"When we wish to describe a single unit of space-movement we can adopt a method similar to that of an architect when drafting a building," Laban wrote. "He cannot show all the inner and outer views in one draft only. He is obliged to make a ground-plan, and at least two elevations, thus conveying to the mind a plastic image of the three dimensional whole.

"Movement is, so to speak, living architecture — living in the sense of changing emplacements as well as changing cohesion. This architecture is created by human movements and is made up of pathways tracing shapes in space . . ."

Countertension–countershaping does not merely refer to muscle tensions that appear in the interplay of opposing muscle groups. It refers also to large configurations that can be described as kinetic, muscular chains, as spatial shapes, and as ordered Effort sequences. They can appear in all the forms that the body can produce: one-dimensional, such as simple standing, or multi-dimensional, such as twisting (spiral, serpentine), etc. They can be symmetrical or asymmetrical.

There can be countershaping in different planes as, for example, upper body moving in horizontal (table plane) against lower body in sagittal (wheel plane). There can be countershaping with different spatial forms as, for example, when the upper body does a complex diagonal movement in the cube while the lower body clearly stabilizes itself with dimensional cross action. There can be different initiations in the countershaping as, for example, a peripheral initiation in the arms against the countertension of a centrally-initiated movement. One can trace the initiation, the renewal and the neutralizing of the countertension/countershaping in the course of the movement. The greater the complexity of the form, the greater is the complexity of body and spatial tensions supporting and sustaining the forms.

These analyses of movement behavior are constantly related to other visible and tactile phenomena, to geometrical forms and to growth changes. Mobile media, such as liquids, illustrate principles that parallel those of human movement: The interrelationship of stability–mobility, form and dynamics, balance and nonbalance. The factors of tension and countertension are always operant; they can be made more apparent when the event is observed from the view of Effort and the use of space. All shifts in tension systems are experienced also as phrasing and rhythm shifts.

As noted earlier, there are states in which one functions without countertension (although internal minuscule countertensions constantly operate). An example of mini-countertension is lying on the floor and folding oneself into a complete rounded shape. Other examples are squatting and crouching. This is very different, however, from a malfunction, such as Parkinson's Disease, causing weakening or loss of the ability to constantly renew counter patterns. Parkinson's Disease is an extreme example which illustrates the complexity of spatial and muscular tension patterns. A patient can be observed slumped toward a rounded body shape, shuffling along the surface of the floor. That this is more than just bad alignment becomes apparent when the patient is asked to push away a

105

Right: *Child Balancing Long Stick*
© Morris H. Jaffe.
Twisted verticality permits Flow
fluctuations and fluctuations
between vertical and horizontal
pulls in the shaping of the hand.

Below: *Girl Imitating Statue*
© Suzanne Fields.
A contrast in upper/lower
countertensions.
Statue: there are continuous
diagonal countertensions from left
leg to right arm and right leg to left
arm.
Girl: the focus of imitation is on the
left arm gesture with curve in the
left hip but without the twisting
countertension through the legs.
This produces a lateral tilt that
cuts off the continuity of the
diagonal, separating instead of
connecting the lower and the
upper body.

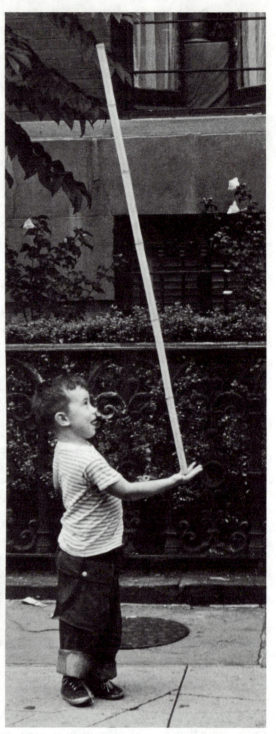

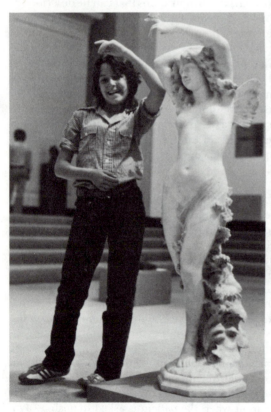

106

heavy piece of furniture or resist the pushing hands–arms of the therapist confronting him. The patient can only lean with his whole body as a total shape toward the object or person. He cannot produce the flexion–extension patterns that create the downward push into the floor against the upward–forward pattern that would serve as a countertension push action to it.

Thus, instead of producing the countershaping of erect pushing forward against an object, the patient will produce a pattern of either total concavity or total convexity (Shape Flow), which leaves him powerless against the object. In addition, with the loss of the downward push into the floor, his gait becomes uncontrolled and goes toward unrestrained acceleration or stops in a frozen rigidity.

In normal functioning, there can be different kinds of countershaping. There can be, for example, right and left countershaping. One arm gathering, the other scattering with the changes of head inclination as a third element. Throughout this process, countertensions shift with the shapes.

Countershaping can be observed in hand skills. In using both hands in an activity, either one hand holds the object while the other handles the tool in action, or the one handling the tool is further supported by the other hand doing complementary shaping movements. In the first case, the countertension is created between a stationary pull and a spatial shaping pull. In the second case, the countertensions are created between two opposed spatial shapings.

Countertensions can be combined in many ways producing various shapes. For example, countertensions from more than one body part creating a one-dimensional path can develop into countershapings when another dimensional pathway is added. In walking forward, we add three other countertensions to the tensions of vertical standing: the forward/backward alternation of the arms, and the right/left alternation of the stepping. What is particularly important is the third countertension created between the arms and the legs. It is the compelling mobility of the diagonal between right arm and left leg (and vice versa) that induces the progression of walking. Meanwhile, the push into the floor in the process of weight transference on each step renews and reinforces the vertical countertension.

Chordic tensions occur when three spatial/tension paths radiate into space simultaneously.

Central, Peripheral, Transversal Paths
Spatial shaping has been described earlier as creating routes of various scales and scale derivatives. It can also be considered as creating trace forms of spatial tensions. The spatial tensions can be ordered in terms of the three primary spatial paths in relation to the kinesphere: central, peripheral, or transversal, or some combination of them. The first travels in radiating pathways from the center of the body, like spokes; the second travels along the outer limits, the periphery, of the kinesphere, creating a sense of edge, always maintaining a fixed distance from the center; the third travels from one peripheral point to another within the kinesphere, traveling between the periphery and the center and, therefore, always off the cross of axes. These are also slightly arc-like. Pulling a fishing net out of the water is a central pulling tension. A Japanese dancer opening a fan, moving it in a half-circle away from the body, moves in a peripheral spatial tension along the boundary of her kinesphere. Pitching a baseball in a wide arc across and up involving the whole body is an example of a transversal spatial tension thrust.

Each path type has many spatial tension possibilities, not all of which involve the total body except as support. Individual limbs or parts of limbs might not follow the primary spatial paths explicitly, but can parallel them. The paths of isolated body parts are still connected to the total body, however, by supportive countertensions from the torso. The tensions that are inherent in each path are affected by the path's directional development in the kinesphere, the path's relationship to the center of weight, and its relationship to verticality, the central axis of the upright body.

Combinations of central, peripheral and transversal spatial/tension paths form more complex spatial shapes and, therefore, more complex tension systems.

107

Spatial Intent

Spatial intent is the key to the difference between body shaping and spatial shaping. It is, therefore, important to be clear about the spatial intent and to be able to identify the spatial tensions that will fulfill it in the total context. For example, one's body creates shapes in the process of breathing: growing and shrinking shapes. As soon as any part of the body relates to a spatial intent, the beginnings of spatial tension occur. General going-toward-or-away-from-the-body movements, for example, simply condense space or disperse it. The degree of spatial tension and shaping in such general movements is minimal. When, however, a specific spatial intent is added, such as a gathering movement of embracing or a scattering movement of repelling particular objects, a new tension is created between the object and the initiation of the movement in the body, and a particular, rather than a general, spatial shape is produced as the movement proceeds.

Renewing Countertensions

The vitality that tensions lend to movement is maintained only insofar as the tensions are permitted to make their subtle adjustments to the moving path in space. They must constantly renew themselves, even in apparent stillness. Attempting to "hold" or "fix" tensions results in tenseness which is static, devitalized, and alienated from the moving Gestalt of its intent. If you change even a finger tension in a spatial chord, for example, by shifting the farthest reach of a diagonal to a different finger, the total shape becomes endangered. The movement no longer reaches fully into its diagonal arc and, therefore, all other directions in the body and limbs are somewhat veering off their clear directionality. The only way to restore the chord is to recreate the spatial intent in all three limbs, which will recreate the accompanying torso tensions — in one adjustment.

Initiation and Center

The opposing pulls of tensions are also reaffirmations of a center as the quintessential balance point between them. In order to control the countershapes, the performer must be aware of the initiation of all pulls of the tensions in relation to the center. Otherwise, the shapes fall apart because tensions lose their central points of reference. This is demonstrated in observations of performances of movement scales and their derivatives and can be discerned in all movement activity by the skilled observer.

The center, however, is not necessarily only a body center of weight and a visible spatial center. It relates also to the balance between various Effort combinations involved in the tension pulls.

The skilled observer becomes aware of initiations of countertensions and the sequences of fluctuations. The center of weight as initiator must be explicit to keep the shape whole as that center shifts to fulfill the long-range intent. For example, when the baby lying on its stomach first tries to lift its head (the beginning of uprightness), the center of active weight for initiation of the movement is in the chest for both the movement head-chest up and its reinforcing countertension of elbow-press down. As he continues toward full uprightness, pulling his legs toward his abdomen to prepare his feet for grounding, the center shifts to the pelvis to support new countertensions between arms and legs.

The centering aspect of tension mobility is exhilarating because it permits maximum play with the hovering instabilities of tension pulls. As in music, more and more departures from tonic structures do not really mean abandonment of structure; what happens is that new structural forms are created with different qualities of centering.

Balanced Tension Shapes

Movements — from simple symmetrical oppositions to complex triadic chordic constellations — should be observed also as total spatial shapes, with inherent spatial tensions. They are spatially stagnant if observed only as predominantly weight masses balancing each other against gravity forces by means of tensing certain muscle groups.

Sometimes, a negative happening will alert a skilled performer to the discovery of his/her body as a total shape. For example, when some part, even a very small or minor part, is injured: a foot, a shoulder, a hand or a finger. It is not only that that part does not work; the injury often engenders an awkwardness that hinders the whole body. The unity of the whole moving body Gestalt is affected in some way.

Shadow Movements

The skilled mover can make many smaller or larger shaping adjustments which the trained observer recognizes as shape changes caused by additional countertensions. Laban called some of these secondary movements accompanying and intertwining with the main forms "shadow-movements" or "shadow-forms." They are like musical overtones with reduced tensions.

Laban observed that when different dynamic expressions were applied to the same traceform, "various accompanying shadow forms appear. One of them will be felt to be the most suitable," to the desired content of the form. They may have a tentative quality but they add emotional content. These finer shades of variations — shadow movements — appear also in Effort and can be observed in such simple actions or activities as picking up an object. The approach to the object may start with a Light/Sudden action, becoming extremely Sustained/Bound as the hand comes closer. But, in addition, several other movements with Effort content may appear in that approach: A frown (Strong/Bound) at the forehead, a squint (Bound/Sudden) of the eyes, an increased Bound pressure in the lips. These are apparently extraneous to the action of approaching. But they convey inner attitudes accompanying the fulfillment of the task: How does the performer apply him/herself? With cramped attention or with the sensuous pleasure that arises from touching the materials? What tangential thoughts or feelings are evoked that may affect precision or impact of the action? Shadow movements may intrude extraneous content by exaggerating fragments or, they may be the beginning of new content that will be integrated into the action.

In mentally ill people, shadow movements may appear as fragmented, endlessly repeated small actions: Tapping on the floor or intertwining the fingers of the hands while talking — reflections of inner life, that, in the absence of more direct expression, can offer key insights into their problems.

Shadow movements may also occur, during the learning process, as tentative, probing attempts to acquire a skill. Many attempts have to be made before the appropriate balance between Shape and Effort is achieved. For example, in threading a needle, one must find the balance between spatial direction, control of Flow, Time and Weight, and one may produce many shadow movements in that process. Trying to imitate someone else's movement, one may succeed in performing the spatial path with some accuracy, but will find it more difficult to get the exact rhythm and Effort sequences because of the influence of one's own shadow movements. Shadow movements add nuances of emotional vitality to an action — negative and positive. They can be the body's warnings of fatigue or illness or they can be openings to expanded possibilities.

Gesture — Posture — Body Attitude

In all these movements we have been exploring, the body parts can be involved singly or in various combinations. And, although the movement of any part affects all other parts, the extent of the effect can vary. *Gesture, posture* and *body attitude* — all of which refer to configurations of body parts usage — describe these effects, but each has more than one connotation in both common and professional vocabularies. These terms are also widely used metaphorically.

Posture and body attitude are most often used interchangeably; the latter generally incorporating the element of expressive content. In common usage, posture refers to total body alignment along the vertical axis struggling with anti-gravity forces. However, in common metaphorical usage, posture also indicates expressive content as, for example, in the reference to "the posture" one assumes with regard to an issue.

Gesture, in common usage, generally refers to the movement of a body part or combination of parts, with the emphasis on the expressive aspects of the move. Metaphorically, this use is translated into allusions to, for example, "a gesture" of generosity.

Laban spoke of *Gebaerde*, which can best be translated as "expressive gesture," or "bearing," or "carriage," referring to the expressiveness of the whole movement form (Gestalt), which, of course, includes stance, movements of the torso and constellation of the limbs.

He did make a distinction in early notation, kinetography, between weight-bearing and non-weight bearing phases of stepping. This distinction has been maintained as notation analysis developed and the non-weight bearing phase is referred to as "gesture." Technically, the difference can be identified in simple step patterns. In order to take a step, the foot gives up its weight-bearing function, its contact with the floor. This non-weight bearing progression (in various ways) to the next step to which the body weight is transferred is called a gesture.

The interrelationship of the weight-bearing phase and gesture and Effort combinations colors the expressive ranges they project. This relationship changes with intent changes; the rhythmic structure and character of the step pattern changes accordingly. For example, a woman enters a room and sees a sleeping child. Not wishing to disturb him, she tiptoes, putting her feet down with minimum impact (Light Weight), and prolonging the weightless (gesture) phase by extreme Sustainment (Time), until she feels her foot touch the floor and then she transfers the full body weight on to the floor. By giving a particular emphasis to the "gesture," the non-weight bearing phase of the step, the original intent was fulfilled functionally and expressively.

Laban introduced the concept of body attitude (carriage) as something that is developing during a movement and/or resulting from it. He termed the four basic forms "pin," "wall," "ball," and "screw." Pin is straight and narrow, wall is straight and spread, ball is rounded, screw is upper body twisted against lower. Each of these forms is not merely an external image of the shapes, but performs a function in relation to space: penetrating, dividing, surrounding (or filling), winding, respectively.

He did not confine himself to those forms. He also observed forms in terms of expressiveness through expansion and contraction. The sunken, shrunk, contracted posture of a depressed person becomes a fixed body attitude in sharp contrast to the expanded, bouncy quality of a "vitally alive" person's expressive body attitude that indicates a readiness to go into action.

The basic positions of classical ballet are also referred to as "postures" and/or "body attitudes." Laban quotes an anonymous 18th century description identifying their expressive content as follows:

First position:	an attitude of attention
Second position:	an attitude of self-confidence and security
Third position:	an attitude of modesty and grace
Fourth position:	an attitude of pride and dignity
Fifth position:	an attitude of artfulness, bodily skill.

Pearl Primus, a dancer and choreographer who teaches African Dance at Columbia University, had a similar identification as noted in the following step positions:

First position:	feet parallel, straight — receptive to taking in, as in meditation
Second position:	feet turned out — pride, arrogance

She thus implied a total body attitude just by requiring a specific change in the leg/foot position.

Judith Kestenberg speaks of body attitude as "the somatic core of the body image which changes with each new developmental phase . . . the way the body is shaped, how it is aligned in space, how body parts are positioned in relation to one another and to the favored positions of the whole body. Body attitude also denotes all the patterns and phrases of movement for which there is readiness at rest. In addition, it indicates the qualities of movement which, through frequent use, have left their imprint upon the body."

In the coding of the Alan Lomax Choreometric project,* a specific definition of body attitude was developed. Recurrent or constant features of the performance of different movements were tabulated to identify an overall body attitude. Thus a combination of torso changes, torso level, torso unit usage, relation to verticality, relation to stance and isolation of segments that were recurrent or constant would describe the body attitude of the performer.

There is a clear relationship between these different applications of the term "body attitude." Different areas of research interpret them selectively for their specific parameters.

Although "posture" is often used interchangeably with "body attitude," Labananalysts also use it in a more specific way, as developed by Warren Lamb, to distinguish it from "gesture," as he defined it. Lamb, a colleague of Laban, developed a specific technical usage of the terms *posture* and *gesture* for particular studies. Applications and developments of it have since been used by others for additional studies. Lamb, himself, continues research to further refine distinctions.

Gesture, here, is any movement of any body part in which Effort or shape elements or combinations can be observed. Posture is not a separate entity; it is an extension of a particular Effort or shape gesture spreading through the whole body. Lamb developed his experience with Laban into an assessment (Action Profiles) method for industrial management, in which the requirements for industrial manager jobs are formulated from studies of Effort/Shape observation. Such profiles can be made for anyone and, although they are still used primarily for industrial management because that is where they are best known, they have also been applied to teachers, doctors, sportsmen and for career guidance in many other job areas.

An important factor in the assessment is the degree to which Effort factors become postural by spreading through the whole body. The degree of this extension is interpreted as an indication of involvement potentiality. Lamb found that compiling the frequency of occurrence of a particular Effort or shape element was inadequate to conclusive analysis. When, however, he observed the spreading of the particular element from an isolated body part gesture into the whole body, he found such observations conclusive indications of full involvement of the subject. He called this spreading into the whole body *postural Effort* and the isolated occurrence he called *gestural Effort*.

In his final evaluations, Lamb found that the proportion of gestural Effort to postural Effort defined the capacity for getting fully involved, like a confirmation of the subject's "courage of his conviction." More precisely, it defines the activity for which the person is internally motivated (i.e., when free of external pressures) as distinguished from activity for which he has no motivation (but may still do if external pressures are strong enough).

Thus, in this usage, gesture/posture differentiates the intensity between two degrees of involvement. In a practical example, Lamb might observe a subject who uses numerous isolated hand gestures that are Direct, but hardly ever spreads that Direct Effort into the whole body. To underline and reinforce the statement of Direct and give it true emphasis, the statement would have to spread into the whole body. Without this extension, the statement lacks impact. The peripheral gestures alone only hint at the involvement. In assessing job aptitudes where, for example, decision-making, flexibility in action, looking for resources play crucial roles, this gesture/posture aspect became a central concept in Lamb's whole methodology.

* *See Chapter 10.*

This usage of the terms *gesture* and *posture*, although defined in a specific way, stems directly from Laban's initial explorations of expressiveness in body movement. Among the other studies to which the terminology has been applied and developed are those of Kestenberg with relation to Tension Flow and Shape Flow in child development, and those of the author and Martha Davis in defining reduced, disturbed or regressed behavior.

Gesture/posture distinctions are sometimes confused with simple shape changes. Such shape changes can be observed when a movement — with minimal Effort involvement — includes the whole body, or a person shifts weight and position — with minimal Effort involvement — simply to get into a new configuration of limbs. Only Neutral Flow is involved in that redistribution of body weight and limb positions. These shape changes are sometimes referred to as "postural shifts." Observations of them are useful in analyses of interaction in groups, as in the studies of psychiatrist Albert Scheflen, and anthropologist Raymond Birdwhistell.

Examples

A Sequence for Comparison of Tensions

1. Start by lying on the floor so that there are no vertical pulls acting on the body to reduce the adjustments to all three dimensions of space.
2. Keep the arms extended and close to the sides of the body and the legs fully extended so that the body assumes the shape of a log. The main experience is length. It is the closest you can come to a one-dimensional experience of the whole body.
3. Now, still lying on your back, try to spread the legs and arms in an even tempo and an even angulation from the shoulders and hips. You become "flat," i.e., two-dimensional like a maple leaf.
4. As you concentrate on the even process of that widening, you may reach a stage where you feel yourself spread into a five-cornered, star-like shape — a pentagram — between the tension points of the crown of the head as the upper end of the midline, both hands and both feet.

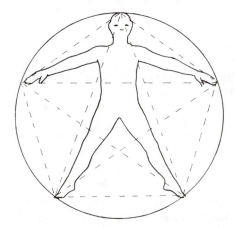

Fig. 32   *Pentagram*

5. As you assume this five-cornered shape in an upright position, the radiating tensions from the center of the body increase, particularly in the now vertical midline axis in relation to the four radiating tensions of the limbs.
6. Additionally, you also become more sharply aware of the spiderweb-like tension at the periphery of the star.
7. Try shifting your emphasis from the radiating central tensions to the peripheral tensions. Different feelings are evoked, shifting between earthy conscious awareness of stability and levels of exaltation as you spread far out.

*   *   *   *   *

Countertension

From a standing position, lift both arms overhead in a wide side/up arc. The beauty and freedom of the movement is reinforced by the shifting countertensions. These countertensions are created by the upward/sideward shaping of the arms against the up/down tension along the spine–neck–head. When the arms are "held" overhead in a slightly open and rounded line, the countertensions are constantly renewed in order to continue the countershaping experience of the original lifting of the arms — the fuller upward/sideward countertensions. As soon as the arms are exactly overhead, they become part of the up/down countertension of standing which creates a more simple tension line, a clear up/down countertension that is part of uprightness. In ordinary vertical standing, the muscular forces in the lower unit constitute a total downward force into the floor against the upward-directed muscular patterns in the upper body, thus creating a countertension between the two forces. In standing, the two processes of pushing into the floor and striving upward are constantly renewed.

*   *   *   *   *

Renewing Countertension

For the experience of renewing countertension, try the following step/arm movement:
1. Stand with feet close together, arms hanging at side.
2. Take a right leg step backward and lift the arms straight backward, without any appreciable countertension between arms and legs.
3. Take a left leg step forward, leaving the arms back. Note the spatial countertension between arms and the stepping legs.

N.B. You will note that if the arms are just "held," uninfluenced by the counterpull of the step into the opposite direction, there will be no active countertension and the body becomes either limp or tense, losing the connection between upper and lower units — shapeless. But, by renewing the spatial intent of the arms as opposite to the step, a new attempt has been made to create a live countertension, which immediately restores the connection between the upper unit and the lower unit. The experience becomes "grounded," and again becomes a total shape.

*   *   *   *   *

The Tensions of a Spiral Shape (Initiating with an Arm/Hand Turn)
This describes a process in which the "space-carving" arm, in this case the right arm, builds increasing countertension between upper and lower body during the turn, which forces tension release through a weight transference (from both legs to one) in the lower body while the arm continues to shape.

1. Stand in a left–diagonal–forward (addressing, with the left arm, the left/forward corner of the room) with weight on both feet, left foot forward, right arm neutral.
2. Start the spiral shape by right arm/hand reaching across and slightly upward (diagonal reach) under the left arm with the upper body contralateral to the lower body. During this process, transfer the weight completely to the left foot as the upper body/right arm leads gradually to a twist of the shoulder/upper body to the left, with strong rotary involvement of the left shoulder joint.
3. A strong countertension is created between the right hip and the left arm/shoulder while the weight is into the ground.
4. When the weight is fully transferred to the left, there is a maximum tension. Balance at this point can only be achieved by including the lower unit in the turn while the arm continues its spiral path. As soon as the lower unit is included in the turn, there is a momentary release of the countertension, unraveling the shoulder/upper body twist and easing the upward shaping of the arm.
5. Now, the normal *neutral* countertension of upright standing is achieved, as the right leg moves into a wide open "second" position.

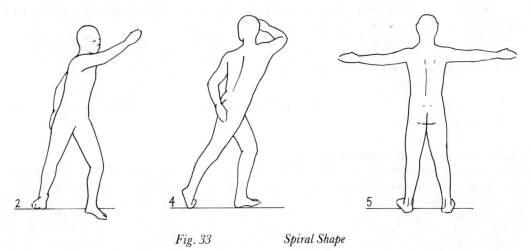

Fig. 33   Spiral Shape

N.B. What frequently happens to a student is that during the reaching across, he might miss the crucial moment of the maximal countertension that occurs with the weight shift. Instead, he merely feels tension in the shoulder and stops the shaping, thereby failing to release the countertension in the lower unit. He has stopped the shaping by just using the trunk to untwist with no connection into the arms or fully into the pelvis. After the turn, his arm is held limp or too fixed across his front, which indicates that the shaping tensions were not carried to the end. He completely missed the tensions of the unraveling of the shoulder twist at the shoulder joint in relation to the lower unit.

*   *   *   *   *

Chordic Tensions

An example of chordic interrelationship of three limbs can be seen in ballet's arabesque: The dancer stands on the right toes with the right arm in a slightly rounded gesture obliquely forward; the left leg is extended in a slightly rounded gesture obliquely backward, and the left arm is fully extended sideward.

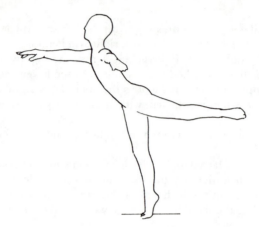

Fig. 34   *Chordic Tensions in Arabesque*

Countertension exists between the three directions of these three limbs (a chordic countertension) with the fourth limb as support. Thus, again, it is a spatial as well as a muscular countertension.

Furthermore, the ethereal character of this balanced stability/mobility is enhanced by the Effort combination of Light Weight/just slightly Bound Flow. This combination of stable/mobile shape and Flow/Weight/Effort in the arabesque gives it its illusory, non-task-oriented character.

*   *   *   *   *

Chordic Tension: Contemporary Ballet

Performance of the contemporary ballet of Paschal Guzman and his company of six dancers. These photographs illustrate examples of calm stability and of exciting mobility. In the photo at the top of the page the six dancers relate to a multilinear, multidimensional sculpture in large spatial poses: One-dimensional, parallel arm gestures either poised on one leg with the other also in clear one-dimensional direction or in sitting or standing poses. Stability is emphasized by the bilaterality of the arms in symmetrical one-dimensional directions and a solid torso. At this moment they seem to be extended in Bound Flow/Sustainment, a calming contrast to the restless winding movement of the three-dimensional spirally shaping sculpture.

In the lower picture, taken outdoors, the five girls are all bubbling playfulness in their slightly off-verticality in space, the chordic tension of their limbs and the detectable Effort elements. The male dancer (again Paschal Guzman) provides a stabilizing element in that frolicking of the girls: the verticality of his body attitude, the bilateral spreading of the arms and emphasis on Strength varying in Free/Boundness with some Lightness while the girls bounce off the floor with asymmetrical gestures off the vertical and with chordic tension in the two arms and free leg. Free Flow is dominant over Bound Flow, Strength in short spurts as accent.

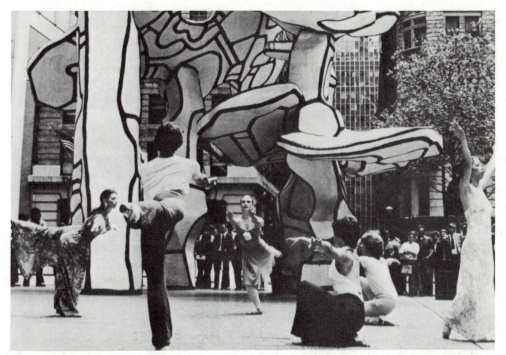

Dancers with Sculpture © Steve Turi.   Courtesy Robert Shuster and Downtown Ballet Company.

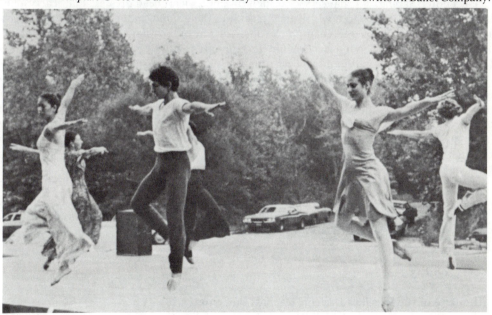

Dancers in Park © Steve Turi.   Courtesy Robert Shuster and Downtown Ballet Company.

*   *   *   *   *

117

Countershaping and Effort

Jazz and Spanish Dance

Different dance styles are identified with different countertensions even when using the same configuration of steps. For example, there is a step that appears in both jazz and Spanish dance. It is a kind of lower leg–toe–heel strutting: The lower leg–foot juts forward toward the floor, touching it with the toes, followed by percussive pressing of the heel into the floor.

The styles are differentiated by countertension differences as defined by the countershaping in the upper body. In the jazz style, the countershaping accompanying the strutting is a lanky, slight inward shaping of the contralateral shoulder–upper arm and a loosely hanging lower arm. The Spanish style produces the countershaping with a convexity of the whole upper body with both arms bilaterally lifted overhead in a slight inward rotation. Each step is accentuated with a renewal of this upward–inward rotated tension of the arms–shoulder against the downward shaping of the thigh also turning in slightly, keeping close to the body, with sharp thigh to toe, thigh to heel accents.

In each case, the Effort sequence is affected, as well as the use of Flow. In the jazz example the lower leg–forefoot is thrust with Free Flow/Suddenness/Strength followed by short Bound Flow Sustainment and a Sudden Bound digging of the heel into the ground. In the Spanish example, the thrust onto the forefoot is Free Flow/Direct/Sudden, becoming Bound followed by a Direct/Sudden/Strong click of the heel on the surface of the floor.

Sudan Dogons Ritual

In the Sudan Dogons Ritual Dance for the Dead, illustrating one of the most complex shapes, a spiral, there is a highly dramatic shift from a lower-unit-induced countershaping to an upper-unit-induced countershaping. The dancers wear high (five or six feet) head dresses. They carry a kind of walking stick in the right hand, which they push into the ground, inducing a high twisting jump which is followed, in the next moment, by a wide swinging of the total upper body twisting into an opposite cycle with a firm countertension into the ground from the legs.

The critical moment occurs in the shifting from one set of shaping countertensions to another set in the opposite body unit. It is the moment when the lower cycle is finished and the upper is induced through a diagonal pull in the body. In Effort terms, this can be described as a high intensity of Weight (Strength), rebounding into Free Flow with short rebounding into Bound Flow and renewed impulsive Suddenness.

It is a demonstration of almost complete abandon and seems to be nearly tearing the body apart. But the tensions of the shape and countershape produce a high degree of control.

*　*　*　*　*

Utmost Mobility

Silhouette of the Russian Dancer, Michail Bartenieff

The silhouette of the dancer Michail Bartenieff overwhelmingly suggests motion; with no arrest nor stillness, we seem to see the very process of "lively" involvement. It was done by E.M. Engert, famous in Germany for his caricatures of well-known personalities and for silhouettes of actors, dancers, birds, flowers.

118

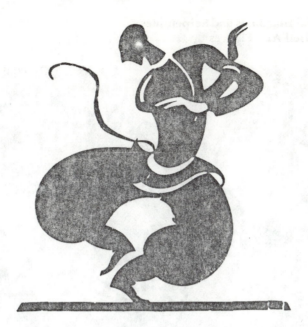

Silhouette of Michail Bartenieff by E.M. Engert.

The slightly caricaturing elements in the black and white presentation of the dancer heighten here the impressions of intense Effort-space involvement. The off-the-vertical balance on the left forefoot, the twist to the right in a diagonal curve to the right of the upper body, the diagonal inclination of the thighs opposed equally by the diagonal inclination of the two forearms suggest utmost mobility.

Additionally, the lines and curves of the blouse, the flying serpentining belt evoke the Suddenness of an imminent turn on a diagonal curve together with the Strong, Sudden lifting of the thigh in that critical moment of change.

The whole picture breathes Flow/Weight/Time fluctuations of the spaceless transformation drive — the "passion" drive. The artist makes one see an "obsessed" dancer, earthy and unpredictable. Because of the many options that are suggested, the dancer must go on.

Effort Description of Bartenieff Silhouette

The Effort indications here are written as a sequence to illustrate the mobility of the action communicated, in contrast to relatively frozen positions of many dance photographs.

Upper body with head

Free/Indirect/Exaggerated Sudden to Bound

Lower body

Upbeat	Free	Free	Rebound
Light	Strong	Light	Bound
	Exag. Sudden	Exag. Sudden	

Flow/Force/Time: the Passion Drive (Spaceless)

119

Effort, Body/Spatial Diagonals and Serpentines:
Three Commedia Dell'Arte Figures*

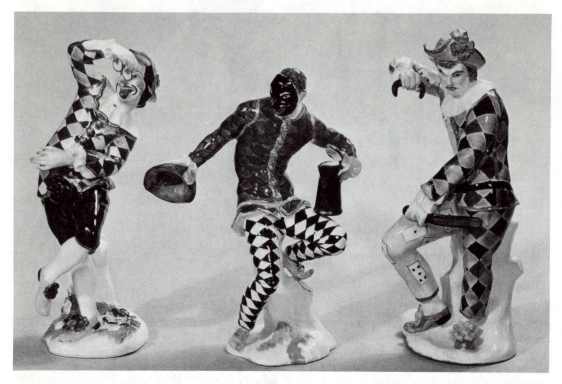

Three Meissen Commedia dell'Arte Figurines by J.J. Kaendler.

These charming rococo figurines, though not conceived as a group, present contrastive poses, costumes, gestures and attributes that strike the viewer as lively, nonchalant, capricious, mobile. Why these adjectives? The overriding quality is mobile: none of the three is fully vertically oriented; each is poised somewhat precariously but fully three-dimensionally between sitting and standing. The middle figure appears as the central figure, a spiral, serpentining tension running fluently through the whole body, dividing the body into two halves with different actions. In the arms the emphasis is on width, somewhat modified on the left as part of a countertension to the sweeping downward outward gesture of the right arm having just taken off the cavalier's hat with Free Flow/Suddenness. The blackmasked face is revealed slightly hunched between his shoulders. With his left arm he holds on to an open pitcher in a rounding, embracing arm–hand gesture (Light/Bound); it is precariously balanced on his left thigh. The spiralling midline of his body, accentuated by the button line of his jacket, divides right and left body halves into a somewhat contracted left and a bulging, widening right, the arms creating a counterbalance by internal rotation on the right and external rotation on the left. It is a peak moment: He is fighting for balance, just about getting a flimsy hold with his left forefoot on the tree trunk, the leg strongly flexed, and he is supporting himself

---

* *Meissen procelain by J.J. Kandler, 1731, inspired by Joullain's etching in "L'Histoire du Theatre" by Luigi Riccoboni, 1728, published in the art magazine "L'Oeil."*

precariously with an almost light touch of the nearly stretched out right leg. An interplay of many spatial tensions, countertensions and different Effort combinations in different body parts can be observed.

The fresh, insouciant harlequin on the left is all sophisticated, whimsical playfulness: tilted off the vertical diagonally and back to the left. He handles — in this impossible carriage of the body — the courtier's lorgnette with the Lightest Indirect touch and an insolent broad grin which displays a floppy tongue. His right leg is firmly thrust into the ground on a steep diagonal while his left leg is bent and lifted in a gesture preparatory to a dancey kick. In every move, in every part of his body he defies the mannered verticality of the courtier by being off the vertical, by contrasting Effort elements — Light/Indirect vs. Sudden/Direct/Bound — in the face and right and left arm–hand and in the whole spatial/Effort multi-action.

The figure on the right somewhat contrasts with the mobile playfulness of the other two. Heavier in body weight, he is more vertically grounded on the left leg. The two arms are in their up–down relationship: the right arm holding the sausage firmly (Strong/Bound) in a rounded gesture, in a fully closed grip in front of the body. The left arm, just as firmly (Strong/Bound) holding the scabbard in a steep forward/down diagonal, slightly across. Both arms are twisted inward toward the body. The gaze of his broad, unsmiling face, sitting on a short stocky neck is directed downward to the left: a gambler, no doubt, but one who holds on tightly to what he got for himself and defends it against any attack. The slight concavity of his torso underlines this holding on to himself; he exudes Bound Strength all over.

*   *   *   *   *

Peripheral and Transversal Sequences in Action: Animal and Human

The characteristics of peripheral and transversal movements and their tensions can be observed in the different kinds of activities and dances which incorporate them.

When props, such as fans, sticks, ribbons are used in dance, the peripheral character of their spatial sequences is predominant. The props frequently complement the costume. The total display is not merely decorative; it represents an attitude toward oneself, one's environment, how one fills the space, how one displays oneself in a role of power or seductiveness or of just playing around themes heightening a festive mood or reinforcing a community ritual, etc.

They are analogues to the display dances in the animal world. Male birds, such as the crane, the grouse, the peacock, display their wings in various degrees of folding, unfolding, with tilting of the body or spreading it near the ground. In some cases, such as the wood grouse, the wings are displayed like fans and turn and twist or shove along the ground on a curved path. It is part of courting, an address to the female; it is not performed by the female. The wood grouse performs often all by himself, accompanying himself with the special song that attracts and calls the female from the distance.

In human movement, some display dances seem to have ancient roots in the texture of the culture. Their spatial patterns contain clear indications of a choreutic order in space. They either outline the cycles of the spatial planes, mainly vertical and sagittal, or go into diagonally inclined arcs and circles. The diagonally inclined curves frequently lead to turning or twisting of the upper body which may be held, perhaps displaying the configuration of two fans.

This peripheral spreading and outlining of space is a cohesive process, progressing with finely graded Flow/Time/Space Effort elements, at times accentuated by centrally initiated stamps or claps of the hand. It may lead to complex intertwining of two partners around a rope and the harmonious dissolving of the complexity. At no time, however, does the peripheral tension become limp; there is a constant renewal of subtle countertensions in the trunk.

121

An example of such choreutic relationships was observed in an Okinawa dance: A group of women, each carrying two fans, stood in a half-circle facing the audience. Remaining in the same place most of the time, they displayed the two fans in various constellations to each other, relating to the other participants in a complementary rather than intertwining display. At one point a turn in the body occurred, led by the right fan outlining the greater part of a peripheral girdle and other choreutically-identifiable peripheral traceforms. The music (played by an orchestra of koto players) supported, with its high tension vibratory sound, the continuity and ease of the peripheral spatial tensions and the subtlety of countertensions in the trunk.

In contrast, transversals can be observed in dances that relate to the martial arts, where weapons such as swords and lances are used. Four volutes of the "B" scale illustrate their functional–expressive possibilities. There are two volutes in each of the examples below. The first example was observed in a filmed version of a 17th-century fight. The second example was observed in a mock-fight dance with wooden swords in a South American folk dance.

1. Starting with the right arm at high/left, "A," the attacker, moves to forward/deep to right/back in a wide transversal sweep that establishes the area "territory" in front and to the right side of the body. This gets the attacker ready for the threatening forward attack, going to deep/left to forward/high in a steeply rising curve that may get at the raised arm of the adversary from below. This same spatial action may occur in a confronting threat even without a weapon. Here, of course, the Effort content would make the meaning explicit, but actually the spatial sweep of the transversal movement will already convey some of the defensive or attacking or threatening intent.

2. Starting from left/forward to high/right to back/deep creates a wide upward-directed sweep that would dislodge any weapon or lifted arm or leg in its pathway and would end in a backward/down crouch. The next move would start from there and go toward right/forward to high/left in an upward sweep towards the left, displacing anything in its way, dislodging a weapon or endangering the balance of the adversary on his right leg.

These examples of spatial sequence patterns illustrate core elements in the expressiveness of human body movement — an implicit order of spatial and dynamic factors which are common to all human communication and which, in some cases, relate to possible animal ancestry.

* * * * *

Work Action: Comparison of Two Construction Workers in Terms of Spatial Shape and Effort Action Interrelation

An observation of a team of two men breaking up a concrete sidewalk for repair of small sections. Each was using a long-handled stone hammer. Note how the Effort/space interrelationship affected endurance, their ability to maintain and repeat the necessary powerful thrusts, and the actual result of the work: maximal breakage of the concrete.

The two men usually alternated actions, each doing a series of thrusts, providing some recuperation for each other. What was observed was how each man organized his sequence for maximal repetition.

The sequence of the process was as follows:
a) Seizing the tool with both hands, right hand leading, starting at the front of the body.
b) Lifting it high overhead (phase one), bearing forward–down to hit the pavement (phase two).
c) Preparing for the next two phases.

One of the team was a slim young man in his early twenties; the other, a more stocky muscular fellow in his late thirties. The obvious difference in working experience invited a comparison.

The Younger Man

Preparation: Standing in a rather narrow stance, he would seize the tool with both hands (the right one gripping higher on the handle than the left) placing it in front of himself, the hammerhead touching the ground.

Phase One: Initiating the action with a Sudden upbeat, he lifted into a clear sagittal arc with Free Flow/Exaggerated Strength, which got him through about two-thirds of the upward path. At the

Transition: level of his neck, he allowed the hammer to be tilted overhead and slightly back, using the momentum of the lift. This produced a short phase of Neutral Flow from

Phase Two: which he bore forward-down, using his whole body and arms with Sudden/Free Flow/Strength, hitting the pavement as the trunk was in a nearly 90 degree forward angle.

Preparation: Preparing for the next action, he made a number of adjustments, changing the grip, pulling the lower body slightly back in a number of Flow changes, maintaining the sagittal plane.

Phase One: He then, with Suddenness, started with Free Flow/Exaggerated Strength as described above. He had to stop after every third or fourth hit.

The Older Man

Preparation: Starting from a wide stance, slightly deflected diagonally left-forward, he places the hammer midway between his two feet.

Phase One: This also deflected his main actions: the lifting and the bearing down. Instead of the clear sagittal arc of the other man, his path was a near steep transversal in both phases so that the whole process was a sort of cycle somewhat between the sagittal and the vertical planes. This introduced a slight diagonal element into both phases.

Phase Two: His lifting in an almost steep transversal upward with Sudden/Free Flow and a crescendo in Strength went, without spatial transition, into the second phase with a Free Flow/Strength downward explosion. He did this almost without bending the trunk. In fact, the countertensions in his wide open, vertical body stance provided a countertension to the limbs' spatial path. This supported the development of his full impact, which produced a much greater amount of broken concrete.

Recuperation: In preparing for the next lift, he maintained his open verticality and solid grounding. He made only a few rapid grip changes that pulled the trunk slightly to the right, getting him on to his cycle of transversals.

Discussion

The young man worked in an almost fragmented way, a sort of start–stop fashion which resulted in contrasts of exaggerated Effort elements or zero Effort and rigid spatial form, limiting his power and endurance.

The older man worked with greater continuity and power because his cyclic action with its diagonal element maintained mobility in space and an uninterrupted Flow pattern allowing Effort combinations to develop without cramped exaggeration.

*   *   *   *   *

Different People Engaged in the Same Movement Activity: Getting Over a Fence

Place: Riverside Park near West 88th Street in New York City on a Sunday afternoon. A broad promenade above the highway is fenced off on the river side by a solid iron fence, behind which the terrain slants steeply toward the highway. Covered with lush greens and small trees and bushes, this slant is used as a downward path to reach the deserted highway, which had been closed off for the holiday, and the river.

Problem: Everyone had to climb over the fence and then walk or slither or run down: young, old, middle-aged; men, women, singles, couples and whole families. The fence, about four feet high, had three cross bars, connecting the vertical rods of the fence which were about five inches apart from each other. The second bar was about ten inches below the top bar and the bottom bar was about ten inches from the ground. Behind the fence was a lamp post that was frequently used in the process of getting over the fence.

Observing for over an hour revealed a panorama of "how to cope." When more than one person was involved, a great range of variations in possible interrelationships was exposed as young couples, friends of different age groups, the elderly or whole families organized themselves around the task of climbing over the fence and making their descent to the highway and river.

It was not just muscular ability that was involved. Temperament, readiness to act and to adapt were all expressed in the movements. Age and/or body weight were only secondary factors. The primary factors determining success in the venture were spatial adaptation and Effort.

Two models of approach emerged:
1. Pulling oneself up to sitting on the top bar and then swinging the legs together or successively over with various kinds of holds, often precarious ones.
2. Trying to straddle the fence from standing on the lower bar, holding on with both hands to the top bar. This involved turning toward the fence while swinging the free leg over the top and reaching the lower bar on the other side or immediately sliding the leg to the ground, finishing the turn while the second leg swung over.

There were, of course, many variations and deviations from these models. There was the group of agile, mobile, independent children in the 8 to 11 age group who, standing on the lower bar, would either pull or jump on the second upper bar or even to the top into an extremely folded squat, then immediately turn and jump on the other side of the ground. The essence of their movement was their tendency toward Free Flow in Effort and the ease with which they folded and unfolded their whole bodies as one action. Out of the Flow emerged clear moments of condensed Strength/Lightness and Suddenness.

There were young men in their late teens to early thirties who had no problem: They galloped toward the fence, jumped up to the top or directly over it to the ground on the other side and kept on running, slithering undaunted to the bottom of the hill. Here, the maturity of their shaping and Effort gave them the advantage over the children: The fully developed sense of readiness to attack — with Flow, Suddenness and Strength fully at their disposal. Here, again, it was not their specifically-trained muscular skill per se, but their intent and drive that motivated their use of Effort.

A number of mature women, soft in muscle tone and non-athletic in appearance, handled the problem with ease by adaptive use of their body weight, Flow, some acceleration/deceleration and diminished Strength, shaping, and using each other with minimal exertion.

Some of the elderly men made it with a different kind of ease using Space Effort, finely graded Flow changes and reduced Weight to provide enough drive and freedom in directional shaping to get over the fence. As they proceeded downhill in light, even steps, their progress was again maintained by adaptive Flow changes and clear right–left weight shifts, using just slight support of the small trees to the right and left of the path.

124

The interrelationships between people ranged from self-reliance to dependency, from restrictiveness and indifference to concerted group effort. Among the young couples, there were some movement statements of equality with neither member asking or accepting help. In another case, a strong young man lifted his girl friend who, quite capably shaping and brimming with Space/Time Effort element fluctuations, allowed this to happen, sliding evenly with a clear space intent out of his arms onto the path where they shared the active descent with carefree rhythm of Light/Free/Bound and adaptive changes from Direct to Indirect.

Among family groups, parent–child relationships were presented in other ranges of variety. One father went over the fence with his two boys and a visitor, while the mother demanded to be helped, making herself very passive in weight, needing support throughout the procedure. In descending on the path, she again leaned on her husband, sending out verbal warnings to the children — be careful, don't do that, etc. — with the result that the children became restricted in their kinespheres and in their freedom to adapt.

Two mothers, each with children: Mother One refused to cross the fence. She was somewhat heavy and constricted in her movement. The girl, about 11, was also somewhat heavy; she protested the mother's negative reactions. She made it over the fence by throwing her weight, awkwardly without any sense of herself, any clear intent in space or any clear Effort. She stood on the other side of the fence, trying to start downhill with her passive weight and lack of connection, turning her head Direct/Bound toward her mother, yelling with a taut jaw, "I can take care of myself. I don't care." The mother did not respond, let the girl go and stood bent over the fence while her 5-year-old sat passively at her feet. There was no verbal or movement interaction between the two.

Mother Two, with two boys in the 8–11 age range, quietly looked over the situation, then suddenly said, "Let's go," as she reached for the first move. The children immediately responded in a triadic concerted action rhythm.

The great event was the Spanish-speaking family, consisting of about a dozen people, representing four generations, with the youngest asleep in its carriage. In an animated exchange, the operation organized itself before the fence: The three younger women, one of them the grandmother of the baby, collected the other four children while the two young men straddled the fence and started to lift the children. The women accompanied the transaction verbally and with little supportive gestures, while the oldest generation looked on. One man lifted the baby carriage with completely even Flow/Strength and set it down with Sustainment/Even Flow. The grandmother was helped, supporting with her own shaping and Flow the action of the two men helping her. One of the young women accomplished the feat with minimal help. Only great-grandmother — small, compact, lively, determined to go — and the mother of the baby were left. The young woman and the two young men, with laughter and chatter, lifted great-grandmother and she responded by shaping her whole body into the supporting hands. With the last young woman climbing over, just slightly assisted, the family started downhill, laughing, shifting supports, developing rhythmic synchronies in a concerted Effort/shape operation. In this large group, the interaction was never interrupted and never monotone. The baby slept through it all.

* * * * *

Right: *Two Dancers in Park*
© Bonnie Freer.
An oblique relationship.
He: Flow/Light Weight dominant.
She: Direct Space/Sudden Time
dominant.
He: more rounded, more on
horizontal plane.
She: more linear in shaping, more
on axes than planes.

Below: *Fishermen Hauling In Net*
© Carol Fenner Williams.
Different shaping for same
activity.
Man left of center: total shaping
initiated from lower body.
Postural Strength/Sustainment/
Bound-Free fluctuations.
Man at center: shaping from chest
and shoulders but with less
adequate support from lower
body. Gestural Strength/
Sustainment/Bound.

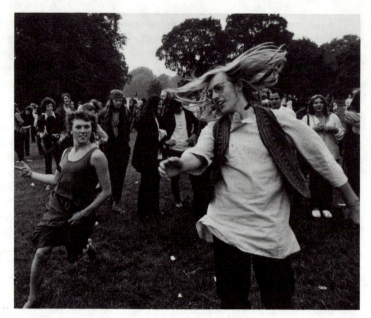

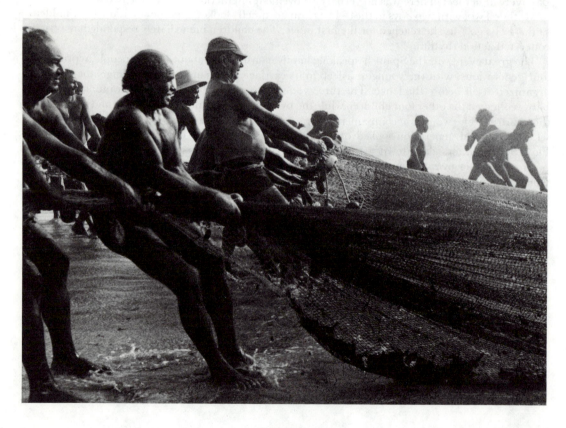

126

CHAPTER 8

Group Interaction

Human unity is the fulfillment of diversity. It is the harmony of opposites. It is a many-stranded texture, with color and depth.

Norman Cousins

Right: *Old Priest and Woman*
© Bonnie Freer.
A contrast in retention of Effort
and shape in aging.
Woman: Effort elements
neutralized. Flow toward Bound.
Shaping also reduced.
Priest: clear directional gestures
even though total body shaping is
somewhat reduced. Right hand:
Direct/Sustained. Left hand:
Light/Sustained.

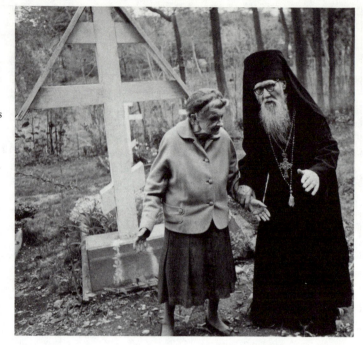

Below: *Group Chanting*
© Bonnie Freer.
Reduction in all Effort elements
and Shape toward Effort and
Shape Flow.

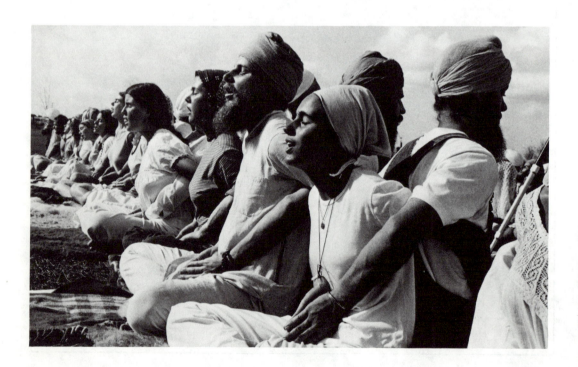

128

Group Interaction

Group interaction can be considered from many different perspectives: number of people involved, the space in which they meet, reason for meeting, relationship before, during and after meeting, extent of interaction or lack of it, the configuration of their meeting, type of confrontation, progressions of variations. Many other factors can also be considered for different kinds of research. The study of group interaction is a discipline in itself, in which nonverbal aspects are a central research resource.

Labananalysis has a particular contribution to make to group interaction studies — directly pertinent to some and indirectly related to other movement research. To this author, the observations of individual body/space/Effort factors could add an important dimension to the field because they reveal differentiations that are often overlooked in the interaction process. The use of space, for example, helps to distinguish the degree to which the participants are self- (body) oriented or other- (space) oriented. The degree to which the whole body is incorporated into the activity can also help define the degree of interaction. For example, are the distal joints included or is an individual cutting off from others by not letting movement go out through the finger tips? Is an individual's anxiety being expressed in a group by holding arms and hands immobile? Or do Effort observations lead to another interpretation of the holding? The Effort fluctuations also help establish group rhythms.

The shape of the group can be observed as an organic structure and identified in terms of the spatial and Effort qualities as a whole from observations of dominant qualities shared by its members.

How the individual kinespheres and action territories are adapted and incorporated into the group also defines qualities of the group. Leadership and other roles are clarified by noting the individual Effort and space factors in relation to the total group. This becomes very clear when one organizes several groups in different ways. For example, one group might be formed with individuals who share particular dynamic qualities, perhaps diminished Effort qualities. If one or two members of each group are exchanged, the change is immediately perceived in both the individuals and the groups. Individual qualities are affected, group roles more or less shifted, and group quality can be modified or transformed.

Whether the movements are synchronic, symmetrical or sequential can be observed and qualities of their Effort rhythms and phrasing compared in Labananalysis terms to help determine individual differences in the group and the components that make the group more cohesive or disconnected.

These factors have all been discussed earlier in this book in other connections and will also appear in Labananalysis applications described in later chapters.

The earlier focus has been primarily on the individual mover. Movements of several people have been discussed in terms of what they might share or how they might contrast with each other or interact each in his or her own way. It is also valuable to make a distinction between how the individual members of a group move versus what occurs in movement terms between them on a group level, as in group spatial configurations. If the observer shifts from watching an individual in a group to seeing also the forms, angles and rhythms between any two members or three or the whole group, the individuals are then seen as parts of a larger body and a whole new world of perception opens up. Some configurations and confrontations with their accompanying Effort combinations are discussed on the following pages.

Right: *Young Woman and Man Talking* © Bonnie Freer. Although there is contrast between the man's wide openness and the woman's horizontal closing in (perhaps culturally influenced sexual distinctions), there is synchrony in the head gestures connecting them. His Effort tends toward Strength and Free Flow; hers toward Lightness and Bound Flow.

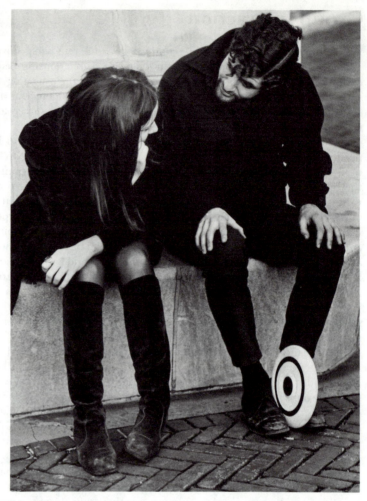

Group Spatial Configurations and Confrontations

Spatial configurations may define relationships between individual people, between individuals and the group and between groups. The configurations outline the territory in which action–interaction develops and communicates what that action–interaction might become. Discussions between two people or around the table of a political meeting, in open mass meetings, parades, processions, dances — all embody spatial configurations that illustrate aspects of the internal relationships. Within an event, changes of group form can delineate particular phases of the event.

The group may be clearly defined or almost formless, compact or loosely scattered, linear, solid, irregular, round or angular. It may have a common front or an unspecified front.

The individuals within the group may be arranged in files, rows or circles or modifications of them. That arrangement will be critical to the nature of their confrontations with each other and of the confrontations of their group with another group, that is, whether they relate face-to-face, side-to-side, obliquely or back-to-back.

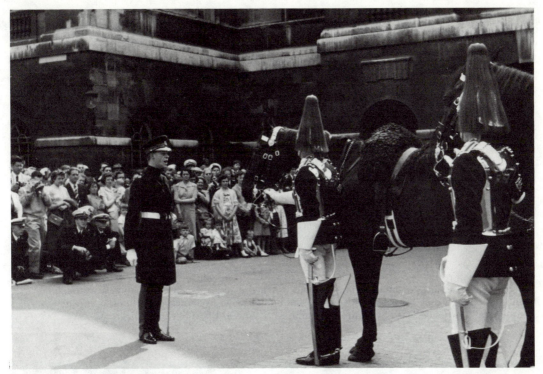

Changing of the Guard © Morris H. Jaffe.
Both officer and guards show Bound Flow, utmost verticality and limited kinesphere action. The officer has Direct Space, Neutral Weight, while the guards show Neutral Space and Strong Weight.

File: The file develops from two people standing behind each other when one simply follows the other or one protects the other. In each case, one of the participants has a somewhat passive role: a father, for example, presenting his young son standing in front of him to friends or a woman showing a pathway to a new neighbor. A file may pick up new participants who will also follow the head person or stand passively, as when waiting for a bus or queuing at a ticket office. Interaction is usually minimal. It is deliberately chosen, for this reason, in grouping prisoners and slaves.

Group interrelation of files consists of passing each other at a distance, parallel to each other or, more actively, coming from different directions toward each other, which may develop into other forms of interaction.

Row: The row originates from a one-to-one, side-by-side formation. It provides an interrelationship of equality, of sharing and being close, having the same focus, possibly sharing the same action. The row is a formation conveying solidarity, advancing and retreating, mutual reinforcement, often forming a wall against an intruder. With its possibility of moving from side to side, a group of rows may envelop an individual or another group. It can lead ultimately to the circle.

There are simple work organizations built on a row: a group of workers unloading packages from a truck that are passed from hand to hand along the row, or a group, in a fire disaster, passing buckets of water from hand to hand.

Two rows opposing each other create confrontation which may lead to a fight or a ceremony of greeting. In a side-by-side configuration, the frontal, potential fighting confrontation is avoided. The confrontation can remain neutral or invite sharing.

131

Circle: The circle can evolve from a file or a row and will have different characteristics depending on whether file or row qualities are transferred. Most often, it evolves from or through the row form with its side-to-side relationship qualities more developed. In a circle, there can be even more sharing because, in addition to the side-to-side contact, there can be a common relationship to the center of the circle when the participants face it and, therefore, each other. This shared relationship with a center makes body, space and Effort tensions more synchronous.

A group sitting around a coffee table in a circle may show synchrony of movement as they, for example, reach for the coffee cups or cross and uncross their legs in unison. The synchrony may also be expressed in other body part actions and in turns from one member to another, where Effort rhythms are shared by shifts in Weight and Time.

This can be seen even more clearly when dancing in a circle where all participants face the center of the circle. Common rhythm in stepping is transmitted from side to side, from one person to the next and to the ones farthest away. In the circle, Effort Flow most easily helps establish the common continuity of the movement and the common order of step directions. A circle thus brings people together; it is one of the oldest forms of social congregation in dance.

Nuns © Bonnie Freer.
The central figure shows countershaping in hands which also appears in her use of total body diagonal. Combinations of Strong Weight, Sudden Time and Bound Flow. Asymmetrical. The others are generally symmetrically closed, essentially vertical, gestural, with reduced Effort in varying degrees.

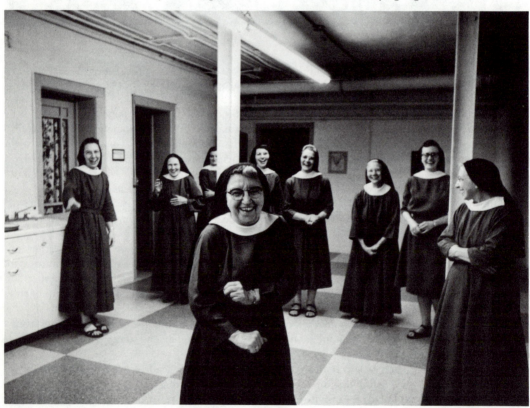

Meeting front to front frequently triggers off a whole series of actions that may lead either to acceptance of each other or to fighting or to an attitude of extreme readiness to fight. Or, one may keep an adversary at reach space distance until a final resolution of hostility enables each to enter the other's reach space totally for an embrace.

Oblique interrelating, a deflection of straight confrontation, occurs occasionally between two participants. It lessens the tendency toward threat and fight because it offers more mobile options. An oblique approach may have a defusing function by combining head-on/forward with the sideward/opening. It allows for a wide territory around and in front, so it is less threatening than if the approach were just head-on/forward. These spatial attitudes are operative even without arm–hand gestures. They are registered by the partner, whether or not he is consciously aware of the meaning or tendency of the other person's movement.

In any interrelationship of two people, there are constant fluctuations between reach space and action space supported by locomotion. When the reach space is shared with particular Effort elements by participants, the hostility, caution, or neutrality can be changed to trust.

Interrelation of three people often results in a dramatic series of internal changes. While the spatial triadic constellation defuses direct confrontation, it may involve a number of different pairings against the third or attempts to involve a very passive third member, so that finally a balance between all three is developed by a synchronous rhythm, by a similar or complementary use of body parts, or by regulating distance, or by spatial and Effort patterns.

Relationships that are established through the reach of kinespheric space are changed when one or both of the participants move from one place to another to extend reach possibility. Action places — wider territory for operations — are thus established.

In all cases, the spatial configurations reflect and help establish the tone of confrontations between individuals and groups. If there is the possibility of eye contact, as, most naturally, in face-to-face confrontations, a critical dimension is added to the relationship. The Effort elements and shaping fluctuations in the movements of approach further color the nature of the approach, how positive or negative the encounter. These approach communications are critical in groups where established role relationships are given, such as parent–child, teacher–student, doctor–patient, etc. The first spatial approach of the dominating figure in such situations may establish how the two will get along, how much trust, give and take, will develop in their interaction.

Spontaneous improvisations often contain elements of confrontations that appear in community dances. Close observation reveals that the improvisation structures reinforce the rules of interrelationships that are acceptable to the whole community; the space/Effort dynamics reflect an order in social behavior. There are times when the intent is recognized instantaneously — almost as precognition — by sensitivity to any one or combinations of the body/space/Effort components of the approach to and the changes within the configurations.

A common Effort rhythm may gradually emerge that will reinforce the solidarity of the group. It could be something like all members of the group moving through a sequence of Free Flow, Strong Weight, Sudden Time and a pause and then repeating the same sequence. The group could also reinforce their solidarity with a successive sequence such as one member using Free Flow/Strong Weight/Sudden Time as another follows with Bound Flow/Light Weight and Sustained Time and all are repeated. In both cases or other variations of them, a socially adaptive order and pleasure may emerge from the shared Effort rhythm.

In studio sessions of movement choirs, spontaneous movement of individuals in groups is used to create ordered dance structures where each participant has contributed his/her individual use of space, Effort and ability to relate to others. The leader may set the theme, then act mainly as a catalyst nurturing rhythmical phrases and group form changes, sometimes by assigning one participant to a different group to change the character of the group. The new member may change the group form from a shapeless clump to a circle, changing the interrelationship of members by not submitting to a domineering member. He/she may introduce changes in Effort combinations infecting the group with a different rhythm. From spontaneous, apparently chaotic beginnings of a number of dissociated individuals, a group form can develop with spatial and Effort interrelationships around a theme that can be identified and that often mirrors the structure of organized, traditional, communal group dances and ceremonial rituals.

A whole set of dances in the western hemisphere, stressing sociability — square dances and quadrilles of America, France, England, Germany, Scandinavia, Russia, etc. — are built on particular spatial confrontations. Couples change from side to side proximity to confrontation; they get involved in whirls and circling, exchange places visiting other couples and, finally, join in a circle and come back to original places in the squares and rows. Configuration of people and use of territory take dominance over complex steps and involved arm–body expression. Other cultures have different types of confrontations.

Greeting behavior in western culture is a confrontation that can be interpreted as a form of fighting behavior modified through Effort or shape changes to a peaceful resolution — a front-to-front configuration, for example, modified to a side-by-side walking off together.

In an early study of greeting behavior done by Adam Kendon, an ethologist, and Andrew Ferber, a psychiatrist, with the author as consultant, a frame-by-frame selection of a whole sequence of a film was examined to observe changing distance, spatial constellation changes, and the presentation of body parts in relation to each other. The study revealed a highly structured, ritualized play with variations when, for instance, a hostess greeted her guests at a party. The different degrees of closeness that the hostess felt for each guest were revealed in the variations within the structured phases of the greeting ritual. The hostess, for example, might rush up to an old family friend and embrace him with total body shaping and then accompany him side-by-side to the gathering place. Or, in contrast, she might greet a more distant acquaintance by standing erect, extending her forearm-hand forward in a linear path.

It would be interesting to add observations of the rhythmical elements of Effort. For example, a warm embrace with Free Flow becoming Bound/Indirectness with short Sustained/Strength is in sharp contrast to a cool greeting of Direct/Bound Flow with minimal Weight and Time. Or, a quite different progression — Free Flow/Lightness going into Neutral Flow or abrupt Direct/Suddenness ending in Bound Flow — might be observed. In general, the absence of Weight and Time or either of these elements would make the greeting cool or reserved or perfunctory in various degrees.

*   *   *   *   *

Examples

Spatial Confrontations

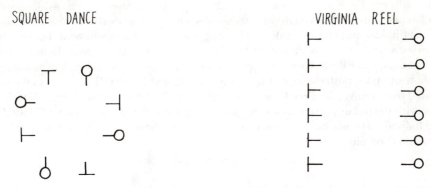

Fig. 35A

*　*　*　*　*

A Configuration of Family Hierarchy

During the historical Samurai period in Japan, the configurations of family hierarchy were structured spatially in such a way that only their desired confrontations could occur. A visit to a home was like a choreographed scene. For example, when a future bride was presented to the master of the house and his family, the spatial configuration between visitor and family and the distance between family members seated in a hierarchical order in the rectangular form was maintained throughout the visit without change.

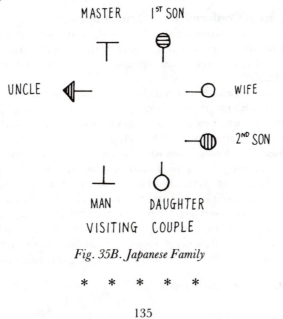

Fig. 35B. *Japanese Family*

*　*　*　*　*

135

Group Effort Rhythms: Exertion/Recuperations

In group activity, when it is important to the continuity of the activity to produce a main Effort action in unison, transitions between the Effort action might also occur in unison, or, they may show individual patterns, since so many different kinds of adequate recuperative transitions are available. These differences can be observed in various cultures where a great deal of work is done in groups and is highly rhythmical, sometimes reinforced by song and drum accompaniment. For example, a crew of four rowing a boat will employ a Basic Effort in unison for the main impact. In the recovery phase, the team not only uses Effort/shape changes recuperatively, but the individual members have greatly varied Effort or space patterns of getting ready for the next impact. They may make exaggerated large spatial trace forms with Free Flow. Some indulge in Free Flow/Sustainment, but they are back each time with the full impactive stroke, as one. The Effort combination is fully recreated each time. Allowing individual recuperative action to occur reinforces the intent, precision and full impact of the unified main action phase.

* * * * *

Observations on a New York Subway Station

A middle-aged man facing two women, literally talked into them at close range with intense involvement.

A little distance away, a young Japanese couple addressed each other on a diagonal at some distance from each other. They occasionally talked, moved in response to each other, slightly turning away or toward each other or just waited, looking for each other's response, establishing their intimate relationship with form and mobility.

On the opposite side, at the edge of the platform, two tall Afro-Americans were side by side looking straight ahead. They were having a great time talking, moving in synchronous rhythms, roaring with laughter, sharing each other without ever looking at each other.

The three groups presented a dramatic contrast in spatial arrangements and the kinds of interactions each configuration enhanced.

* * * * *

Duet in Canon: Problems of Conformity*   A Student Report

"My partner and I recently had a performance where we danced a duet in canon. She choreographed the piece, and I learned the movements. The movements themselves were easy, but because we use our weight so very differently, our weight quality and phrasing differed. It was important in this canon for our dancing to be alike.

"I have been in group pieces before where conformity is important and accomplishing consistency difficult. It usually takes much time, trial and error, and intuitive guessing about why, although the movements are the same, it doesn't look right. Knowing exactly what to correct, let alone how to correct it, seemed in the past a rather impossible task.

"We were able to observe each other, see what we each were doing (in comparison to what we thought we were doing) and compare results. Let me use one turn as an example. Basically, it was a full circular pivot in plié to the right. Torso, head and arms were tilted right at initiation and finished toward the left. She used a central initiation and a sensing of her weight which carried her in Shape Flow to the left. I most naturally used a quick peripheral initiation in my hands, which carried me around in Lightness and Bound Flow, arms shaping transversely until I finished left. Knowing what I preferred to do, I was able to emulate her movement by initiating centrally, really getting into my plié with a swing phrase and more Free Flow, allowing my weight to carry me around. Although she

* *Diana Schmitt, Dance Notation Bureau student project.*

tended to Shape Flow while I [tended] toward a more spatial orientation, and although we both used our weight differently in many places during the piece, we were able to key into our breath and work on the important initiations and phrase accents so that the piece held together as a unified duet . . .

"I was amazed at how easily and how fast we were able [through Labananalysis] to pinpoint problems and go about correcting them. Pinpointing was easier than correcting. Correcting often meant going back and working on basic movement qualities [adding more Labananalysis to intuitive explorations]."

In this case, defining individual differences became essential to understanding the difficulties of performing synchronous group action.

* * * * *

Observations of an Actors' Training Class
Students started with preparatory exercises designed to evoke images of live sculpture by going through the body's articulations. It was done in anatomical sequence, going through the articulations in a successive way of almost uninterrupted moving in an improvisatory style: flexing/extending, rotating, lateral bending and cycling (head, upper trunk, lower trunk, whole trunk). There was great emphasis on the successive use of articulations in the upper body and on alternate use of central impulse as initiation and peripheral isolation of body parts.

The movements in these exercises were essentially isolated, self-oriented. The object of the next exercises was to explore alternations between sharing one's space and returning to one's own space for the experience of relating to self and to others.

What was not made clear to these students was the difference between physical and emotional sharing of the same space. The students, although physically sharing the same space, still appeared isolated and self-related. What they lacked, except for brief accents, was spatially directed movement within that space that would have connected them emotionally, adding an awareness of each other in the space and spatial tensions they shared.

This unawareness of spatial intent was also accompanied by limitations in their use of Effort. There was a nearly complete absence of the Space Effort. They stayed continuously with Weight/Time/Flow, the Spaceless, "passion" drive, with recuperations only into the Free Flow combination of the drive. High intensity Sudden/Strong/Bound Flow prevailed, which created a kind of intense agonized mood that rarely found relief. Some of the students never reached this peak mood; they stayed most of the time in Flow, with little clearly defined Weight or extremes of Time.

Since they lacked awareness of the distinction between body-oriented and space-oriented movement, they limited their ability to relate to each other — a crucial problem for actors. Also, with the nearly total absence of the Space Effort, their communication was confined to expression within a repertoire overcast by a sameness in quality.

* * * * *

Movement Behavior Analysis from Videotaped Group Session
As part of a symposium on group therapy analysis chaired by Jay Fidler at the 1969 convention of the American Group Therapy Association in New Orleans, a Labananalysis* of group movement behavior seen in a videotaped session was compared with verbal analysis of the session.

The Labananalysis focused on postural shifts, Effort dynamics of each group member and subgrouping patterns. The session was divided into six episodes which were identified by the principal speaker's participation, i.e., each time he spoke, a new episode appeared to be established.

One young woman, who actually spoke very little, nevertheless — through her manner and

_____
* *By the author and Martha Davis.*

nonverbal behavior — emerged as the chief activator with the greatest ability to relate to others. Another woman, who talked a great deal, vying for the attention of the therapist, made impact only with her voice and the sharpness of her words, while her body dynamics were actually very low in variation and intensity. Such discrepancy between verbal and nonverbal behavior can often be observed and systematically documented.

Unfortunately, many films and videotapes are made as the one used for this symposium — with poor lighting and an ever-shifting camera focus that only exposes part of the group at a time, severely limiting one's observations of the movement behavior.

*　　*　　*　　*　　*

"Authentic Response"

"Authentic response" is a term sometimes applied to that movement which is initiated entirely by the performer without any outside structured stimulus.

The author observed a group in a community movement session based on "authentic" response. It was the last of twelve sessions for the group, which was about 60 percent female, 40 percent male, its members ranging in age from fourteen years to mid-fifties.

The structure of the group was extremely loose; music was used sparingly. Each person found a place — sitting, lying or standing — for himself/herself. It was not until about the middle of the session that some had a "feeling" for body "stretching" — the first activity.

The first task was to "find relationship between body parts, hand, foot, etc., to rest of body." This produced isolated movements, i.e., confined to the individual; many group members still did not participate.

Next, the task of relating to people produced sub-groups, a greater amount of level changes. Gradually more Effort elements, such as Weight, Time and Flow appeared in the movements which were then supported by music. At one point, an attempt was made to stimulate discussion about the movements produced.

A Nubian record brought intensive involvement within small groups. The vibratory rhythms of the music elicited more sequencing and communication in the movement. As the music stopped, rhythm died down and participants drifted into sitting and lying on the floor, some gently rocking.

A short discussion followed which could not be heard by the observers but there appeared to be a synchrony of feeling. However, to this observer, the most astonishing impression was the near absence of relationship to space, while body aspects related primarily to the giving in to weight. Furthermore, Time and Weight, the predominant Effort elements, had very little range variation.

The leader hardly participated in the movement. Her constant concern with empathy kept her in a neutral state expressed through some body weight and Flow, occasionally some Flow with Time. Her weak Space Effort further defined her role as supportive rather than stimulating or leading.

In later meetings with the leader apart from the group, the experience of combinations of Flow/Space and Space/Time was a revelation to her, as were the large patterns of the icosahedron scales. She studied the "A" scale as a means of expanding herself in space and also as an activating stimulus to working out conflict through the resources of dance, symbolic representation and metaphor.

The weakness of the group experience could be traced to a too literal, too rigid adherence to the principle of waiting for the "authentic" response. Leaving the structuring of the event totally to generalized tasks and to chance happenings between people is too limiting. With the introduction of imagery, crystallization of Effort/shape elements into common group use, there is much greater possibility for the evolution of a dance or a ritual that can transcend the personal experience into a group experience. Both are important.

The concrete language of Labananalysis provides a vocabulary around which such group experi-

138

ences can crystallize, without psychologizing or over-choreographing, by picking up themes, phrases, interaction statements, metaphors, and working in a group through them. The movements themselves will provide the stimulus, insights and resolutions.

* * * * *

Movement Choir

Between 1920 and 1933 Laban and his collaborators, Albrecht Knust and Martin Gleisner, developed what he called "movement choirs" throughout Germany. Such choirs were often created with labor and other organizations. He worked with as many as 500 people for a single choir performance; their emotional power became so striking that they were eventually banned in Hitler's Germany. Laban considered them "playful structures with a very special significance . . . a form of religious art of dance of the kind that has existed in many forms in the past and in many religions."

The emphasis was on the experience of "the joy of movement," in groups. "The dancer in the movement choir," he wrote in *Gymnastik und Tanz*, "expresses himself, but purified, more enhanced and nearer to an archetypal ideal. From the depth of his being he draws a newly awakened sense of movement and anchors it durably and solidly in his system through the enthusiastic and dedicated act of performing movement." Specially trained dance leaders gave dance stimuli within a structured framework that permitted the participants to move from their own spontaneity. This play led to creating dances together that were performed at festive occasions. By giving form to the improvisations of the individuals and the groups, the performance became repeatable because it was anchored in reaffirmation of a common experience.

Marian Chace and others have utilized similar dance productions in dance therapy programs with hospitalized psychiatric patients as part of the last phase of the patients' recuperations — one of the links to the outside world with its various demands on initiative and responsiveness.

Developing one's own vitality and resources by moving in a group sharing the pleasure of movement satisfies a deep communal need. Some people may start with a vague idea of finding exercise for their tired, tense or flaccid bodies that will not be as boring as mechanical exercises or as "cute" as "dancey" exercises. The movement choir takes them beyond that. In the communally-oriented movement group, body control can and should be practiced in conjunction with exploratory, expressive work. There are many themes that can be used as points of departure — space themes, Effort themes, music, poetry, legends, sounds, singing, props or rhythmical instruments.

The sensitivity of the leader is constantly tested and challenged, not only by what he/she can bring to the experience, but by what he/she can perceive and incorporate from the performers. The core of the experience may originate from very simple movement forms. Breathing, simple opening and closing of the arms and the whole body, the discovery of spatial and Effort rhythms may set off long forgotten feelings that have been buried under frozen spatial or Effort tensions. Images are evoked through moving. This is the beginning of creating a dance together. A structure develops that allows individual variations and sharing in one's own terms.

Labananalysis lends itself to providing the needed structure and variation to the group improvisations. Out of these first improvisations, relationships and themes begin to crystallize into rhythmical forms. Frequently, in the groups' first physical contact and intermingling, moments of high aggression — chaos — may occur. At these points, the introduction of a new or additional spatial theme may diffuse that high tension and stimulate the search for new movement resolutions.

From these experiences, the leader as well as the participants may make important discoveries about themselves: their potential as movers and interactors, and, even more crucial, the contribution of each member in the group. In some cases there are clashes of individual dynamics within one group and/or between two groups. Aggression at these points can very often be transformed by suggesting a change in spatial or Effort themes. A skillful leader can facilitate this process.

One of the aims of the movement choir is to arouse the unresponsive members of the group. For example, in one of the author's groups there was a woman who complained that she could neither "feel" anything in the movement changes nor contact anyone else in the group. She stood vertically erect, immobile, touching other group members only peripherally and remained nonreactive, throughout her whole body, to approaches by others. We decided to introduce a new group theme: each individual was to go quickly into a triadic constellation of head–limbs–body and then to change it to a completely new triadic relationship and then again to a third, entirely different, constellation. After initiating several such changes, we introduced the theme of change in one limb only at a time, suggesting that the group members savor the new constellation for a few moments before changing the second and then the third limb in the same manner. When we tried this in the group, the woman who had earlier experienced such difficulty in sensing the movement changes and in making contact with others, registered for the first time an intensive change. Her personal experience of her own body began to be transferred to her experience of others' movements around her. She became able to sense the variations and respond to the approaches of the others in the choir.

Each group experience, however, does not have to lead to such a synchronic, harmonious resolution in sharing. The meeting of distinctively contrastive groups — or contrastive movement in members of one group — also can provide a richness in which all shades of movement expressiveness are evoked and maintained in dynamic balance.

This kind of communal dancing has, of course, ancient historical precedents. All folk dances represent community creations that were preserved in structures and allowed individual variations. They survive because they reflect core feelings and attitudes. Unfortunately, they too often become so frozen in their structures that the spontaneous expression becomes limited. This is especially true when performed outside the context of their respective cultural life styles; they are often depleted of their meaningful intent. What we often see has lost its character and innate tensions.

New movement choirs need to be created for expression of the particular tensions and feelings of particular periods and environments. Today, movement choir forms serve in the search for new balance between over-individualistic, self-centered and often sentimental expression, and the rediscovery of vital resources for moving together. They enrich both professionals and non-professionals moving beyond mechanistic, simple strength–speed oriented dance. Another dimension is added to dance by directing individual expression to a specific communal expression.

Laban, in *Gymnastik und Tanz* (1927) wrote:

"The main emphasis of modern artistic body culture should be directed toward movement choirs at festive presentations and community performances to reveal the joy of dance experience on a healthy, strong and durable body/mind/spirit basis . . .

"Whoever becomes aware of the terrifying lack of the sense of movement in children's schools, universities and private courses for children and adults, and who then becomes convinced that this lack of the most natural, most beneficial forces of man has to be eliminated, could only turn to one means: the art of choric dance . . ."

Referring to the choric dancer, he wrote:

"In this case, one does not need to deal primarily with how the body dance training can and should serve the dance presentation on the stage, but rather the reverse: how the participant may gain from the experience of aesthetically-oriented body training, how new values can be awakened in the process of preparing and presenting choric movement works . . .

"In dance — especially in choric dance — it is enthusiasm or its primeval source that swing together with depth of feeling and clarity of comprehension . . . the urge to create choric dance works poetic in character, can lead way beyond utilitarian considerations of purely functional exercise to human values . . ."

CHAPTER 9

Dance Therapy

> If psychoanalysis brings about a change in the mental attitude, there should be a corresponding physical change. If dance therapy brings about a change in the body's behavior, there should be a corresponding change in the mind. Both methods aim to change the total human, mind and body . . . .
>
> *Trudi Schoop*

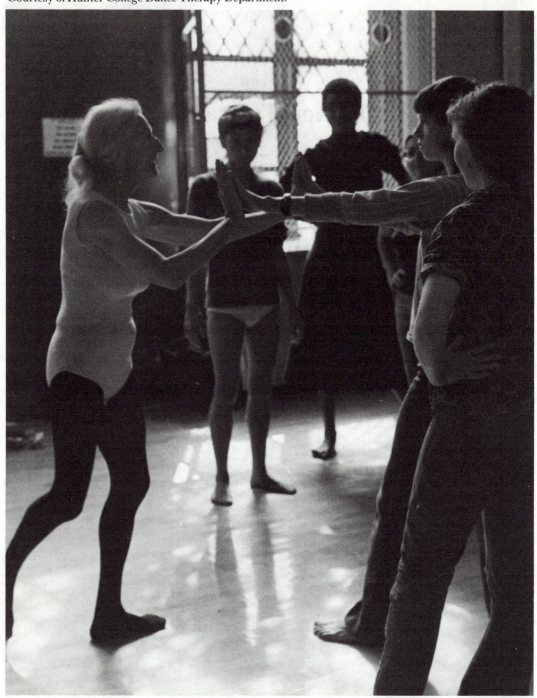

Dance Therapy

The resources of dance — for pleasure or art or therapy — crystallize qualities of ordinary movement and behavior. Therefore, the study of dance movement is a study of human movement possibilities, both functional and expressive.

Dance therapy requires observation based on movement analysis and, always, the possibility of producing change. Even if the change is minuscule, it is significant because each shift reverberates throughout the whole Gestalt. Research in any behavioral science can be given new perspectives by the therapists' observation skills and the questions they raise.

Dance therapy, from its small, highly individualized beginnings in the fifties, has developed at a dizzying speed since the 1960's. This acceleration started with the formation of the American Dance Therapy Association (ADTA) under the leadership of Marian Chace, who brought together the eastern and the California core groups of Trudi Schoop, Mary Whitehouse, Alma Hawkins, Franziska Boas and Lilyan Espenak. ADTA defines dance therapy as "the psychotherapeutic use of movement as a process which furthers the emotional and physical integration of the individual."

Many factors contributed to the enormous increase in the number of dance therapists and to the growing stature of the field. The cultural and environmental concern with body–mind interrelationship created a receptive milieu. And, in the field of mental health, the work of the psychiatrist, Wilhelm Reich, provided a forceful impetus to body–mind treatment of mental illness which had wide repercussions.

Simultaneously, there is increasing interest in oriental healing and meditative approaches to health and therapy such as yoga, T'ai Chi Ch'uan and others, with varying levels of understanding, practice and integration of these influences among dance therapists.

The pioneers of dance therapy in the United States, with very few exceptions, were led into working therapeutically with dance by profound changes in their lives as dancers and/or from earlier work with dance for children. Almost all of them describe their starts in a hospital as "accidental" or "near-accidental."

Though they differed in personality, background and approach, they had in common a belief that it is possible to reach people's feelings through the exciting, enlivening and calming power of dance. Wherever they became established, they found sympathetic understanding among some psychiatric staff members in the institutions where they worked, even though they were targets for disdain by many. The understanding frequently led to some form of coordinated team work which gave dance therapy a chance to grow.

By the time ADTA was formed, its pioneers had already trained a number of students as co-workers or therapists who had then to go out on their own to find affiliations with institutions or clinics. ADTA also attracted to its membership others who had independently developed movement therapy approaches.

A whole spectrum of dance therapy approaches evolved from movement as a recreational, socializing activity to a therapeutic tool with a great variety of psychological, psychiatric orientations by the practising dance therapists.

It is still a wide open field, with continuing discussions to clarify its differentiations from other therapeutic tools and approaches to mental illness and health. Only the fact that it concerns body movement as one of the inherent tools distinguishes dance therapy consistently. But even here, there is debate about the emphasis on the resources of dance or other modes of movement. In addition, there is a continuing attempt to develop a common vocabulary.

Labananalysis has a particular contribution to the field because it provides an objective vocabulary and a notation for recording observations of movement. It allows for exploration of the great range of dynamic shades making up the wholeness of the experience and describes functional, expressive changes in relation to the movement process itself.

The training in visual and kinaesthetic perception prepares the observer to perceive concretely the integration of physical muscular levels of activity with feeling, thinking levels of behavior in terms of body, Effort and space. These components are experienced by the therapist and the patient with a common vocabulary to share and deal with the components simultaneously in objective terms that are tolerable to the patient. Thus, another level is added to the patients' awareness, which gives them "handles" to greater control over their own lives.

Some of the on-going questions to which dance therapists address themselves are: 1) The role of dance as a specific resource; 2) The role of Bartenieff Fundamentals as a specific resource; 3) The incorporation of other techniques and disciplines; and 4) The role of Labananalysis as a key resource. We shall consider each of these in the following pages.

The Role of Dance as a Specific Resource

The extent to which the objective structural resources of dance per se should be utilized is often juxtaposed to the importance of subjective expressiveness in movement. These are questions about what is an acceptable degree of "structure" in the work. Does structure inhibit or release freedom? Such questions lead to the even larger questions about the nature of freedom, the relationship of permissiveness to freedom, the differences between freedom and license, the degree, if any, of manipulation that is necessary or acceptable in educational methods, parental controls or lack of them, the therapist's responsibilities, and others. These are not new questions, but in recent times opinions about them seem to be more polarized than at other periods.

Too often, there is a misconception that freedom should be identified with any outburst of feeling at a given moment. In fact, such moments and series of such moments are more like touchstones to freedom, rather than freedom itself. For, to be free, one needs to feel that his/her whole person is at the center of such expressive moments, rather than have them be fragmented moments that can tear his/her center apart.

For the dance therapist, the resources of dance itself offer stabilizing structures within which the moments of subjective expressiveness can occur autonomously and fully, with a simultaneous internal and external relationship. When the focus is entirely on the subjective, internal expressiveness, even its outward manifestation is disconnected from the environment. Sometimes a therapist becomes so preoccupied with making the patient aware of internal feelings that he/she fails to observe the most subtle visible movement indication of them and thus overlooks the opportunity to — through movement — extend or transform the feelings into another level of external relationship. Since the primary function of the therapist is to help a patient find an acceptable identity and satisfying mode of behavior for himself and in his society, it is important to maintain a context of flow between both internal and external as active as possible.

When the focus of the therapist is only on the subjective, isolated, body level without any relation to space or the possibility of structure of any kind, there is a great danger of getting the patient stuck in single aspects of his/her problem and increasing the fragmentation of his/her movement activity. An emphasis on internal awareness *divorced from spatial context* can be self-defeating and immobilizing and cut the patient off from experiencing interaction with others. This is especially dangerous in the therapeutic situation which is always, in some form, colored by an existing fragmentation of the patient.

The resources of dance offer both subjective and objective expressiveness and activity. By projecting feelings into space through the body, the movements themselves are immediately communicative. Images and metaphors can stimulate the imagination with minimal verbalization. The experience of building one's own organic structures in space can subtly build confidence in one's self. To do this with others helps to develop a sense of supportiveness from the community and an ability to make adaptations for the interdependence of that support.

The Role of Bartenieff Fundamentals as a Specific Resource

Resolutions of the "duality" problem of body and mind functioning have, of course, been explored from many points of view and will, undoubtedly, continue to be. Trapped in the polarities, emotional functioning gets torn between the two.

Dance therapists must particularly concern themselves with this problem because they deal with the resultant disharmony of that emotional trauma. The therapist deals with all levels of functioning — encompassing body, mind and feeling or emotion — and has the responsibility to modify the pulls toward opposite extremes in order to avoid increasing fragmentation. Therefore, the effort should be made, not to minimize any separate aspect, but to understand more about all aspects so that their interrelationship can best be understood.

This author — to the dismay of some of her colleagues — insists that her dance therapy students study in detail the functional level of body activity and sharpen their perceptions of the expressive content inherent in that activity. One is not the "symbol" for the other. The functional and expressive contents of movement are two sides of the same coin. They can be described by the Labananalysis vocabulary, and when the observation abilities of the therapist are highly developed, he or she can identify what is seen and empathize with and analyze directions which might be strengthened, modified or changed.

The dance therapist's vocabulary includes references to specific anatomical functional aspects of movement — center of weight, connectedness, muscle tension and relaxation. It offers a wide range of options for dealing with body awareness and feeling.

For example, when starting a movement session on the floor, the patient's awareness of self may be developed by helping him/her focus in three ways: On breath, on body weight, and on initiation of action. First, in stillness; then in action.

The patient can be aided to feel the rhythm of breathing as changing the "inner" space of the body, the body cavities. The cavities become "full," growing in shape, or "empty," shrinking in shape. With these alternations, the feeling of body weight is gradually perceived with its center localized in the pelvis. There is a feeling of increasing heaviness with the feeling of being empty, exhaling. There is the feeling of diminished weight with being full, inhaling.

As the patient becomes increasingly aware of his/her breath, weight and center, a readiness to shift the body weight from its center to initiate an action is experienced. This may lead to rolling over, getting on to hands and knees, and toward other changes, with an increasing connection to the concomitant feelings.

Exercises that involve two people can be very important at the appropriate moment. The "Seesaw" exercise,* for example, is an exercise in which the rhythm of muscle tension and relaxation is experienced in relation to breath and in relation to a partner. What is important is that the awareness is developed from the actual experience rather than from initially intellectualizing about the experience. The latter tends to fragment the experience and thus can add to the existing disturbance of the patient.

In the "Seesaw" exercise, the partners rise and sink in opposition to each other. Their muscle tensions and relaxations, therefore, create countertensions between them. Thus, they are, in a sense, affecting each other's breathing. Each is aware of his own heaviness with breathing out and sinking,

* *See Appendix B.*

145

and of lightness with breathing in and rising. This increasingly builds an automatic rhythm, which gradually eliminates a conscious attention to breathing and muscular activity.

Such exercises enable the subject to experience the rhythmic relationship of breathing to muscle activity and feeling in an organic happening that occurs without immediate conscious instruction such as "This is the way to breathe." It can be experienced as a continuum — without fragmentation. In therapy, this is particularly productive. After the experience, discussion of the details is possible.

The origins of Bartenieff Fundamentals and their relation to Labananalysis concepts are discussed in Chapter 1 and the Appendix. The six basic exercises and their elaborations are not a set of prescriptions. They are a means of becoming aware of some primary experiences of the self and being led from that to a clearer feeling of oneself in relation to others. Deviations from maximal body movement function appear in varying degrees among the "healthy" and the "sick." If the therapist is aware of significant points inherent in the material, she/he can make them as tangible as possible for the patient. Therefore, the therapist might try to experience and recognize, for instance,

1. The integration of the upper and lower body into one unit, with distinctively diverse roles: The upper unit's manipulative communicative role; the lower unit's emphasis on weight, sensing body weight and, through it, connection to the ground (groundedness) as an anchor for the upper unit; the role of weight transference in locomotion.
2. The central importance of initiation and intent in movement.
3. The development, from a state of non-struggle with verticality, lying on the floor, to full uprightness. That movement experience will first concentrate on the body aspect with Weight and Flow Effort elements and then develop with full responses to Effort impulses and to the demands from the environment. This can provide the possibility to re-experience early phases of the patient's life.

One does not achieve "groundedness" and "integration" just by practicing the exercises and their elaborations. They develop along with an awareness of the body in motion and in apparent stillness, its shape and relation to space, and the Effort dynamics that enliven its expression.

Thus, for the therapist the Fundamentals are tools for re-experiencing, renewing, refreshing and expanding both the therapist's and the patient's resources.

The Incorporation of Other Techniques and Disciplines
As techniques are added to the repertoire of the dance therapist, it is vital that the implications of the techniques be absorbed along with their mechanical facility.

The pioneers in dance therapy often worked intuitively and developed personal approaches to body awareness. Some of their approaches became more structured by their followers, but, unfortunately, the structure sometimes became fixed and out of contact with the initial intuitive insights about the actual body function.

Marian Chace, the leading pioneer, who had developed and established dance therapy in St. Elizabeth's Hospital in Washington, D.C., was an extraordinarily intuitive therapist. One was immediately struck by the power of her personality. In her work with patients, she had an uncanny ability to relate to emotional frustration and she had power, as an overwhelming matriarchal personality, to support her patients. She was an artist of great sensibility and empathy with buried anger and frustration.

Although she worked intuitively, as an artist, her intelligence enabled her to quickly grasp the professional concepts and language of the psychiatrists with whom she worked. She knew, as a modern dancer, about Laban's work, but she never incorporated his vocabulary into her intuitive analyses of expressiveness. Although she had a profound influence on her students and co-workers, it was not so much by teaching techniques as by the example she set and the force of her own personality, which made students face elemental facts about themselves. Each student had to translate Chace's approach and demonstration of certain principles into his/her own personal style.

Other therapeutic styles and approaches were also explored and introduced by a number of dance therapists. The emphasis is always on reconciling body, mind, feeling splits. Neurological research increasingly supports such reconciliation.

The approaches of other cultures — particularly the oriental — are also gaining widespread popularity. Uninterrupted traditions in these cultures have produced body–mind approaches to serve various purposes: Preparation for defense-attack, healing, meditation for the liberation of the mind, specific training in various bodily skills, and others. In each approach the body sensations, the feeling and mental processes are interwoven to serve their specific purposes and the general well-being of the subject. They are often associated with dance and, in some instances, with the mystic core of a religion.

Methods such as the Alexander technique, a means of guiding the individual to lightness and expansion through subtle touch, and the more vigorous manipulative Ida Rolf technique, and others, are increasingly incorporated into body–mind therapies through deeper understanding and efficiency of the body movement experience.

Any source that offers materials useful to therapy has to be seen, understood and experienced within its own and the larger context. It is dangerous to casually include some other technique because it does something special for a specific condition or individual. Therapy cannot be given to all, like a pill, for instant results. It is possible, however, to integrate into the therapy new or foreign approaches to movement. But it must be done with intelligence and authenticity if they are to be truly integrated and not just tacked on like fragmentary appendages.

A Positive Example

A positive example of cultural integration is illustrated by Al Chung-liang Huang in his book about the essence of T'ai Chi. He uses the personal experience of his oriental roots and his full exposure to western society to work through the content of the traditional form of T'ai Chi to the universality of its core qualities. He transmits these core qualities to the student in such a way that the student can integrate them with his/her own self within the T'ai Chi form.

This working through the two orientations sets his approach apart from the fragmented popularization of other exotic accommodations to western tastes. Obviously, to just read his movement book is inadequate; one must work directly with the material (ideally in one of his workshops) to experience the exchange of traditions and their integration.

A Negative Example

An example of the danger of superficial appropriation of new materials can be observed in the frequently fragmented, indiscriminate use of yoga. This is quite widespread and can be traced to casual teaching and studying that is irresponsible and promotes misunderstanding and misuse of a valid discipline. The misuse frequently results in diminished movement responses instead of full harmonious balance of action and non-action.

In Labananalysis terms, the possible results of such misinterpretation can be described as follows:

1. The movement Flow becomes either Bound or Neutral, rather than maintaining natural fluctuations between Free and Bound Flow.
2. Instead of clear Effort elements of the Indulging type, such as Light (Weight), Sustained (Time) and Indirect (Space), the Effort elements are unclear, neutralized.

147

3. Instead of using the whole kinesphere, space may become restricted.

4. Instead of a clear spatial intent, there is a preoccupation with pushing the body into the shape apparently desired by the teacher.

5. A generalized tendency toward passivity is observed, particularly in the initiation of action and of Flow. This differs sharply from the goal of a guru, who uses his physical and spiritual energy to produce clear initiations and fulfilled body shapes.

6. When the positions are executed sloppily, the tensions and countertensions inherent in them are distorted. Thus, instead of balanced tensions that produce relaxation, the performer will experience abrasive exertions or muddy non-tension. Since the tensions and countertensions of each position have specific body/mind effects, sloppy performance will also limit those effects. Thus, the therapeutic goals are defeated.

The Role of Labananalysis as a Key Resource

As with all dance therapy techniques, it is essential that the application of Labananalysis be understood in its entirety to be utilized responsibly. It is not just a theory or a notation system with stultifying prescriptions and parameters. Its comprehension enables the therapist to meet unexpected challenges to think, feel and act in terms of movement process in multiple ways that are discriminating, precise, and responsive to changes from fighting to yielding, from simple rhythms to complex spatial and dynamic structures. It can also be used to describe other movement approaches, not for value judgments, but in terms of specific insight to certain movement factors.

Some students of movement behavior, while acknowledging the basic unity of body/mind factors, then proceed to tear it apart in the course of their investigations, assuming that the fragments added to each other will make the whole. That is an oversimplification. The factors must be considered together as constellations, not as fragments. Laban's holistic view that movement is a process that is always part of behavior involving body and Effort and space preserves the constellations even as it describes variations within them. In therapy, sudden critical changes, as well as gradual changes, can be understood at their various levels as part of the reintegration process of the patient, even while there may be no verbal acknowledgement by the patient.

As the therapist perceives the body/Effort/space constellations of the patient's movement behavior, particular areas of imbalance may be identified. For example, a patient's Effort profile may reveal an absence of Directness in the space Effort. At that point, the therapist should *not* isolate the absence as a localized deficiency and focus on it with, for example, Directness exercises per se. If the absence of a single Effort is a deficiency, it must be dealt with in its multi-level context rather than in point by point prescriptions.

Therefore, the Directness deficiency in this case should be treated in the context of the patient's whole organization of Effort combinations and the accompanying spatial shape actions. The therapist may first start to explore all combinations of the patient's repertoire, such as Flow with Weight (Strength or Lightness), Flow with Time (Sudden or Sustained) and soon, from there, the therapist may gain access to the use of Directness in combination. It is important at this point to recall that the Inner States (two-element Effort combinations) are identified in pairs of opposites. Therefore, if, for example, the therapist is working with Flow/Time, he/she may be able to reach — as a sort of recuperative action — the combination of Space/Weight.

The "Directness" that the therapist wishes to revive in the patient's repertoire may be elicited as a recuperative state from activating the Flow/Time that was already in the patient's repertoire. In each case, the Effort combinations are vehicles for feelings. Instead of restless flitting about (Free Flow/Sudden Time), the patient becomes steadied, anchored (Strong Weight/Direct Space). Again, this depends greatly on the skillful introduction of such combinations.

There are other routes that can be followed to retrain the missing perceptions of certain Effort elements. To continue with this case, the fact that spatial perceptions are associated with attention and precision can be utilized by playing games that stimulate attention and exactness. Again, the therapist must be on constant guard that he/she not limit him/herself to a single approach and especially to avoid over-repetition of any one combination.

There is particular danger in repetition of a prescription, such as singling out one type of action with the same verbal accompaniment to serve as a module for changing a specific aspect of behavior by reproducing the sequence over and over, day after day. The action may, sooner or later, become a conditioned response (as in behavioral modification), but the loss may thereby be greater than the gain. For when the response is merely a "conditioned" response, the *intent* of movement dynamics is no longer a fresh movement impulse arising from the given momentary body/mind state. Instead, it becomes mechanistic and isolated from the live and constantly fluctuating process of the whole organism. It may become frozen out of the multi-level process.

Sometimes, traumatic, shocking experiences are stored as fixed, isolated gestures or symbolic representations of an experience. Dance therapy can sometimes release these fixations and, sometimes in conjunction with verbal therapy, expose and help to dissipate their cause. The verbal associations, usually after the experience, may be minimal or they may become major aspects of the total recovery.

The therapist serves as a movement catalyst, creating an environment in which the patient can relate — in movement — to others, from whatever level is possible for him/her, and then grow toward an expanded level, and eventually, work through immobilization and out of it.

Skilled movement observation resulting from experience and the application of specific resources, such as Labananalysis, can also crystallize seemingly "intuitive" recognition of meaning in movement behavior. There was the case of a woman with an almost constant sudden convulsive turning of the head and back, for which no organic or neurological basis could be found. The movement could be described as Free Flow/Indirect upbeat going to Strength/Suddenness/Bound Flow, an abrupt ending. On later analysis, it occurred to the author that the combination of Weight, Time and Flow central to the movement was recognizable as an internalized Drive, the Passion Drive.

At the time, the movement was noted by the staff as an aberration; specific movement analysis of the meaning was not pursued. The doctor directed all his attention to his verbal, emotional relationship with the patient. Watching from the observation room, it was immediately apparent to the author (an "intuitive" recognition) that the gesture expressed sudden terror — turning away from something frightening. The psychiatrist then directed his attention to the movement, which led to the patient's recall and revelation of her father's violent attacks on her mother. As the patient was encouraged to make the verbal and physical association, the "tic" gradually disappeared.

Fixed isolated gestures or sequences that appear in exaggerated and often apparently inexplicable form in the movement behavior of the mentally ill can also be related to symbolic representations that accompany various rituals in "normal" lives. Rituals are attempts to structure, through visible action, both terrifying and life-affirming experiences so they can be recalled and restated, sometimes alone, sometimes with a group.

Because they are so apparent — often in bizarre ways in mental illness — rituals may be used both individually and in groups in dance therapy as pathways to reconnections with recovery. They play regulatory roles in attempts to bring order into the chaos of many lives.

They appear spontaneously in the games that children play when they enact the terrifying aspects of life and death. They appear in more structured forms in weddings, burials, and other "rites of passage" and festivals.

Ritual actions (symbolic representation) are the source of many folk dance themes, such as weapon dances and work dances and they appear spontaneously in dance improvisations and/or are choreographed into professional dance.

In all these cases, the source of the symbolic action or sequences is used to re-affirm and strengthen certain shared feelings and cooperative actions in the community. Access to the power of the ritualistic happenings has to be maintained so that the therapist may not miss some of the deepest, most complex, feeling aspects of the human organism. Since these ritualistic happenings often become aspects of dance, they can therefore, through dance therapy, be regenerated, re-experienced, to lead back to their sources. In group dance, the feelings and imaginative associations are shared in the expressiveness of the group — whether the participants are disturbed or "normal" — when a community of people move together for a special situation or occasion. Only highly developed observation skills enable the therapist to appraise and empathize with connotations of the events and work with them in specific situations.

To modify repetitions and ritualistic activity, props can be used; they are excellent resources for expanding the movement repertoire of some patients. Different kinds of props require varied combinations of movement factors, evoking varied expressiveness.

In the context of Labananalysis, the differences associated with different props can be explored within specific treatment plans at appropriate stages of individual or group sessions. They should not be considered as external or decorative movement elements, dissociated from the patient's problems, even though the patient may have the experience of just playing. As classic devices of dance — from ritualism to festive community displays — props have been used for their evocative, symbolizing power or simply to underline the enjoyment of moving. Particularly in the work with children, the mentally retarded and the aged, playing with these devices can become a learning experience.

When the therapist is not involved in the activity, he/she should take every opportunity to observe patients' movements wherever possible out of the context of therapist/patient interaction. From the movement alone, with no sound, the Labananalysis vocabulary can be used to transmit perceptions that might otherwise be lost or that reinforce other diagnostic possibilities.

Another key aspect of the Labananalysis orientation is that it can sensitize the therapist to the quality of his/her physical touch of the patient. The quality of the therapist's touch can be critical to the patient–therapist relationship. Touch can vary in shape and Effort elements from a fleeting Light/Sudden poke to a constricting encircling two-dimensional grip to a supportive reassuring Sustained/slightly Bound/Indirect enveloping hold. Touch should be a form of three-dimensional shaping which is supportive rather than a form of more linear impositions such as poking, unless for a specific purpose. Some children (and adults) may never have been held in a three-dimensional shaping way that is initiated from the body center and is also transmitted through even peripheral touch. No touching by the therapist should be made without this awareness.

Essentially, the Labananalysis vocabulary's value is two-fold: As a tool for identifying the patient's individual expression and interaction with others. And as a device that enables the therapist to observe the patient outside the confines of therapist–patient immediate relationship. It is a vital resource for the development of dance therapy as a discipline.

Some Conclusions

What is most important for patient and therapist is to keep both intellect and feeling accessible and functional without fragmentation. The dance therapy discipline should not be permitted to deteriorate into amorphously indulgent self-expressiveness. Nor should it become so structured by mechanical measurements that the parts become greater than the whole. The delicate balance between structure and permissiveness must be gently maintained because either extreme becomes destructive. So, also, is this true for the delicate balance between the degrees of subjectivity and objectivity a therapist can bring to the patient's problems. Continuous research in refinements of observation techniques must be examined, experienced and evaluated.

Dance therapy stresses changes in the learning experience. Sensory, kinaesthetic, and feeling experiences are developed through movement, instead of repetitive, mechanical rote-learning. And the movement processes themselves are expressive — statements of feeling and thinking.

The problems of healing and restoring mental, emotional health are not confined to pathological extremes. There are differences in degree of mental health, rather than kind. The current explorations in healing oriented toward "restorations" of wholeness — some ancient and some apparently new — are reflections of the wide-spread concern with problems of personal and community wholeness and survival. They are intimately related because what is accepted as appropriate functioning by the individual is dependent on the society in which the individual lives.

Dance therapy is one of the avenues of exploration of these problems. It should be integrated with other art therapies and conventional psychology, psychiatry, anthropology and sociology as well. What it attempts to offer are many physical paths toward the restoration of the creative use of the self, individually and in the community of others.

151

Examples

Individual Patients: Movement Therapy

Catherine: Catherine, an elderly woman psychiatrist trained by Freud in Vienna in the early thirties, was a client of the author for several years. As a therapist she was a particularly empathetic listener to her patients, to the extent that she literally gave up her own action impulses. She loathed any physical task or activity, though she verbally acknowledged the need for psychotherapists to get physically involved to counteract the hours of sitting and listening. She was overweight and lacked tone and easily gave in to indulging in passive treatment.

The author worked with simple exercises first but introduced stimuli for spontaneous responses: playing with balls of different sizes and weights to arouse Effort and spatial responses to deal with attention and readiness to adjust to moving objects. This worked to some extent and she showed great interest in the theoretical aspects of the author's work — but it stayed always a struggle between passive indulging and awakening her sense of playfulness.

Ann: Ann was an elderly psychotherapist of Freudian orientation whose relationship with the author extended over twenty years. She first came to the author in her late fifties. She started on a long road, from not acknowledging her lack of vital basic body dynamics to a discovery of them in her work and life, at different degrees of complexity.

All through her very active adult life she had all kinds of complaints of pain, of weakness, hypersensitivities to hot, cold, touch. She had been constantly involved with various medical specialists for some minor and more serious disturbances.

The first impression of her was of a tall, erect woman with an exaggerated tense and twisted use of her head–neck over a flaccid body. There was a generally low muscle tonus, especially marked in her feet, which lacked tonus almost completely in the small muscles that give a foot shape, mobility and strength. She was aware of the new trends in body movement training and had already tried relaxation and breathing with a breathing specialist. The intense conflict with her body made her at times demanding and constantly watching her symptoms and looking for effective cures.

We started on a therapeutic body level, using the German connective tissue reflex massage in conjunction with simple specific shaping movements. In spurts and relapses changes gradually occurred; she began to discover connections between body and limb segments and articulations that brought some comfort over increasingly longer periods. She became very dependent on "treatment," as she called the sessions, though still pursuing other medical resources. She did the structured exercises faithfully, with a strictly cerebral attitude — they were mechanical actions to her. Change in attitude occurred very gradually. Her way of reacting to life and work was to regulate it by conscious effort, not allowing sensation, feeling to arise from her body experiences. There were interruptions of the movement sessions by surgery (among them a hip bone replacement). For a long time she did not respond to either Effort or space qualities or concepts, but her sensitivity to experience with her articulary functions increased. Subtly, gradually, new insights into her attitude toward her body developed. She became a sort of engineer of her body. A greater independence from "treatment" developed; it became a cooperation. She was able to pinpoint the problem, taking initiative, trying movement sequences and work under supervision of the therapist. In spite of her conflictive relationship to her body, her initiative overcame some of the former fighting attitudes and mellowed the demanding tendencies.

It is interesting to note that both these professionals — intensely involved with human beings — never accepted the use of the Effort/shape vocabulary. They were aware that they had been exposed to a multifaceted approach; they acknowledged the changes that occurred to them, and incorporated their new insights in their own language.

152

Rachel: Rachel, a secretary in her fifties, had for years been a high speed typist in well-paid jobs that, however, gave no sense of fulfillment or physical pleasure or challenge. She came to the author having never "exercised" in all her life because, to her, exercise was just mechanical means of keeping body weight down and improving posture. The idea of having pleasure through movement, being animated into liveliness, was completely closed to her. Everything in her life was mechanical: the running of the household she kept with an unloved husband, buying the pretty clothes she felt she needed mainly for appearance's sake in the offices she worked in. There were no other interests she shared with her husband and friends. In the first sessions she expressed some of the disgust with her life, her husband and, foremost, with her typing jobs.

She started with very simple floor work. Her reaction for weeks was constantly complaining that she could not understand what she was asked to experience. She demanded endless explanations and was unwilling to try some of the movements by herself; she might just do them "wrong." Exposed to many variations of "feeling" her body, her body weight, rolling around on the floor, changing her "size," lengthening and shortening, widening and narrowing, she slowly evolved sensations: Relaxation that made her burst into tears, "feeling so strange" or talking about her sad, empty life. Her demand for explanations gradually was replaced by feeling "energized" by moving. She discovered swinging the arms–shoulders in space and began to enjoy figure 8 and other spatial forms, introducing discernment of large and small reach space. She came very regularly and stayed an individual student, although we suggested joining a movement class. Intensity of her participation in her sessions increased. She made changes in her personal life, finding resources of enjoyment and new relationships to people.

It seems that in almost all cases the primary experience, by whatever approach, has to be establishing the center of the body in relation to the floor, in relation to space, and in stimulation of reach space, out of which Effort usually develops spontaneously as a feeling for acting "alive."

Gloria: Gloria, a young ballet dancer, had her own dance school together with a woman partner, an elderly M.D. and psychiatrist in private practice.

Gloria had a medical history of back problems of several years standing. It was finally diagnosed as a slipped disc, but without fusion of the spinal segment. When she still complained about pain and inability to fully do her passive and active trunk–leg stretches, a second operation was suggested. Instead, she decided to try gentle manipulation and specific exercises.

She came to the author's office, a thin, blonde, blue-eyed ballet dancer, in appearance and movement almost adolescent. Strictly ballet trained, her movements were extremely linear, lacking almost entirely in Effort qualities, particularly in Flow fluctuations. She was more of a weightless elf than a young woman in her mid-twenties. Her main concern was with her pain and the ranges of flexion/extension of her legs, arms and trunk. This exclusive concern with her articular functioning lasted over two years, during which she followed the author's prescriptions while continuing to teach ballet techniques. She even made her partner attend some of her treatment sessions to become her efficient supervisor.

The pain had diminished during the first few months, after which progress seemed to slow up. Several times during the second year it was suggested she join some of the Effort workshops at the studio. There it became most apparent that she shied away from any dynamic contrast or intense response to an Effort challenge. She would either shorten her participation in a session or not finish the course because she felt "uncomfortable." Her main quality stayed Light, with no fluctuation in Flow or other Effort components or combinations emerging. At one point she seemed ready to sign up for the whole training program but she stayed away at the last moment. She continued sessions with the author but there was no change toward establishing a central support of weight, nor any attempt in spatial and/or Effort vocabulary. Particularly spatial tasks or experimenting only confused her.

153

Then the author sent her away, telling her that she no longer needed therapeutic sessions for pain, that only her own initiative toward becoming a creative dancer–performer could get her off the plateau of working for technical progress only. At almost the same time, several crises occurred in her personal life, as she was struggling with the challenge the author had presented to her. She initiated several external changes: leaving her partner, making plans to go to another city, changing her apartment. Then very suddenly her mother died. What had been a conflicting relationship became a profound shock. The author saw her a few times during that period of uncertainty and loss, without physically working with her. Over several months the uncertainty of plans persisted and the tension between herself and her partner mounted.

About six months later she went back to her partner and her school. She had joined a group of circus acrobats studying various skills, particularly acrobatics. She had found her centeredness in these activities and had acquired a very appealing, still-childlike liveliness, full of Effort combinations. She succeeded in doing extremes in acrobatics, radical back bends. This latter fact is significant. She dared to take risks, endangering her scarred back, and discovered in the process a whole range of Effort and Shape dynamics. She was by now around thirty years old, and she felt she had a new existence. Labananalysis had been a catalyst in that process.

* * * * *

Phrasing

A young woman joining a group therapy session appeared more lively and dynamic than most newcomers to a group. With the sound system turned off, we therapists, observing through a one-way screen, were recording clear Effort elements and clear Flow changes and directional movement in the group. But I observed a peculiar organization of this patient's movement phrases: Every phrase ended with an abrupt cutting off with Bound (Flow)/Direct (Space), Sudden (Time)/Bound (Flow), or Direct/Sudden becoming Bound. The overall impression of this repetitive rhythm ending made me exclaim, "She is destructive; she is suicidal." Suddenly, the sound system was turned on and her harsh voice was heard, telling the group that she wanted to poison herself. Her particular organization of sequences as sharp linear path changes accompanying abrupt Effort changes produced a "moment of truth" in movement behavior. The experience also pointed out the importance of phrasing observations to convey critical messages about underlying, prevailing moods.

* * * * *

Working with props

In working with bedridden children (age 7–11) at Blythdale Hospital for orthopedically handi-capped children, we used ribbon dances with the girls. We involved the children in the whole process from making paper ribbon sticks to using them as props in snake, dragon and wave dances or exploring the many spatial possibilities of the figure of 8, circles, and other forms, traveling in the kinesphere. Often, this was accompanied by music. A couple of sticks (about 10 inches long) were used to create rhythm sounds as well as spatial patterns which, when used by a group sitting in wheelchairs, could involve the whole group in different relationships, such as two rows facing each other or a circle relating to a center person. This activity would also be connected to the work of the art therapist, painting and decorating the sticks, so each child recognized and selected her own stick when they were distributed for the session, which helped to establish her personal identity in the anonymity of the hospital environment.

One six-year-old girl, who was bedridden because of hip disease, had almost completely retreated from contact with other children and did not react to either story telling, music or anything we tried individually with her. We then moved her bed into the art room where she was offered paper and crayons just to scribble. The movement therapist started her on her own piece of paper and gradually a "dance" with crayon lines developed which was the beginning of access to movement and to imaginative activity and feelings that accompanied movement. Playfulness had to be restimulated; it was one of the ingredients of the rehabilitation process, during which the therapist could identify, in movement terms, the emotional problems.

In work with the mentally retarded, props became an even more specific tool for the stimulation of sensorimotor, sense and functional experiences. In defective functioning, there are additional problems in integrating often deficient sensorimotor abilities with primary internal body relationships and the surrounding space. Work with props served to develop the rudiments of grasping, holding and handling objects and, through them, relating to other people. There are two kinds of props that particularly lend themselves to this goal. One is balls of different sizes and weights, the other is the hoop (a plastic ring of about 30 inches in diameter). These props offer innumerable possibilities for sensory, Effort, spatial and rhythmic experiences, in addition to developing focus and arousing attention toward the outside world. Both are, of course, universal playthings, but they can also provide very specific learning experiences about weight, size, thrusting and rolling, distance and selection of goal and other combinations of Effort elements. Passing the ball in various ways from one person to another or playing with it individually also develops rhythmic awareness.

The hoop offers another spectrum of differentiating experiences: Tactile, spatial and dynamic. The use of the hoop can systematically provide all the spatial relationships necessary for awareness of the environment: Pulling toward and away, turning, twisting, up–down, right–left, inside–outside, piercing through and going around, the many possibilities of using various body parts.

* * * * *

Art and Dance Therapy

We were asked by a psychiatrist, interested in both art and dance therapies, to observe a patient working on a picture with the art therapist. The patient was a young man, about twenty years old, who loved both dance and painting. The art therapist, Lynn Flexner Berger, had been struck by the fact that the patient was very sensitive to fine shades in color but that he frequently would cover the picture at the end with charcoal lines or circles.

In the movement observation, we saw him first using wavy and round shapes in delicate shades of light colors, covering the major part of the paper. This was done with Light touch/Indirectness and slight fluctuations between Sustained and Sudden. Then, as he took a look at the nearly finished picture, he took a piece of charcoal and in vehement circling motions — Strength and Exaggerated Suddenness with some changes between Direct and Indirect, with the greater emphasis on the Direct — he covered the center of his painting. The contrast was striking and reflected his conflict, as described by his psychiatrist: He was afraid of his gentle, seemingly feminine side, which he kept trying to annihilate. What is significant here is that the movement observations would have clearly revealed the conflict even without seeing the art work produced by the movement.

It was interesting to us that in the dance therapy sessions, he moved with great ease, although at times with Bound Flow that had few fluctuations. Although his power had never erupted as it did in the painting, the Bound Flow in contrast to the facile quality of his movement was a clue to inner conflict. In this case, the patient was not with us long enough to follow up with additional research. Since some patients respond more easily to one art medium than another, it is invaluable, in the interest of the patient's most rapid recovery, to have evaluation communications between the different kinds of therapists so they can program from shared information and goals.

* * * * *

Post-Partum Psychosis: 20 Year Old Woman

The case of a young woman in a post-partum depression after her first baby. In group therapy sessions, we observed peculiar squirming movements in the lower trunk. Our observations are noted on the chart below:

Effort Characteristics

Flow: Rita had a very frequent trunk movement which started Free, then Bound to exaggerated Bound, a pause followed by a sudden release into Free Flow which was immediately arrested in Bound Flow.

Space–Weight–Time: In the first days of her hospitalization no Effort qualities appeared except for Suddenness in her head movement. After the first week Sustainment, Indirectness appeared with the Effort Flow pattern described.

Spatial Characteristics

Flow: Either Shape Flow in–out or gathering shapes as in cupping both hands close to her face while eating or sitting for long periods in a gathered shape.

Lateral–Vertical–Sagittal: The repetitive trunk gesture described was an upward gesture held momentarily, then dropping in Free Flow. This was not spatial movement rising and sinking but a body "stretching" upward. During the first weeks there was little spatial movement but primarily Shape Flow (in–out movement limited to single planes). Within a few days however, rising and sinking became distinct and some narrowing, advancing and retreating appeared.

Characteristic Patterns

The repetitive trunk gesture predominated in the very restricted movement repertoire of Rita during the first days of her hospitalization. It was a Bound "pulling up" of the torso, starting with contractions in the pelvic region, spreading to the torso with increasingly Bound Flow, then dropping with Free Flow and immediately caught with Bound Flow and gathering. Shaping at this time was primarily gathering as when she ate and would cup both hands to her face. There were indications of fragmentation in that her movement was limited to single planes. Her facial expression was rigid; she would look furtively and erratically around the group. Her movement in walking and dancing was largely gestural with back and pelvis held immobile.

After several observations it became apparent that the repetitive trunk gesture was somehow the key to her present state. On careful evaluation it occurred to the observer that it resembled distorted labor movements: muscular contractions in the pelvic region held and then released. However, this arresting of the movement in Bound Flow suggested she was not fully releasing. It appeared to be a re-enactment of giving birth in which she was still "holding on." She had in fact a difficult delivery some three weeks prior to hospitalization, and from her very limited movement repertoire it appears she had limited resources with which to cope with such a traumatic experience. Under certain overwhelming stresses, the traumatic experience may be fixed into a ritual movement or re-enactment of the original event. Rita's movement mainly appeared to be different forms of "holding on" — there was little outward-directed movement.

It is possible that the birth, which was an especially difficult experience for her, was considered a loss of a part of herself. Another factor was the absence of her husband, a sailor, when the child was born, which perhaps added to her feeling of wanting to delay the birth, to "hold on," to "freeze" her behavior.

During the two months of observation, she participated in dance therapy sessions, as well as group sessions. The physical contact in the dance circle, the particular concern that some of the older women showed — dancing with her, following her suggestions as to the music to be used — seemed to calm her and give her a feeling of being mothered. A climate was created in which she began to enjoy the physical activity and respond to a variety of movement relating to the other patients. She also began to verbally express her frustration. Gradually, the bizarre contortions disappeared and she got interested in the baby, whose existence she had almost completely negated before her hospitalization.

*   *   *   *   *

Movement Analysis of Hospitalized Patients*

The patients observed were three depressives, two males and one female, and one schizophrenic male. A summary of the movement observations identifies three different types of depression and suggests their prognosis, and a chart compares core qualities of the two male depressives with those of the male schizophrenic.

Case I, Male No. 1: It was the segmented use of the body limbs, the lack of participation of the trunk, the near neutrality with complete absence of Space Effort, the absence of postural Effort, the near absence of Shaping and extremely short phrases with long pauses, low rate of eye contact, monotone of voice that added up to an impression of a patient in a state of passivity, cut off from life, from initiation and motivation.

Case II, Male No. 2: Though he was also extremely passive, notably in body attitude, limbs and trunk, he differed from the first patient because of some rudimentary phrasing in his head and hand gestures. In the ongoing activity of his hands were some clearly defined Effort elements: Lightness, Indirectness and some reduced Time. In functional activity such as lighting a cigaret, he showed clear Direct/Indirect variations. There was some eye contact, though very little change in facial expression. Talking about his family, his gestures became Indirect/Bound with some reduced Suddenness (Weightless/Internalized Drive). He seemed passive in feeling and initiation of action, suggesting a state of general exhaustion rather than being cut off from life.

Observation of the second interview a few weeks later showed quite dramatic return of Effort and Shape qualities, relating to the interviewer and variations in phrasing and voice quality.

Case III, Female: She was in complete contact with herself and her environment. There was considerable range and variation of all Effort elements, including postural Effort, clear sequencing without pauses or fragmentation. Her low mood showed mainly in a slight rigidity and tension in her upper body (chest–shoulder) and occasionally some limpness in hand gestures. This increased when she spoke about the problem of her son. It was this very real grief that seemed to have somewhat dampened her natural vitality and her ability to respond to the environment and initiate action.

---

*   *These observations were made from video tapes of interviews at a hospital. The interviewer was not visible.*

Comparison between Two Depressed Male Patients and One Schizophrenic Patient in a Severe Psychotic Episode

Note the marked differences in core qualities between the two male patients in depressive states and the male schizophrenic. Only qualities of marked difference are listed.

Depressed	Schizophrenic
1. Body Attitude:	
the body heavy, almost limp in one unit, near collapse	somewhat rigid, partially limp
2. Body Parts:	
Patient No. 1 uses limbs somewhat segmentally, limits the use of arm to forearm/hand and head	random use of body parts, perhaps starting with one segment of arm, and continuing with another body part quite distant. Hardly ever finished any movement
Patient No. 2 reduced use of limbs and head	
3. Simultaneous/Successive:	
mostly simultaneous	diffuse, not discernible
4. Space:	
extremely limited kinesphere, more shape flow than shaping, some directional, relating to in and out	extremely disorganized in shape and direction; starts vaguely peripheral, never clearly into direction or shape; in and out vague, no gather/scatter
5. Effort/Flow:	
greatly reduced in variation and in clear formulation of Effort, often nearly Neutral, interrupted by pauses, Intent reduced, transition jerky or neutral	almost complete absence of Effort and unvarying even Flow, fleetingly punctuated by extreme Bound or extreme Free with no transition
6. Phrasing:	
very short, predominantly two phasic with frequent long pauses	extremely diffuse, no discernible initiation, or transition or ending in either Effort or Shape
7. Eye Contact and Face:	
avoiding or fleeting, mostly turned inward, looking down	turned face to interviewer stays immobile, completely smooth with the eyes wide open, slowly blinking and staring without seeing

*   *   *   *   *

Vision, Spatial Awareness, and Mobility

Shortsightedness, focus difficulties, unilateral eye deficiencies not only affect the range of moving in space, but also reduce general mobility and, particularly, the initiation of action. The relationship of vision to expressive movement becomes especially apparent to the Labananalysis observer.

For example, X, extremely shortsighted, who had worn very strong glasses since childhood, came

158

to one of our body movement classes. Through most of her childhood and adult life, she had stayed away from almost any form of physical activity. Now, married, she had two very lively young children and was having difficulties in handling them.

She did not appear tense or stiff; she was just reluctant to move. The simplest spatial task in exercising frightened, almost terrorized her. We worked with her individually, in addition to the group work where she enjoyed the contact with other participants.

In one of the early individual sessions, we asked her to reach with one arm across her body and toward the back. She stopped as she reached the left hip with her right hand; in fact, she was "stuck." It was as if she was hitting an impenetrable wall at the opposite side of her body and there was no mobilizing flow of movement to carry her beyond the limited area to turn her toward a new focus. We immediately saw that this was not a matter of insufficient range in her shoulder due to muscle weakness or stiffness.

She had the physical ability to do it. However, because of her limited vision, she had cut off the possibilities of the maximal use of what was possible even with her limited vision. She had eliminated the possibilities of side and back of her reach space and thereby limited her spatial intents.

We began to develop all kinds of movement combinations — without forcing those movements that she wasn't capable of — and tried to involve her in the classes in groups with more than one partner so she had to relate to right and left. These new situations so terrified her that her ability to change had to be developed very gradually.

We also had her explore space harmony scales in order to enrich her spatial differentiation and focus her spatial intents.

We worked on the grounding of her body through the Bartenieff Fundamentals. This gave her an awareness of her center of weight so that she could connect it to her spatial intents and be grounded as she pursued them.

The fundamentals and space harmony work also gave her more initiative in working with the group because they strengthened her ability to extend and vary her visual focus.

Her visual limitations contributed to her generally soft and passive quality. She began to be aware of that passivity as she participated in group improvisations. She recognized that she would choose the role of the one being supported or enveloped most of the time; she also realized how difficult it was for her to take initiative or lead.

Over a period of two years work, she began gradually to change. Her new awareness of her weight center gave her more courage to release the mobility of her flow to fulfill her increasing spatial awareness and the potentialities of her kinesphere. The ranges of her Effort elements expanded with greater intensities and variety included. She formed new relationships with people, began to vary her spatial focus and her spatial and Effort responses.

After she left the classes, we did not see her for two years. When she returned, her body attitude on entering the room indicated a responsive ease and she initiated movements toward the group that confirmed it. In her daily life, she was participating in a number of physical activities including, to her great satisfaction, playing physical games with her children. She had also, incidentally – perhaps symbolically – replaced her heavy glasses with contact lenses. (Glasses tend to restrict the use of lateral space more than contact lenses.)

In our training programs, we frequently encountered dramatic relationships between vision and the whole use of space and Effort. It seems to evidence itself most specifically in relationship to the use of the horizontal plane, right/left and forward/backward as illustrated above. In general, the horizontal plane is the least well-developed, especially in western body movement, but it becomes particularly neglected when there is concomitant visual limitation.

*　　*　　*　　*　　*

The Use of Core Qualities in a Child Development Study

As part of continuous research for innate constitutional factors that can be traced throughout childhood and adulthood, an early study by the psychiatrist Margaret Fries produced a series of films of three children that included short episodes from the first five days of life to the age of twelve years. Each child was seen in the same situations at the same ages.

In her original study Fries had defined three types of children by a gross, quantitative estimate of how much activity occurred in a startle reaction *during the first five days of life*. She differentiated them as "active," "moderately active," and "quiet."

During a colloquium of psychiatrists on child development, this author was asked to observe films of the three children and to comment with more specificity, if possible, on the classifications. The shortness of the episodes and the film's flattening effect on three-dimensionality limited the selection of movement parameters to be traced through observations. In addition the films selected for the meeting were not edited specifically for this purpose so there was a concentration on the moderately active child with only selected clips on the other two.

However, six "core" parameters emerged that seemed most suitable to the situation. By observing their constancy throughout the film material available, it was possible to identify greater or lesser adaptability of coping with the environment as reflections of constitutional factors.

The first three are observable in the first few weeks of life; the last three become evident as sitting posture and locomotion develop. All six are operative throughout childhood and discernible in the adult.

The six factors were selected from Labananalysis:

1. Differentiated vs. less differentiated use of the limbs and their segments, head/trunk, and constellations of trunk and limb.
2. Dominance of asymmetrical over symmetrical use of limbs. Asymmetric use stimulates greater mobility and develops greater selectivity and range in pattern.
3. Use of areas of reach space (personal kinesphere) around the body before full uprightness vs. limited use of reach space.
4. Flexible or fixed use of verticality.
5. Development of verticality and full use of kinesphere into a territorial space (locomotor space) vs. limited use. This becomes visible in the sitting stage.
6. Organization of activity patterns into phrases — ordering, combining, alternating, elaborating — vs. short monotone flexion/extension actions.

The active child, a boy, was shown only in the startle reflex. In that, he showed twenty-three to twenty-six different gross movements of limbs, body, head with a variety of selections of different symmetrical and asymmetrical body-limb constellations, variations in head movements and bounces of the whole body from right to left, gradually coming to rest.

Mary, the moderately active child, showed a multi-use of all limbs, fifteen to eighteen changes with a variety of body parts used and emphasis on horizontal use of limbs in upper and lower limbs, shifting the body from right to left and varying symmetrical and asymmetrical use of limbs.

Anna showed only nine changes, stressing mainly flexion/extension ranges, the length axis of the body, and fixed constellations of limbs. She ended in the same rigid constellation of limbs, actually a postural reflex: upper limbs flexed, lower limbs extended. There was a definite emphasis on symmetrical use of limbs.

There were two more startle observations for the period of the first three months that confirmed the first gross evaluation. Anna always ended in a symmetrical position, usually upper flexed, lower extended, while Mary ended in asymmetry, not always using the same constellation.

Beyond the initial startle film, the comparisons could only be made between the two girls because of insufficient film of the boy's development in the colloquium presentation.

At nine months, the difference between the two children became more marked. Mary, sitting on the couch handling toys, was "all over the place" as she attempted to let herself down on the floor in a sequence, rolling over horizontally, turning into widening, and ending on the floor in a wide stance.

Anna sat on the floor slightly bent forward with both legs completely straight. She handled toys when they were offered to her in a tentative way, close to her body; there seemed to be no relation to the kinesphere.

At two years, Mary blossomed as she mastered walking, climbing, chasing pigeons, meeting children in the playground. Wherever she was, she occupied space for her vigorous actions. Mary's predilection for asymmetrical differentiated use of body limbs and space as well as territory had her organizing longer action sequences in her 18th-19th months episode. She experimented with various ways of climbing a fence using sagittal as well as horizontal approaches and asymmetrical right/left balance. In climbing stairs, she varied with alternate stepping, one foot stepping and reversing to creeping. She ran, climbed through a fence, ran to chase pigeons and stopped before a group of children — all in one prolonged series of activities.

Anna was seen playing in the playground. Her mother took away her toy. She became frozen, standing with her legs close together and straight, the arms in extreme elbow flexion, held close to her body.

At four, Anna and Mary were shown sitting in a clinic side by side being undressed by their mothers. Mary sat very upright, using her elbows in vigorously spreading herself and resisting the pulling off of her clothing. Anna sank slightly and retreated with pulled in elbows to protect herself from her mother seizing her clothing. The attitude was reminiscent of her early startle response: flexed upper limbs, high tension extension of the lower.

The filmed material included various other episodes of clinical visits and test situations. Mary showed some dampening of her initiative and immediacy of response to the environment which were related by Fries to particular difficulties with the child's mother, and probably temporary. Anna developed in a steady way with a limited kinesphere, lack of a varied Effort/Shape range within which there was a clear emphasis on precision with Light touch in handling small objects and in movements.

This study, for all its limitations of materials and hardware, revealed valid perceptions in terms of Effort/Shape elements and combinations, consistent with the psychoanalytic follow-ups of the cases. Mary showed a tendency toward adaptability, the left end of the scale established by the six parameters, while Anna showed a stronger tendency toward rigid non-adaptability at the other end of the scale.

What is important for the movement specialist is 1) the significance of core qualities which reflect interrelationships of movement behavior elements and 2) the significance of pattern roots that appear in the early startle behavior and are crystallized into later behavior patterns.

*   *   *   *   *

Dance Therapy (Labananalysis) for Mentally Retarded

An example of another possibility for therapy through movement is the work done with the mentally retarded. In Bronx State Hospital, the author participated as a consultant for research in a project headed by Y. Taketomo in a unit for severely retarded adults.

It was started with severely defective people of a wide age range from adolescents to old age. There was also a wide range of deficiency: brain damage, mongolism, senility, retarded or arrested development.

Susan Brainard, a performing modern dancer trained in Labananalysis, was the therapist in charge. She was then one of the few people so trained who committed herself to work with the retarded and had a special talent for it.

She worked first with individual therapy, which preceded group therapy. Each participating patient was started on gym mats on the floor in a small treatment room. The therapist worked with the patient through the functional levels of lying, sitting, rolling over, creeping to standing, and then responding to a partner — the therapist or another patient. Physical contact and props were used to induce action.

Work with these patients helped to confirm the effectiveness of Bartenieff Fundamentals as a baseline for getting around, functioning, communicating on even the simplest level. However, they were not presented as exercises. They were presented, in this case by a dancer, in any way that they might serve as stimuli for rhythmic reactions to the environment. The therapist also was fortunate in obtaining volunteer help from some of her Labananalysis students, so she didn't always have to work alone. The work moved very slowly and required extreme patience. A special section in heavy gymnastics requiring more dynamics and maximal use of the whole body was introduced for the male adults, who were, in general, more physically intact. The special sessions were led without music, but by verbal command and were very much enjoyed by the participants.

Within the work of two winter/spring terms, a picture of changes emerged — obviously, an uneven one. But there were changes in general motility, in improved speech patterns, in locomotion, and in social ability. The outstanding feature was that a more human communicative atmosphere had been established. Physical therapy and very sensitive occupational therapy were also used as preparation for manual skills. In some instances this concerted effort resulted in "graduating" some of the patients to general wards or sheltered workshops.

An Example of a Group Therapy Session for Mentally Retarded Adults

The therapist would start by moving herself. She would give verbal encouragement, enlivening commands, such as "Stretch as far as you can," or "Move your toes", "Let me see it," to activate the patients who were passively sitting in a circle (6 to 12 participants). Slowly, they worked through the whole body, bending and stretching, etc. Then, everyone joined in a circle, standing, sometimes free, sometimes holding hands.

Very gradually, a theme, such as stamping or rocking or clapping, would be introduced and pursued until the majority could follow it. Almost always, toward the end of the session, a common rhythm, a steady pattern, a firm grip on each other were established out of chaotic, fragmented, individual gestures.

Of course, there were patients on the ward who were unreachable by any therapy practiced then, but it was perhaps only the limitations of time and trained personnel that closed off their possibilities. The Labananalysis approach to dance therapy suggests additional means of identifying a level at which the patient can be reached to initiate development — however minute — to another level. It also suggests a variety of approaches to the next level.

* * * * *

Working with the Aged

In Bronx State Hospital, the author also had the opportunity to work for a few months with aged men and women who had neurological/psychological problems. Experiences there were limited, but they reflected the experiences of other dance therapy colleagues who have specialized in working with the aged. It is an area of increasing concern and attention and it is hoped that more research will focus on some of the following observations:

1. The effect and vital importance of physical and, particularly, physical/rhythmical activity in affecting depressive moods and the reduction in physical function that often accompanies depression. Aged people in general have a much greater physical and mental potential than is usually assumed by their doctors and associates and — what is even more important — by the aged person her/himself.

2. Physical rhythmical activity, particularly in dance or dance-like form, reinforced by music brings out the latent ability to socialize and to enjoy play activities and games, using balls and other props. This childlike ability to "play" should not be confused with senility. It is a genuinely childlike state available to older persons who are no longer pressed by the responsibilities of their early and middle lives. It is the quality that so often links grandparents with their grandchildren, sharing, playing together and communicating their enthusiasm and playfulness.

3. Other exercise is equally important in maintaining and improving function and greater physical self-confidence and to diminish fear of falling and injury. There are also functional exercises than can minimize actual physical disabilities by relating the exercises, in conjunction with walking, to stairclimbing and the use of walking sticks and crutches.

4. In dance therapy for the aged, the role of the therapist sometimes has a different emphasis than in groups of younger people. With the latter, the therapist often serves primarily as a catalyst, but with the former, a more active role in initiating new stimuli to movement and creating relationships among the group members and with the therapist may be more often necessary.

5. The resources of the Labananalysis vocabulary, particularly in the use of Space and Effort dynamics, could be directed toward special studies of the problems of old age. Through such studies there can be much greater refinement of the distinctions between, for example, reduced dynamics as opposed to defective or total loss of dynamics and the distinctions between physical and mental disabilities.

*   *   *   *   *

163

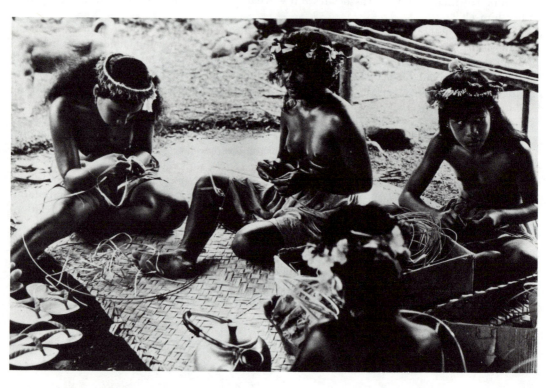

Three Girls Weaving © Kim Bailey.
An activity of the forearm and hand in a limited kinesphere. Girl on left shows full postural Effort while the other two have gestural Effort.
Girl on left: Flow/Direct/Light touch.
Girl in center: Flow fluctuations, slight Strength variations, no Space.
Girl on right: Flow and shaping guide task.

CHAPTER 10
Ethnic Studies

In certain epochs, in definite parts of the world, in particular occupations, in cherished aesthetic creeds or in utilitarian skills, some attitudes of the body are preferred and more frequently used than others . . .

The selection of and preference for certain bodily attitudes create style . . . but it is in the transitions between positions that an appropriate change of expression is made, thus creating a dynamically coherent movement style.

Communities seem to regard a certain uniformity of movement behavior as indispensable for safeguarding the stability of the community spirit. They also tend to stress a common ideal of beauty, very often connected with a utilitarian value, especially esteemed in the community of a particular epoch . . . This subconscious evaluation of people's movement is practiced by almost everybody.

The finer shades of style will be understood only after a thorough study of the rhythmic content of the attitudes in which a definite series of Effort combinations has been used.

Rudolf Laban

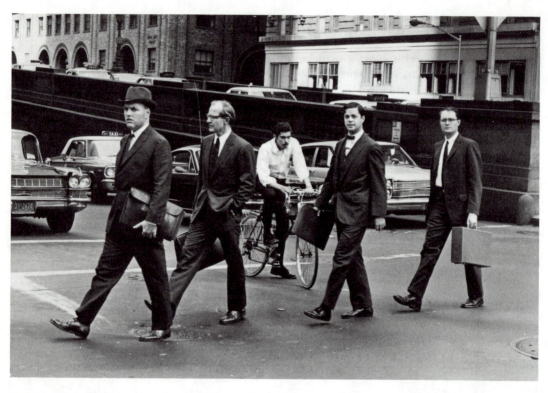

Four Businessmen on Park Avenue © Bonnie Freer.
All in general phase of weight transference, all show pronounced verticality. Second from left most distinctive (also most unaware of camera) because anticipatory twist in upper body accompanies his Free Flow, Sudden Time, and Direct Space, which is in contrast to the more Bound Flow and Neutral Effort of the others.

Ethnic Studies

In recent years, research in ethnology, anthropology and folklore has been expanded beyond the documentation of artifacts, language study, social customs, anatomical body typing, to include more psychological and sociological factors. Most recently, detailed body movement phenomena have been included. Pioneering research in these areas has been produced by anthropologists, sociologists, psychologists, and movement specialists such as Gregory Bateson, Ray Birdwhistell, David Efron, Edward Hall, Margaret Mead, Mantle Hood and others (see Bibliography).

However, the movement observation resources have not yet been fully tapped. Even as recently as 1973, a Dance Ethnology Inventory* with a vast file of sources and cultures, revealed a startling ignorance of the extent of actual movement observation resources. Twelve aspects of dance are identified, of which "movement" is one. Under movement, the references are to formation, enumeration of activities, such as step, throwing, stamping, clapping, solo performance or group performances. In short, very generalized, non-differentiating activities, with no analysis of structural, functional, expressive, rhythmic elements.

It wasn't until 1972 that a conference was organized (by CORD, the Committee on Research in Dance), for the first time, to bring dancers, behavioral scientists and anthropologists together to address themselves to more interdisciplinary research. CORD's intensive efforts in the last five years to stimulate support research is sorely needed and invaluable.

At their International Conference in Honolulu in conjunction with the American Dance Guild in the summer of 1978, there was a new depth of mutual understanding between western and oriental participants. The individual presentations sparked a readiness to absorb cross-cultural influences as stimuli to their own development. In this enormously accelerating process, Labananalysis may play an important role.

Studies of movement behavior in ethnic, cultural contexts can no longer be regarded simply as studies of "foreign" behavior, but rather as explorations of the wide range of possibilities of our own "human" behavior. What makes ethnicity "foreign" to many is not just departures from what is familiar, but a lack of awareness of the components even of the "familiar." That ignorance obscures the common threads between the familiar and the foreign.

Ethnic studies of movement behavior also raise questions about delineations of normal and abnormal behavior. For what is normal in one culture may not be so in another. And distinctions must be made between what is an acceptable movement within one culture (though aberrant in another) and what is not acceptable even within a culture.

Laban himself, as an artist, had always been searching beyond what was considered "typical" style or "typical" beauty. Interested in all the deviations and variations of movement, he made distinctions between what was typical for a community, a social class or an historical epoch in order to most accurately perceive styles and individual spontaneous characteristics. He also challenged aesthetic biases of the west by pointing out how relative value judgments may shift within a group, a culture or a period. He particularly underlined the importance of Effort combinations as distinguishing characteristics of styles.

Some very basic research in ethnic dance had been done by Gertrude Kurath, ethnomusicologist, and her co-workers in the nineteen forties, when they worked on categorization of dance and recognized the potential of Labanotation as a tool for study. Kurath worked together with Nadja Chilkovsky, dancer and choreographer who at that time headed a branch of the Dance Notation Bureau in Philadelphia.

---

* *An archive at Harvard University established by George C. Murdock, now professor emeritus at Pittsburgh University.*

Looking at movement itself as observable behavior in ethnic and cultural anthropology studies is still rare, in spite of pioneering studies by Kurath and Joann W. Kealiinohomoku, ethnologist and anthropologist. Kealiinohomoku is currently writing a new ethnography with dance as the organizing principle.

Since the forties, Kinetography Laban (the European term for the notation) has, through the impetus of Albrecht Knust, Laban's early colleague in notation, made major inroads into ethnology and folklore by extensive notation of folk dances. Knust worked in Hamburg, Munich and, finally, since the 50s, in the Folkwangschule in Essen-Werden, where the director, Kurt Jooss (a choreographer), established a notation center for him. By training a number of folklorists in Hungary, Poland and Yugoslavia, he contributed to the creation of comprehensive archives in those countries.

In those countries, government supported studies used Kinetography Laban over a period of more than twenty-five years, covering whole provinces and smaller regions and producing folklore movement archives that are invaluable to comparative studies of rhythm, variation, phrasing, sequences and music–dance interrelationship. The Hungarian folklorist and folk dancer, Martin Gyoergy, and his co-worker, I. Lanyi, set a record by having covered 280 villages. Although filmed records have been added to this documentation in the last ten years, they have not replaced notated "kinetograms" of dances and their variations in Hungary or in Poland.

A whole literature of notated dances for the folk dancer teacher and textbooks for teaching have since appeared in Hungary (Maria Szentpal) and in Poland (Roderyk Lange). The influence of kinetography in folklore extends also to the professional dance in Hungary. Notation is used in the education of professional ballet dancers at the opera, starting when they are children. Reading materials for these children include folk dancing in kinetography along with Bartok music for children derived from folk music. (Emma Lugosy, who teaches movement and notation to children at the Budapest Opera House, is a well-known Labanotator, trained by Albrecht Knust.)

In comparison to this monumental body of work collected in state archives, other notation efforts in the ethnic field are scarce and scattered among individually-initiated works in the United States and abroad. This is all the more regrettable as traditional materials are fast disappearing in Europe and all over the world.

Among these scattered attempts to use Labanotation for documentation of ethnic material are several books in which it is used as illustration. Carl Wolz, head of the dance division of the Department of Theatre and Drama at the University of Hawaii, has published a book on the Japanese Bugaku (the Japanese court dance of men). His illustrations include pictures, scholarly notes, and Labanotated examples of basic steps, arm movements, motifs as well as one whole dance in Labanotation. The selection of notated steps and larger motifs was made according to the codification of Japanese tradition. This introduces the reader to what is considered by the Japanese themselves to be "basic" style elements as perceived in their culture and, therefore, may provide a key to understanding the structural units that make up the core of dance experience within a specific culture.

Another example of the use of Labanotation as a tool in ethnic data collection is the work of Adrienne Kaeppler, an anthropologist and curator at the Bishop Museum, Honolulu, Hawaii, who did a structural analysis of Tongan dance. In her study, she focuses on the relationship of specified units in dances, relates them also to verbal texts of accompanying dance songs, and differentiates their purposes according to their hierarchical roles in society. She uses Labanotation to identify the basic units and motifs on which these dances are built.

As the world becomes more accessible to everyone, professionals and non-professionals explore new experiences through dance and are affected by an increasing multifaceted, cross-disciplinary interest in ethnic dance, its meaning, structure and social implications. The modern dancers and choreographers have new attitudes toward body techniques and expressions of non-western cultures.

They study yoga, t'ai chi ch'uan and other body–mind oriented movement techniques; they go to foreign countries to study with indigenous teachers instead of being satisfied with secondhand versions offered locally. There are growing numbers of imported highly theatrical performances as indigenous groups are brought over from parts of the world previously accessible only to the scientific explorer. They attract audiences curious to relate to ancestral pasts and "alien" cultures apart from their own provincial prejudices. All of this is a far cry from the "chinoiserie" outlook of the baroque and rococo ballet which lasted through the 19th century.

The present surge in folk dancing has added a new dimension to its revival in the early 1920's when Margaret H'Doubler, teacher of physical education and dance at the University of Wisconsin, recommended it as a healthy, vigorous, pleasurable, rhythmic activity. Now, folk dancing is also part of the search for deeper understanding of dance as a cultural and universal experience, a search for the common, as well as the different elements in apparently foreign cultures.

However, refinements of ethnic distinctions in movement can be used as raw materials for research only when their qualitative components are communicated. It is not steps that distinguish ethnic authenticity, but the qualitative process of arriving at them.

Choreometrics

Labananalysis became particularly significant to current ethnic movement studies with its contribution to choreometrics in the Alan Lomax anthropological studies at Columbia University in 1965. Choreometrics is a dance–work rating system developed by the ethnologist Alan Lomax, with Irmgard Bartenieff and Forrestine Paulay, a former student, and colleague at the Dance Notation Bureau, to differentiate movement style cross-culturally. It is derived from kinesics, communication theory, Labananalysis and cultural anthropology. For the purposes of the Columbia studies, focus was on cultural patterns rather than individual variations within the culture.* Later studies set up other parameters for which rating scales were developed, more or less relating to choreometrics or other Labananalysis methodology.

Already existing was Mr. Lomax's survey of music performance, as analyzed from a coding sheet, listing a number of features that could serve by computerization as cross-cultural differentiators.

The specific task of Paulay and Bartenieff was to develop a rating scale which would make use of the existent ethnographic film and which could define movement performance features to help differentiate one movement style from another cross-culturally. This could be of great value to the field work anthropologist. The rating scale was to be developed within the framework of the cross-cultural survey of other systems of communication, the relationship of its features to each other and to factors of social structure.

The coding sheet was developed without access to the Lomax music study so that each communication system could be studied separately. It had also been stipulated that we, Bartenieff and Paulay, not be anthropologically trained, so that we could work as "pure" movement specialists.

In the course of two years, we viewed hundreds of ethnic films that were varied in photographic quality and in selections of subject. We soon found that the specifics of Labananalysis observation were too detailed for the assignment. We had been notating individual movement patterns which did not identify differential movement features shared by the majority of the culture members being observed. This led us to a new way of observing.

---

* *This observation and recording system was in contrast to other methodologies that incorporated a Laban orientation. For example, Warren Lamb's method for management selectivity observed and immediately notated individual changes in the process of moving that would add up to a rather detailed profile of either a skill or a specific type of behavior.*

What was necessary was to learn to rate the relative dominance of patterns observed as selected movement components, some of which were derived from Labananalysis. The ratings were then computer analyzed and produced differentiating constellations of shared movement features which were called the "core" quality constellations. This coding sheet was labeled "Use of the Body."

The first part of the coding dealt with the description of how body part usage is observed. It enumerates the body segments and tabulates frequency of usage as segments or as whole units. In addition, the coding sheet provided for the observation of use of space by the body and/or its parts. There was, however, only a slight reference (11 out of 63) to dynamic accents, the rhythmic features of Effort. For example, although tempo and speed were noted, the Time Effort elements of Urgency or Sustainment and the Weight Effort elements of Strength or Lightness were not noted. This limited the observation of the rhythm and feeling of what might be called temperamental coloring. For full Labananalysis application, all three components — body, space and Effort — must be noted in order to assess individual distinctions in their interrelationships.

In the choreometrics project, with selective Labananalysis, the results are profiles of differences in complexity as to body parts usage and use of space that indicate how members of the culture cope with their environment in terms of work and dance. A socio-economic cultural style, rather than interpersonal relationships, is distinguished in accord with the intention of the original project. Later, several additional sheets were developed to deal with group behavior, roles of female and male and other interaction features.

Studies can be developed to identify cultural temperaments in addition to socio-economic styles if another set of parameters are defined with an emphasis on Effort observations. In-depth studies within cultures that may or may not be compared to other cultures can be developed.

The methodology could use the same computer processing for individual observations to obtain the cross-cultural constellations. However, the observations would be of Flow, Space, Force and Time Effort elements which would reveal common rhythms and melodies of phrasing, indicative of emotion and temperaments. These emotional, temperamental factors can be correlated with the other findings of the choreometrics projects.

Some of the findings from correlations of the choreometrics project, which were made between features of the movement styles and other cultural factors such as song, orchestra, speech, child rearing, economy, political organization, family structure are paraphrased below from a recent conversation with Alan Lomax.

a. Profiles of dance and work from samples of cultures produced patterns within individual cultures that closely resemble each other.

b. From the profiles of several hundred dances clustered by the computer, a taxonomy of dance is emerging, which markedly resembles geographical classifications separately established for culture pattern and for song performance.

c. It is possible to characterize many world regions and sub-regions of dance in terms of contrastive profiles, that is, sets of movement characteristics whose frequencies vary significantly from region to region.

d. Since certain movement traits or sets of traits have been established as distinctive of certain culture regions, it is possible to trace the spread of culture tradition historically by noting the spread of these patterns. Thus, the movement patterns of single cultures can be seen as variations and adaptations of the patterns of more extended traditions, such as American, Polynesian, Black African, etc., as can be seen in the Eskimo/Iroquois/Micronesia examples described below.

e. Some movement style indicators can be more correlated with indicators of socio-technical development. Others are more related to sex role, others to climate, others to patterns of social organization and interaction. These factors can now be seen as clear influences on specific aspects of movement as exemplified in dance. Thus we begin to have a view of the important role of movement in human adaptation and in the evolution of culture.

f. Many aspects of movement formerly considered to be either genetic in origin or individual can now be seen as parts of cultural language that has socially valued significance and can be learned.

g. The choreometrics measures of group patterning show that dance choreography reinforces and reflects the main features of group organization — as observed in the work teams and other groups of society — so that we may now speak of a sort of social choreography.

The choreometrics scales continue to be tested for their reliability in description, for their usefulness in classifying and characterizing movement styles cross-culturally. Only those that prove serviceable in comparative observation and in the contrastive characterization of culture are retained or left unrevised. The present form of choreometrics was reached after numerous major and minor revisions.

The choreometrics project has been published in detail and in the even more compelling form of films, which instruct others in using its measures, and to illustrate its theses with examples from all over the world. Each film is a sort of world map of cross-cultural models of movement behavior. More such audio-visual reports and teaching films are in various stages of development.

Choreometrics opened new possibilities for cross-cultural studies by analyzing aspects of body movement style and relating them to cultural styles. With additional Labananalysis parameters, studies of intra-cultural movement styles can further identify cultural temperament distinctions. Workshops in 1974 and 1976, organized by Lucy Venable at Ohio University have developed additional detailed rating sheets for dance style analysts. In addition, individual studies by Dance Notation Bureau graduates, the Laban Institute of Movement Studies and programs of the Institute for Non-Verbal Communication Research provide resources for new directions in basic research of ethnic studies of movement.

Examples

Choreometric Profile*

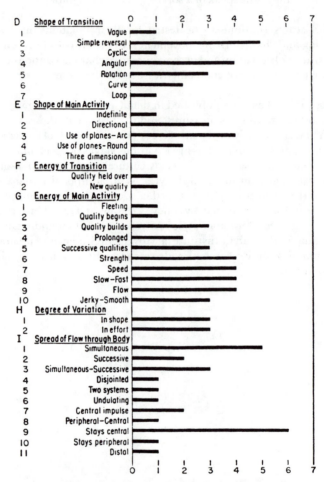

Eskimo drum dance. The four body parts used are the trunk, whole arm, forearm, and whole leg. One-unit body attitude: frontal plane with right-left stress.

* * * * *

*   *See Bibliography: Alan Lomax*, Folk Song Style and Culture.

A Cross-Cultural Example:* (from choreometrics project)

A study of Eskimo, Iroquois and Micronesian movement showed a strong similarity between Eskimo and Iroquois movement and marked dissimilarities between Eskimo and Micronesian movement. Indeed, the overall statistical similarity between Eskimo and Iroquois is 87 points out of a possible 100. Although the formations and steps employed by the two cultures are considerably different, choreometrics discovered and specified the underlying pattern that animates both their expressive and practical activity and that marks these two cultures as Amerindian.

The Caribou Eskimo confronts his cold environment from the vantage of a wide frontal body stance. His compactly held torso provides a firm base for the straight thrusts he delivers with club and spear, in his swift and energetic actions. Whether seen killing a seal with a single blow of his fist or, in a more relaxed fashion striking the edge of a drum head with the drum stick, the Eskimo organizes his movement with simultaneity. Simultaneity is the term used to describe those actions in which all body parts move in unison, a mode of action which produces maximum power. The Eskimo moves through his environment with straight linear actions and changes direction with sharp angular transitions. Thus, his application of Effort is accompanied by economy in the use of space.

Like the Eskimo's, the stance observed in films of male dancers in Micronesia is wide. The movement is dissimilar, however, in other important respects. The rhythmic up and down motion of the pelvis and legs establishes a pulsating base for the more intricate use of forearms and hands. One notes a slight rocking motion of the chest and waves of movement rising from the center of the torso and flowing segment by segment into the outstretched arms. This successive, rather than simultaneous, use of the torso occurs again in the bodies of men constructing a canoe. It permits a serial involvement of body parts, along with smoothly flowing motions and curving spatial patterns. Straight line reversals are notably absent in this Micronesian activity.

Thus, in the paired profiles of work and dance from the Arctic Eskimo and the tropical Micronesian, there are two contrastive style sets, each suitable and presumably functional in its own environment. The Micronesian movement has a higher load of features found most frequently among complex productive economies. The Eskimo movement, on the other hand, has lower frequencies of those qualities and higher occurrences of traits found in the behavior of the simpler technologies — hunters and collectors, for example.

Where the coding sheet allowed for rating general variation, it was noted that the Micronesians had more variations in spatial patterns and more variations in ranges of Time Effort and Weight Effort than the Eskimos. Such variations occur at an even higher level of frequency in Eastern Asian movement. Indeed, statistical studies show that such variations increase directly with productive and social complexity.

* * * * *

---

* *Taken from I. Bartenieff, F. Paulay, "Dance as Cultural Expression," in* Dance in Academe, *edited by M. Haberman and T.G. Meisel, Teachers College Press, Columbia University, N.Y. 1971.*

An Independent (I.B.) Intra-Cultural Example: American Indian

In a study of two different dances from the same ethnic culture, a broad range of the culture's movement behavior possibilities are illustrated. The style features are ones that were found to be differentially significant in choreometrics. To them were added the Effort/space concern for affinities and for phrasing and sequence.

The Yaqui Indian Easter Ceremony is performed at Tucson, Arizona. Since 1634, these Indians have had their own form of Catholic Church.

From the Saturday before Palm Sunday until Easter Sunday, three groups of Yaqui Indians, who gather every year from different communities, perform. Each group performs particular roles in the ceremonial ritual. There are two main groups, the Chapoyekas and the Matachini. The former are men of all ages wearing drab trousers and shirts, carrying wooden daggers and wearing masks. They represent the dark forces — evil. The latter group, the Matachini, are children, young people and women, dressed in ordinary summer clothes, without masks or props. They represent goodness and innocence. In contrast to the earth-bound, alert qualities of the Chapoyekas, the Matachini are light and carefree.

During the week, there are also performances by solo dancers known as Deer Dancers whose sacred dances represent the Indian spiritual tradition within an Indian/Christian version of a Christian Passion play. They transform the qualities of the deer, whom they represent, by intensifying them to a near-trance accompanied by rattles and bells.

The two dances — Matachini group and deer dancer solo — are analyzed below. The Matachini dance was performed in the afternoon after they had been threatened by the Chapoyekas. They form an unstructured rounded group in the middle of the open air performance space before the church.

As privileged audience to these ceremonies, the author had agreed not to take any notes. Therefore, a number of "core" qualities had to be mentally recorded and the chart was developed hours after the performance, from memory. In reviewing the notes made immediately after the event, although they did not provide a full description, the author found that she had recorded the most essential features, in both number and kind, of the Yaqui cultural style as later defined.

The chart below shows that both the Matachinis and the Deer Dancer were oriented to clear dimensions of straight up/down, right/left, forward/backward. However, they differed in their spatial and Effort emphases: They represented opposite ends of these dimensional ranges and of the Effort elements related to those ranges.

The Deer Dancer digs downward with downward spatial intent, into the ground with Strength and speed, with Bound Flow in the whole torso, leaning slightly forward and predominantly upward. His high-speed grounding steps are accompanied by constantly renewed downward accentuating circling of the gourd rattles. The constant renewal of all these tensions results in high intensity vibrations that reverberate through pelvis, thighs and legs.

In contrast to the high-speed ground steps of the Deer Dancer, the Matachini use off-the-ground, frequently bouncy steps, accompanied by light vibratory shakings. They use the same vertical but with emphasis on upward spatial intent to bounce off the ground with Light, Free Flow at high speed. Instead of high-intensity lower body vibrations, theirs are more delicate shakings.

As always, Effort/space observations of patterns that appear and may recur help to describe the moods and roles of the performers.

Comparing Style Elements (Similarities and Differences) in the Dances of the Matachinis and the Deer Dancers

Style Feature	Matachinis	Deer Dancer
BODY ATTITUDE	upright, slightly concave knees slightly bent	straight torso leaning forward and upward into space, knees and hips bent at sharp angles
STANCE	predominantly narrow	narrow with some excursions into width
RELATION OF FOOT TO GROUND	bouncing off ground	digging into the ground with high force and accelerations building up to explosive leaps
USE OF SPACE	linear, directional with frequent vague transitions	always linear and angular in transition
USE OF EFFORT Main Elements	Strength, together with Suddenness rebounding into Lightness	exaggerated Strength, exaggerated Suddenness, constantly recreated
ORGANIZATION OF EFFORT IN SEQUENCES	1) Light arm gesture, holding twig: Free Flow Strength developing into exaggerated Suddenness being neutralized into Light very Bound Flow	1) arm—hands using rattles: arm held straight forward—down or close to body flexed at sharp angle; rapid, small circular wrist shakes from the wrist with constantly recreated high Strength—Suddennesses, building up into Bound vibratory shaking
	2) step: Free, swinging lower leg gesture becoming Bound immediately followed by Strong touching of ground ending in Bound Flow	2) step: digging step — small progression, digging into ground while sliding forward with high Strength—Suddennesses constantly recreated in a crescendo of Bound Flow, causing vibratory reverberations through whole leg and pelvis stalking step — exaggerated quick, Free Flow upbeat, moderately strong contact with floor, pause followed by head gesture Sudden Bound
INTENSITY OF INVOLVEMENT Gesture/Posture Predominance	alternate gesture/posture emergence	short gestural upbeat followed by long series of postural movement

* * * * *

175

Blackfoot Indians: Intra-Cultural Analysis

Ethnic analysis is not, of course, confined to dance, although dance crystallizes qualities that appear throughout the life of the culture and there is a consistency between those qualities and other movement within the culture.

A non-dance analysis (intra-, not inter-cultural) was made from a short piece of film showing two Blackfoot Indians telling a story in their sign language, followed by a scene where some men of this tribe sit and talk.

They are seen only sitting throughout the film. What strikes the viewer is the extremely vertical center lines of their body attitudes, with focus on the high front area of the kinesphere, the clear use of pure directions: up/down, forward/backward, more rarely side/side; the angular transitions when changing directions; the simultaneous, solid use of segments of arm/hand, forearm/hand; the absence of successively spreading movement; absence of any rounded, shaping movements; and the high intensity of Strength, Suddenness, Directness. There are shorter or longer phrases; they always build up to a major accent. There are clear fluctuations between Free and Bound Flow, with accents of Sudden/Bound, Strong/Sustained, Sudden/Strong, Direct/Sustained. The sharing of qualities with the Yaqui profile is marked.

*   *   *   *   *

Effort and Style

The use of Effort as a major factor in defining style has also been illustrated by Judy Van Zile, a dancer and ethnologist. Although she used the term "energy," rather than Effort, the dynamic aspects of her observations can be made much more specific and clear when analyzed as Effort.

For example, when discussing the teaching and learning experience of east–west exchanges, she described a Javanese dancer studying American modern dance. The dancer mastered the form and pattern, but still looked Javanese in performance, and thus bypassed the meaning of the American dance.

An Effort analysis would identify the Javanese cultural style by its specific handling of Flow fluctuations: They are very small, giving the Flow an evenness that only gradually changes to a fluctuation of Bound to Free to Bound, etc. In contrast, the American modern dance style often has abrupt changes from highly Bound Flow to Free Flow. Thus, the underlying cultural Flow style of the Javanese dancer affected the proper forms and patterns that he mastered in the American dance in such a way that the expressive meaning was changed.

Judy Van Zile has also commented on her own study of Korean dance: She was unable to follow her teacher's instructions or understand the rhythm and meaning of the dance until she discovered the subtle (Effort) accents in initiation and transition in what had originally appeared to be simple linear movement with little variation in Effort.

*   *   *   *   *

176

Japanese Kabuki Dancer and Western Ballet

The Japanese Kabuki dancer illustrates particularly the relationship of dance Effort/space observations to non-dance activities. He operates his fan with spatial peripheral countertension. With the same quality of shaping and countertension of the whole body in relation to the arm–hand that holds the fan, he creates an incredible number of illusions. The fan becomes a weapon, a cup, a brush. For instance, in depicting the rising moon with his fan, he creates a countertension in his body by maintaining the straight center line in the front torso, while leaning slightly forward and up. The arm–hand, holding the fan, travels along the periphery of its reaching space, as the high vertical restrictive countertension develops in the chest and spine. The performer thus creates a "feeling" and illusion of distance between himself and the prop, which illusion is perceived by the viewer, as a wide, distant horizon.

The martial arts represent another aspect of spatial expressiveness — transversal shaping. This is observed when, from a wide diagonal stance, a large three-dimensional action sphere is opened around the body for the use of Basic and Full Effort combinations in manipulating the weapon in wide, powerful slashes and sweeping hits.

This range in the martial and theatrical arts is consistent with the traditional Japanese daily movement behavior: Conventional gestures in daily exchanges of talking, greeting. Ceremonial uses of implements at home contain a great deal of peripheral countertensions, which give a self-effacing quality to the gesture, while the many forms of body techniques and the adaptation of western sports, their prowess in fighting, incorporate the transversal shaping as well — altogether a wide range of spatial and dynamic expressiveness.

Incidentally, the port-de-bras of the western classical ballet makes a similar peripheral use of midline-centered tension of chest–spine against the rounded opening of the arms in front and to the side, led from the hands. The same tension appears in arabesque movements. Here, again, the peripheral countertension supports the "illusion" of overcoming weight and gravity, reaching into an unearthly dimension. The distinction between these constellations and those of the Japanese described above lies in other factors, such as, for example, body attitude, in which the Japanese has a straight back with a slight forward inclination, while the ballet dancer is completely vertically aligned; center of weight, which is in lower (pelvic) area for Japanese and in upper (chest) area in the ballet; and grounding, which is, for the Japanese, earthbound, even with great jumps related to the lower body, while in the ballet, the quality is heaven-reaching, off-the-ground.

* * * * *

Teaching Ethnic Dance

Because Labananalysis, particularly Effort/Shape aspects, identifies qualitative components of movement, Jean Erdman, chairperson of the dance department of New York University, invited me to teach students of ethnic dance at NYU Performing Arts School. Student classes, with an "authentic" representative of a cultural style as teacher, were videotaped. I was to teach Effort/Shape analysis, through theory and movement sessions, supported by the use of ethnic films concentrating on the dance and other cultural activities of the particular style taught. It was hoped that the use of Labananalysis concepts would hasten the process of getting to the essentials of the style, getting to the core meaning or "spirit of the dance."

Two central problems for the students arose: Resistance to giving up an imitative approach to learning and resistance to giving up their artificial division between technique and expressive, creative, inventive performance. Resistance to giving up imitating the teacher exclusively was based on their notion that once the steps and gestures were grasped and executed correctly, meaning, spiritual content, the "style" would be forthcoming. The ethnic performer teachers, themselves, stressed that the purely mechanical imitation of steps, without feeling the spirit, or meaning, or the human communication of gestures, negated the essence of the expression. We hoped to provide a vocabulary that could gradually connect the technique and expressiveness in the teaching process.

Most students and teachers underestimated the importance of the whole cultural baseline of daily life and spiritual tradition from which the meaning of the dance evolved. After the class saw films of activities other than dance, which showed the same movement features as the dance, they began to identify baselines of common behavior and expression in the individuals of the culture being studied. Then, when they saw themselves on videotape next to the ethnic teacher, they began to compare differentiating movement features in the teacher and themselves. It became clear that it was not mere clumsiness or technical inability that had delayed their learning process, but the failure to see that the constellation of qualities, not the single features, determined the essence of a particular dance.

We then explored with the students what movement features are essential to define a particular style. First, one must identify the features that appear in an event simultaneously as constellations. Then, as those constellations recur, it is possible to identify what can be called the core of the style.

Ten categories (from Choreometrics and Labananalysis) were selected as the basis for their observations in the organization of their learning experience:

Body Attitude, Stance
Body Parts Used
Simultaneous and Successive Movement
Use of Space
Use of Spatial Transition
Use of Effort; Identifying Dominant Elements
Dominant Effort Combinations
Organization of Effort in Sequence
Use of Flow
Use of Territory

Rather than just imitating details of a movement — struggling with slow learning and quick forgetting — they worked with the constellations as core qualities to learn the movements, with particular emphasis on the individual dynamics that would fulfill the intent of the culture. This gave them the Gestalt of the style within which details could be identified and integrated much more rapidly and then refined as part of the whole.

For example, when the students were preparing to study a dance from India, the teacher was in a starting position which the students were mechanically imitating. The teacher's position was a total body attitude that related itself to the ground and space in a particular way; the students' positions were mechanical configurations of limbs. Not until it was pointed out to them that the position had the particular spatial tensions of a rhomboid did the students actually experience themselves in space and with the quality intrinsic to those tensions. Only then could they move within that space appropriately.

To further identify style, we emphasized also the phrasing of Effort elements and spatial paths and their combinations. Characteristic phrasing can be identified in the organization of the rhythms of a culture as well as of an individual. That does not necessarily mean that all individuals in a given culture have the same phrasing, but that individuals have characteristic phrasings and groups of varied individuals can produce "cultural" patterns of phrasing similar to the rhythms of speech.

*   *   *   *   *

Same Task in Different Cultures: Polishing a Metal Bowl
North African and Scandinavian Women

Simple everyday activities reflect the characteristic shaping and Effort element preferences of the culture in which they exist. Thus, polishing a gourd or round bowl in the African movement style will show a dominance of curved, figure-of-eight or serpentine shapes in the action of the hand holding the cloth, with corresponding countershaping in the supporting hand. The predominant Effort elements will be Free Flow with small fluctuations toward Bound Flow; Indirectness sweeping over the surface; emphases on Time with Suddenness constantly re-created and embedded in the progression, the emphasis on shaping rather than Strong Effort.

The Scandinavian uses the action hand with a linear approach, staying in one plane with inward-directed small circles; the supporting hand holding the bowl on the working table. Instead of countershaping, there are slight interruptions of surface contact as the action hand moves to another place, and the supporting hand re-establishes itself in the accompanying static support. The Effort distribution will emphasize Flow fluctuation between Bound and Free; Time fluctuations between Neutral and Sudden; and more marked fluctuations of Strength and rebound toward Lightness.

As can be seen, the whole process is less smooth, less cohesive in shape, more energized in contrast to the easy flowing spatial mobility of the African. Both are highly efficient. Their Effort/Shape differences are consistent with other cultural adaptations to their environments.

*   *   *   *   *

179

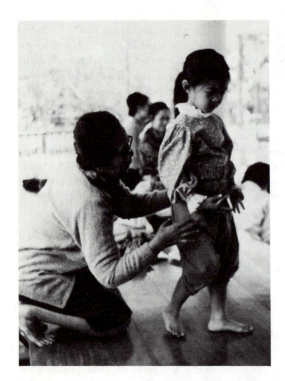

Thai Woman Teaching Child to Dance
© Stephanie Krebs.
Use of body shaping to
communicate limb constellation to
student.

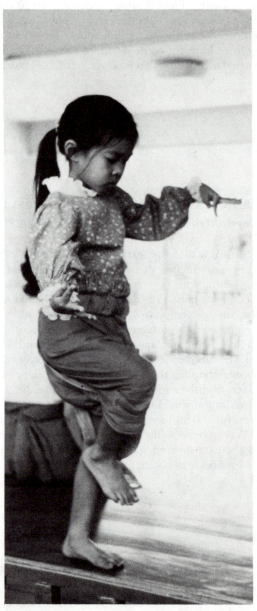

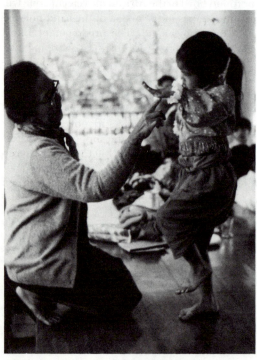

CHAPTER 11

Additional Applications

An observer of a moving person is at once aware, not only of the paths and rhythms of movement, but also of the mood the paths in themselves carry, because the shapes of the movements through space are always more or less colored by a feeling or an idea. The content of ideas and feelings which we have when moving or seeing movement can be analysed as well as the forms and lines in space.

Rudolf Laban

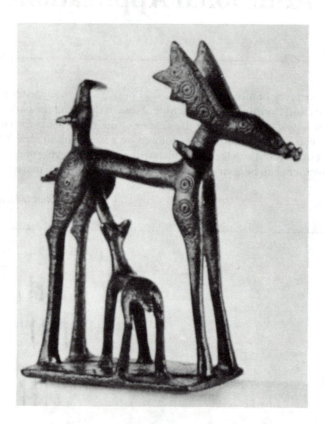

Deer and Fawn (Greek 8th century B.C.). Courtesy of Museum of Fine Arts, Boston, H.L. Pierce Fund 98.650.

Additional Applications

Animals, Territory and Labananalysis

Animals also differ in their use of space and Effort. The complexity of that usage is increased with prehensile differentiation. In fights for survival, the spatial relationships and the ordering of Effort elements are especially crystallized.

The outstanding difference between such ordered sequences and human spatial approaches is, of course, the difference in uprightness, which is both positive and negative. Positive in the extended range that it offers; negative in its more precarious balance. Uprightness permits more continuous three-dimensional movement selections, while the quadruped has only excursions into three-dimensionality. On the other hand, the quadruped has a greater ability to go sharply, instantaneously, from high intensity in Effort and crystallized spatial precision into a state of relaxation.

The combinations of Effort and space elements rather than any single factor determine adequacy to different situations. In the examples below, the animals have been observed in fighting, nurturing and play.

Mare and Foal

In an experiment* to condition newborn foals to human touch, six or seven foals were observed during their first session with the woman who would stroke and fondle them for a certain time and later repeat the sessions over a period of weeks or months. In that first session, the mare, held by the head reins, was kept nearby while the foal was handled on the lap of the experimentor.

Some mares would get somewhat restless. A dramatic incident developed with one particular mare. When the foal was placed on the lap of the woman, the mare became quite excited. She pulled away from the stable boy and confronted the woman holding her offspring. It looked as if she would step on her. However, as she came very close, she abruptly turned to her right in a quarter of a turn, which left her left flank exposed to the woman with the foal. With a swift, gentle, sideward reach of her left foreleg, she lifted/ pulled the foal out of the woman's lap and placed it between her forelegs. Holding tightly on to the foal, she shook her head–neck in a dynamic gesture — a serpentine upward curve with Free Flow/ Strength/Suddenness — that reverberated through the whole body.

The whole sequence of approaching, then focusing on the foal and seizing it, was clearly ordered spatially in relation to the foal. The seizing was a horizontal encycling of just the foal — a clear choice not to have a head-on attack with the woman.

* * * * *

* *Recorded on untitled film. Footage made for Institute for Inter-Cultural Studies by William Mitchell and Sandor Kirsch. Shown at American Association of Anthropological Science meeting, Washington, D.C., 1968.*

Fight Between Mountain Lion and Wild Boar*

A TV wildlife program included a filmed fight between a mountain lion (prehensile ability) and a small wild boar (no prehensile ability). Their differences in use of Effort seemed to make for a most uneven match but each animal had compensatory strengths that made the outcome unpredictable. The body of the large cat and the use of its reach space was more three-dimensional than that of the little boar, which seemed almost flat and compact, supported on four thin legs with little differentiation of knee and foot in contrast to the well-articulated forepaws and hind legs of the cat. The cat could, therefore, pounce upon and seize his victim with his claws. His whole body fully changed its shape from a condensed curling up to a wide and spread elongation.

Lying low, crouched near the ground, the mountain lion was condensed into his curled up shape, while the boar stood turned in a way that offered his whole naked flank to the enemy. For quite a while, they seemed to just mock each other, retreating and advancing in various ways and at various speeds in their individual territories, changing their front angles of confrontation and returning to the initial confrontation described above.

In these changes within their individual territories, it became apparent that the boar — by the high speed of advancing and retreating, turning and circling — was well equipped to meet challenge or evade it. In the course of these mockfight challenges, they began to use an increasing amount of territory, with the boar always succeeding in outrunning the lion.

Then, in one of the direct confrontations, the cat made his first pouncing attack, attempting to jump on the boar's neck. With a high speed turn, the boar warded off the attack, and, using his massive head and body in a total piston-like head and trunk action, he lashed out at one of the cat's paws, as he (the boar) was ready to run off. The boar, after several such encounters, outran the lion, who finally gave up, fatigued.

Analysis: The boar, though little differentiated in the use of his limbs and body — there were no major body shape changes, no indication of spatial shaping in the four limbs which moved almost one-dimensionally — relied primarily on defending himself by using the territory for flight and by quick changes in spatial orientation towards his enemy.

He attacked in short spurts. With exaggerated Strength and Suddenness, he would lash out with his whole body, led by the head, but never losing his readiness to go into immediate flight, or to circle with Suddenness, away from the lion. He had the ability to use his flat body with his muscular neck–head as a thrust in the attack, supported by the bony stable legs that were able to maintain a lightning speed in the actual attack and an undiminished endurance in his escape run at that speed.

Labananalysis would summarize the fight as follows:

In terms of Effort, the boar had exaggerated Sudden Time and exaggerated Strong Weight, with little variation and only occasional lapses into neutral Time and neutral Weight. There was no discernible Space Effort. The boar's head thrust hitting the lion's paw appeared to be the result of a generalized spatial pattern rather than of a specific spatial goal. This subtle difference is one that the author has frequently observed as a distinction between human and animal use of space. In cultures where human skills are rudimentary, a similar undefined attitude toward space can also be observed.

There was also no clear shaping of the boar's body. He maintained the same total body shape most of the time, but compensated with the high intensity of his Time and Weight Effort combinations to flee over a large territory.

The lion's body shape had much more adaptability: In the pursuit for food, he was winding his way through the high savanna grass, sniffing, constantly adjusting his body to the ground while trailing signs for a possible victim. He would pause on a high rock, sitting on his hind legs, scanning the

---

* *NBC–TV program, "Wild Kingdom."*

territory around, looking into a distance. As he descended from the rocky hill in loping jumps, there were constant adjustments also in the use of his forelimbs, with part or full support in adaptive changes that spread through the whole flexible body. He prepared for an attack by retreating into a curled-up body shape, close to the ground. In the attack, he would use his forelimbs, aiming at his victim as he pounced down in an attempt to seize him. His movement traced a clear grasp-like, enveloping spatial shape, while the boar depended primarily on flat, compact body shape.

The lion's Effort combinations in attack were Free Flow, Strength and Suddenness going into Bound, Diminishing Suddenness and ending in a neutralizing of Effort as he desisted and retreated into his rounded shape, waiting, building up for the next assault. His repertoire in Effort, though not greater in number of Effort elements used, had greater variability in combinations than the boar had. But, again, as with the boar, there was no discernible clear Space Effort.

From other observations of animals (mammals and, particularly, monkeys and apes), this author comes to a tentative conclusion that full development of the Space Effort may be linked to the more complete uprightness of the human species.

Uprightness makes the space of the full kinesphere around the body available to human movement in contrast to the half-kinespheric space of the quadruped. Thus, the human has three-dimensional shaping possibilities that are not possible for the quadruped. The Space Effort seems to develop as an aid to dealing with the increasing complexity of spatial choices in the full kinesphere.

*　*　*　*　*

Functional Rehabilitation

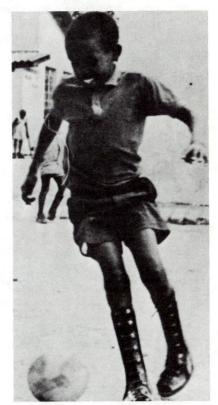

Right: *Handicapped Boy Kicking Ball*
© Rehabilitation International.
Unusual total involvement in spite of the marked disability in the left leg. Total spatial intent toward the ball. Struggling against generally Bound Flow which is heightened by the disability, he cannot produce the shape he wants to support his Sudden/Direct Effort combination. He compensates with the upper body diagonal twist supported by Light Weight/Sudden Time about to go into Free Flow. This will enable him to throw his whole body around, rather than depending on his leg alone, to kick the ball.

When teaching a patient with massive but not total paralysis in the lower unit to walk with long leg braces and crutches, one can observe the weakening or near absence of countertensions. When there is some residual muscle power in the lower limbs, the patient can be started in a standing position within a set of parallel bars that are waist high. The object is to develop in the patient's arms the downward tension which is provided by the active legs of a healthy individual. This is done by having the patient push down on the bars with his arms, so that, eventually, crutches can be used and whatever patterns are possible in the lower body can be activated.

The downward *pushing* tension of the right arm toward the floor induces a *pulling* of the left lower trunk-pelvis-hip forward — a contralateral tension.

However, what frequently happens is that the patient, holding on to, instead of pushing down, the bars, pulls his body toward the arm into a total rounding shape. He then has no countertension into the floor. If this pattern cannot be corrected, the patient cannot be taught to walk with crutches in a contralateral pattern. Instead, he has to be taught what is called a "bilateral swing through," which means the two crutches are advanced, the arms produce the downward push into the floor through the crutches and heave the whole body forward between the crutches. There is, then, no possibility to develop upper–lower countertension. Instead, an extraordinary feat of strength in just the shoulder girdle is required. The patient has to bear down on the handles of the crutches with his full body weight using only the muscles of the upper chest, upper back, scapula and arm muscles — a great condensation of muscle tension.

In contrast, the contralateral crutch walking produces countertensions of right–left, upper–lower torso, so that the body becomes totally involved by balancing tensions rather than partially involved by sheer muscle strength of isolated areas. One spatial pattern against another forms counteracting forces or shapes in different segments of the body which relate to each other, thus distributing the patterns of tensions and countertensions throughout the body and increasing the possibilities of mobility.

* * * * *

Contrast Between Two Musicians

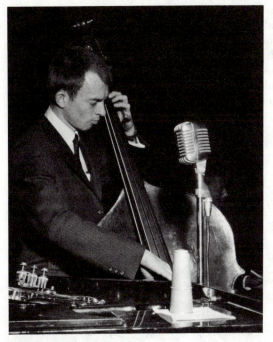

© Popsie

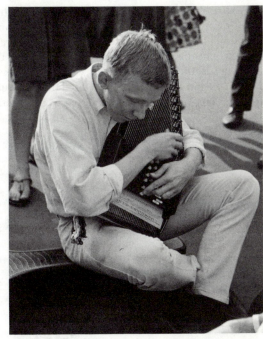

© Nat Norman.

Even to the untutored eye, a movement contrast is clearly apparent in these pictures of two musicians. Labananalysis can also point out the following observations although, of course, they would require confirmation from live performance observations.

Both musicians are shaping their bodies to their instruments, but the bass player's shaping is more total because of the countertensions. In contrast, the autoharp player's shaping is almost passive.

Bass Player: Total body shaping to instrument in Bound Flow with Free Accents. His body shaping is very much defined by the countertensions of left–in–up against right–out–down/forward — countertensions that go through the body. The left hand gathers; left arm has Sustainment; fingers Sudden/Sustained fluctuations of Light/Strong. Right arm scatters. Emphasis on Strength with Light Rebound/Sudden Time.

Autoharp Player: In contrast, he almost passively embraces the instrument with his total body shape with minimal countertension. It is as if he totally gathers to himself in contrast to the other who both gathers and scatters. The tensions are concentrated in forearms and hands — between the plucking of the right hand and pressing of the left hand — almost without going through the body. Free Flow with some Bound accent is predominant with more giving into his weight rather than crystallizing the Weight Effort. His Effort elements are diminished, less clearly differentiated than those of the bass player. The Time range between Sudden and Sustained appears hardly contrastive. Left hand is Sustained with diminished Strength. Right hand appears more Sudden with Lightness and Bound Flow — all somewhat diminished.

*   *   *   *   *

187

Martial Arts: The Japanese Way of the Sword (Kendo)

The martial arts of China and Japan have deep historical roots in both countries. They include the use of many types of weapons as well as "freehand" fighting, such as boxing, wrestling, and other weaponless forms of self-defense. Regional differences and the contributions of masters at different periods of history have added many variations in the techniques. What is common to all these forms, however, is their stress on the mastery of sensorimotor experience, spatial awareness, breath awareness and Effort — all embedded in a spiritual, religious ethos and attitude about dealing with an opponent. Laban studied these arts in great detail to learn basic principles of movement embodied in them.

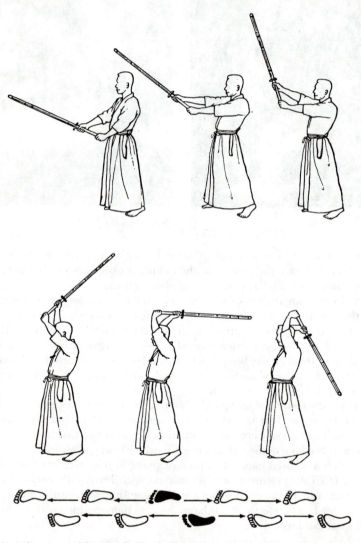

Above: *Kendo: Suburi*. Courtesy of Charles E. Tuttle Publishers. (From *This is Kendo: The Art of Japanese Fencing*, by Junzo Sasamori and Gordon Warner.)

The art of the sword and of archery are considered the highest of the martial arts. In Japan, Kendo, the art of the sword, is associated historically with the aristocratic Samurai as an example of powerful noble conduct for the whole country. The Samurai looked upon it as training in knowing how to die which taught them how to live. Throughout his life a Samurai would continue the pursuit of higher perfection in his art and life styles. In that sense, there is some similarity to medieval European chilvalry, but the difference in conception of body skills is reflected in the difference in armor, which was considerably lighter for the Samurai. Although some body parts were armored for protection, the primary focus was on perfecting the art of attack–defense with full freedom of movement and the ability to react to every move of the opponent by *anticipating* it. The arts are practiced currently with renewed intensity as a sport and for self-realization with a philosophical attitude that emphasizes the control of passion by means of impersonal use of skills. The pure form of Kendo, *Kata*, is distinguished from modern Kendo in that its total purpose is to improve and maintain the technical purity of the art.

Cultivation of the attitude of respect and courtesy is constantly practiced and a strict code of etiquette prevails throughout the Kendo encounter.

There is a great emphasis on the beginner's need for guidance and all phases of training and teaching are regulated by extensive codification of all the elements of the process. Heedless action or being carried away by emotion that would over-ride the observation of proper etiquette is con-demned. Constant evaluation, correction, and polish are demanded. The cardinal virtues in attain-ing mastery are hard work, understanding, practice and, above all, patience.

The ego is suppressed and the Kendoist uses his whole being, all his faculties of sensory and spatial awareness and quick responsiveness for meticulous execution of strokes. He knows every aspect of his weapon from the curvature of the blade to its thinness and sharpness and its fit into the handle. He respects all the properties of the leather scabbard from which the sword can easily be drawn and slipped back without the use of the eye, when the "feel" of the operating hand of its master is perfectly trained. The perfect tool and the mastery of speed in space and body can bring a quick end to a fight that will express respect for the human dignity of the opponent.

There is a Kendo saying about the basic attitude toward fighting that can also be described by Labananalysis vocabulary: "Eyes first [Attention: Space Effort], Footwork next [Weight transfer-ence], Courage third [Time Effort and Spatial Initiation] and Strength fourth [Weight Effort]." Significantly, the massive Weight Effort comes last in the enumeration.

All actions are perceived as parts of a whole. Therefore, all the details are related to each other: the position of the feet, the grip of the sword with right and left hands, drawing the sword out of the scabbard without losing the visual focus on the opponent, the rhythm, etc.

The basic practice exercise is called *suburi*. Positions of both hands and feet are precisely chosen, the involvement of the total body and unwavering eye contact are crucial. After a specifically prescribed procedure of entering the arena or stage, acknowledging the god and the presence of each other and following a sequence of positioning themselves and their swords in particular relationships to themselves and each other, the Kendoists assume positions in which they are facing each other with swords directed at each other's throats.

The body attitude at this point is absolutely stable and vertical with the weight evenly distributed on both feet. The backward foot is slightly behind and to the side of the front foot, and parallel to it. This places the heels in a slightly diagonal relationship to each other which opens the reach space all around and also allows readiness for quick turns. Through a series of attacking and defending strokes in quick succession of changes from attack to defense to attack, the adversaries may change distance between them and occupy a larger section of the space.

At the end of each form, they return to the original confrontation, crossing each other's swords at the prescribed angle. This core confrontation sets the sagittal orbit for a number of basic strokes. The maximal orbit leads from forward–high to vertical–up with the sword pointing a clear backward–high. Although, during some phases, both horizontal and diagonal deflections occur, the most massive strokes of attack are on that sagittal orbit and are executed with both hands.

The two hands holding the sword are in a diagonal relationship — right slightly ahead of the left hand in a right–forward diagonal. That grip is related to the whole body stance. The two hands grip the sword in the planar direction forward–high in relation to the midline and center of the body. Thus the sword points to the upper forward corner of the sagittal plane at the throat of the opponent. The "correct" grip and use of the sword combining spatial and articular principles, is developed as follows:

Left hand (action hand) grips from below and leads.
Right hand (steadying hand) grips from above.
Rotary factor operant as right and left hand are slightly rotated inwardly against each other.
Thumb Positions: Inside of the grip for right hand on top.
Bottom inside for the left hand.
This creates a slightly diagonal countertension, again, stability with readiness for mobility.

As the sword is lifted for the sagittal arc, the left hand leads with the right hand steadying it as it goes through the whole arc. Deviations from the arc will incline toward different specific points of the opponent's body. In practicing these different inclinations, the student recites the body parts they are aimed at. There is extraordinary spatial and Effort precision. In some strokes, speeds of 125 miles per hour are momentarily reached in turns and jumps with the striking sword.

Labananalysis Observations

1. Kendo is a total Effort and space involvement. Though every detail — body part and segments, foot position, exact verticality, the exact planes of strokes, the transference of weight — is studied minutely and meticulously timed, the concept of the whole is never violated.

2. As in the defense scale there are ordered sequences through which vital points of the opponent's body are aimed at and reached in the attack (in Kendo: head, throat, wrist, chest) and codified with maximum precision and economy.

3. The training develops Suddenness in defense as well as in attack. By knowing the points of greatest vulnerability, the defense can either bar the weapon or deflect the intended stroke, letting it occur in space outside the kinesphere.

4. Awareness of the articulations of the bodies of fighter and opponent and of the spatial areas and the spatial axes of each other make for very clearly defined action space, great mobility and absolute precision of weight shifts.

5. Great stress is placed on the use of breath. Impact is always accompanied by sound on the exhalation phase. Sounds are released according to the combination of Suddenness/Strength or widely sweeping Flow/Strength.

* * * * *

Dance*

Laban defined dance as an art "when human movement creates compositions of lines in space which, from a definite start, show a structural development, a buildup leading to a climax, a solution and an ending. Such a dance work has a representative, exhibitive value. It is filled with a uniform mood and expresses things that cannot be expressed unequivocally and in all details by spoken words; it has a meaningful, understandable content." Gymnastics, on the other hand, "always serves the specific purpose of strengthening the body and controlling limb movement in the surrounding space" without reference to expressive content. In both dance and gymnastics, the mastery of the body "is, of course, based on skill and order, especially the rhythmic order."

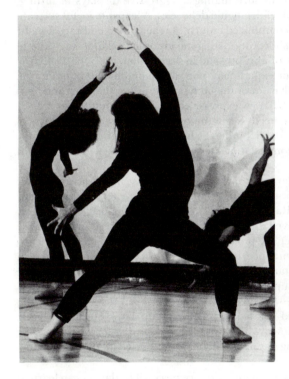

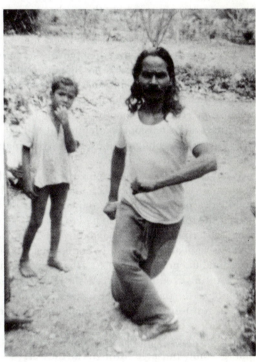

Dance Class led by Carolyn Bilderback © Liza Stelle.   *Indian Dancer in West Bengal* © Judy Van Zile.

* *Note: Application of Labananalysis to dance serves an obvious purpose for dancers and choreographers, but it also serves the observer from other disciplines as an exploration of components common to all movement process and, therefore, to human behavior.*

191

The choreographer "captures the expressive content of dance movements. Thus, the mover is given a dance-like stimulus. A variety of such stimuli can be used. They can be selected from those spatial/rhythmically-structured gestures that the dancer uses as the language of his art. The dancer has an alphabet of definite and harmonically performable spatial swings. He knows the interrelationships of those swings and spatial paths. He knows that one combination may be more harmonious and another one more dissonant and grotesque. He develops this harmony and grace or the dissonant and grotesque into really powerful expression. . . . In this sense, one can go even further. One can give the participant pantomimic ideas . . ."

The dancer is constantly involved with tensions and changes leading to *transformations* of movement. He/she changes size, width, depth, extends, recoils, embraces, resists. Moods can change from sluggish awakening to gradual perceptions of surroundings. Aggressive displays of hitting, pressing, compressing strength can change into playful, languid delicacies. A leap into joyful staccato can be followed by sinking, falling, rolling into a compressed crouch. A reach out to embrace may be followed by a retreat into oneself. There may be short contrasting moods or long elaborate stories of conflict and explosions that dissolve into serenity or abruptly end in destruction.

Without tension, there is no change, no life or experimentation, no communication, no dance. There is a zero state of emptiness. Tensions evolve out of the body/space/Effort changing relationships in their various configurations to maintain balance, expressiveness, and continuity.

The dancer, transformed by changing tensions, needs to continuously renew his/her awareness of the causes of the tensions, both internal and external: How he/she breathes through the movements, their initiations, configurations, Effort combinations, spatial intents and relationships to the physical and emotional environment.

What is it that makes one remember a particular gesture or movement phrase in a dance or theater performance as one remembers a melody or a line of poetry? More than ten years ago, the author attended a performance of a dance drama by Rabindranath Tagore. Udar Shankar, the dancer, played the role of a king who had to ban his beloved queen from the palace and the country because she had been unfaithful. He stood very erect over the prostrate figure of the queen. He bade her to rise: His right arm in a slightly Bound/Sustainment opened the gesture into a wide upward arc with a Sustained fluency, Weightless. There was a hesitancy, an almost supporting, encompassing gesture as if wanting to embrace her. As she rose with a supplicating gesture — lowered head, her two hands touching at the palms pressed against her chest — he extended his majestic open verticality, starting with a gesture, palm down, whole arm inward rotated. Strength/Bound Flow/Sustained Time increased as he directed his arm forward and down with Sustained, compelling forwardness. The clarity of space, the intensity of Effort, evoking sadness and majestic power at the same time, unforgettably pulsated through the theater.

Such Effort combinations are intrinsic to the basic themes of dance pieces. The dancer can learn to recognize what Effort elements are active, which of those are dominant and, even more important, where combinations appear, how they are phrased, and which Effort rhythms seem to be characteristic. The linking features, transitions in the phrases, the distinctions between fully realized Effort elements and diminished ones are also important. Effort accents can be differentiated in a particular body part from overall maintained Effort elements or combinations. All these factors help to identify the core of the dance which gives continuity to the performance with all its component variations. The whole texture of a work is colored by the Effort attunement to its spatial shaping — the use of directional, planar, spiral spatial patterns, spatial transitions, transverse and peripheral paths — and the use of floor patterns.

From a baseline of sequence observations, the dancer can explore characteristic rhythmic organization in different dance styles as they relate to tension systems common to movement and music. For example the differences in dances of east and west include different relationships to the

192

floor and to the Weight/Flow factor in initiation. The east, low slung from the hip–pelvis, "sits" into the ground, a position from which the dancers get central initiation for their strong and sudden discharge of Effort combinations in straight kicks and roundabout transverse shaping leg movements. That initiation adds strength, width, and action space openings into all directions, resulting in "connected" rounded shapes and sharp piercing lines. The west, in contrast, uses the floor to bounce off from or press into from above. Or they resist it or fall on it and rise high above it. They initiate from a slightly higher center than the east. Scottish dancers, for example, are high and light on their toes, in spite of large bodies, while the Chinese, Japanese and Koreans dig their heels into the ground, turning and progressing from below with complex arm–upper trunk shaping.

Dancers and choreographers can use the Laban scales to explore such differences and as points of departure for improvisational modes with spatial/Effort variations. From the "A" and "B" scales of the icosahedron, for example, they can create mobile spatial chords as triadic tensions by isolating every fourth transverse inclination from either "A" or "B" scale and by performing each transversal with a different limb. Four chords can be derived from the "A" scale as three limbs perform the movements listed below simultaneously — each limb selecting its own sequence.

	Limb 1	**Limb 2**	**Limb 3**
Chord 1	high/right	back/high	right/back
to	to	to	to
Chord 2	back/deep	right/forward	high/left
to	to	to	to
Chord 3	left/forward	deep/left	forward/deep
to	to	to	to
Chord 4	deep/right	forward/high	left/back

The more stationary arabesques of classical ballet use the directions of the dimensional scale.

The dancer will find that the selections are not arbitrary; the sequences support balance and the choice may be made according to the quality of tension compatible with the performer's intent.

While the ballet arabesque can be considered a modified *directional* chord built on the stability of the directional cross of axes, the transverse chords are built on modified *diagonals* and, therefore, are more mobile.

The modified diagonal is initiated from the corner of a plane, that is, off the vertical axis, which will establish the mobile quality of the developing chord. For instance, one arm may start at one corner, high/right of the vertical plane. The natural sense of balance would guide the opposite arm into left/forward of the horizontal plane and either the right or left leg into back/deep of the sagittal plane.

The chords that can be derived from the "A" and "B" scales are extreme models of mobility. Therefore, they almost require a partner to provide stable countertension to their fullest expression. Such combinations open up a whole area of choreographic exploration in partner work where three-limbed chordic tensions can be developed with a high degree of mobile balance and minimum external supportive structures.

"In the process of moving," Laban wrote, "the limbs describe certain sequential counter-directions and even other secondary spatial directions . . . . One can follow one movement with another in two ways: Either by changing into its counterdirection or leading back to the center of movement . . . . One can also follow one direction by another along the periphery, so-to-speak reaching for the goal by groping/touching along the edge of the movement sphere, which would mean making use of secondary spatial directions . . . .

"Rhythm is the law of gesture which makes the gesture proceed at one time with a flightly quality and at another time less so . . . . through the changes between tension and de-tension . . . . with a sequential progression in space that is more or less eased or hindered . . ."

Dance Training

There is at present an eruption of dance activity on many levels reaching a wide range of increasingly receptive audiences. New York City can fill three big theaters with major competing professional companies. The versatility of the repertoire of these large companies makes new demands on the creative performer. Where before a company would present programs based on the established tradition of ballet with new creations by one or two choreographers to give the company its individual distinguishing mark, now any number of different choreographers may be called in to stage a new work experimenting with unusual movement groping for new styles. Classical ballet groups take dance works from choreographers of modern dance. Modern choreographers are skilled in ballet; the dancers are faced with interchanging challenges. Experimental dance groups of various orientations and individualities are constantly contributing new attitudes toward movement expression and some of their unusual experiments have been picked up by the large dance theatres. Versatility is more than ever in demand and only the fittest survive.

These new trends influence the education of dancers toward more sensitivity training and more differentiation of movement perceptions than exclusive rote learning and imitation provide. There is a great need for a common vocabulary for such differentiating perceptions. With so many different styles offered, the experienced and inexperienced student and performer frequently spend a great deal of time sampling various techniques and styles without being able to integrate them, to make them accessible resources for creating or interpreting dance. Labananalysis may play a role here that could affect all dance education — professional and non-professional, company and individual — for choreographer, performer or community group leader.

Dance teachers in private studios attract a great many people who do not want to become performers on the stage but enjoy dancing with others as a form of expressive communication. This is an important trend and specific approaches are required that are not diluted forms of modern stage dance but are more related to Laban's movement choirs in Germany in the twenties and early thirties. The creative talents of too many people are buried under continuous mechanical practice and overstress on fragmented technical demands.

Individual dancers, by understanding more specifically what their bodies are doing both physio-logically and spatially, can make corrections more economically and extend their creative possibili-ties. Some, unfortunately, still suffer from the mystique that understanding cuts off creativity. In fact, whether the understanding precedes or follows the experience, it is a decisive element in the dancer's growth as an artist.

One dancer in a fundamentals class discovered the importance of finding his own personal breathing rhythm after experimenting with various breathing areas in his body in the performance of different movements. He experienced the difference between letting a relaxed style of breathing take the leg or body in movement as opposed to gripping the abdominal muscles and using more energy for poorer results. For all the corrections he had given and received in ballet classes, he had not really known what the connections were anatomically, because his anatomy class was not directly related to movement. In the fundamentals classes he learned "the principles of conserving energy," by moving with minimal strain and maximum output, understanding the interrelationship of weight, shape, initiation, the importance of spatial and Effort transitions, the concept of "groundedness."

Another student had great difficulties with any "initiation" of either center of weight or Effort exertion, and particularly with all shaping and reaching space. It was as if she could do nothing with space, especially all areas behind the body and head; space was impenetrable. Her movement revealed neutralized shaping all the time, near-absence of clear Effort combinations, a peculiar emptiness a non-readiness to communicate. In contrast to another dancer who constantly went toward dissolving action into Zero Flow, this woman was arresting her Flow in high Boundness. In both, breathing was arrested around the ribs and absent in the lower abdomen.

The student's problem appears to be the result of, among other things, *misuse* of a technique — in this case, Yoga. For the past two years, she had been practicing Hatha Yoga "stretching" and "relaxing" her "overstretched" body to counteract her six hours a day dance practice. She felt it had done a lot for her, but, in fact, her practice had become so compulsive that even her voice had become metallic, lacking any fluctuation in timbre.

Her problems became apparent to the author in a week-end workshop. In so short a time, one could only suggest a long-range remedial program, which, in practice, could be adapted to the student's responses. Her breath flow and initiation might be awakened through work with sound, at first, rather than movement. At the same time, through work with fundamentals, one would try to heighten awareness of basic connections to center of weight, chest and shoulders. Movement rhythms might evoke images that release her flow of breath and the rhythmic accents might help her awareness of clear initiations. Only in practice could one know how a particular student's blocks may be loosened, whether the damage observed is a passing stage or whether the malfunction is irreversible. Problems of devitalized dynamics are often observed as results of drug experiments and radical overconcentrations in some techniques. The restoration of differentiating dynamics requires highly individualized attention.

In another example, a woman in her forties, a mixture of South Florida Indian and Spanish gypsy, participated in a course on Effort in Ethnic Dance. She had danced for over twenty years, mainly in night clubs doing Spanish dancing. With her impulsive abrupt intensity, it seemed at first that we did not reach her at all in terms of the specific Labananalysis vocabulary. She seemed confused, often at a loss as to what to make of the teaching. But she kept trying to do the improvisations and follow the demonstrated examples.

During the last two weeks, she began to ask questions that showed that Effort concepts made some sense to her. She was the first to hand in a picture notebook. Her observations were mostly centered on Effort which, to her, meant identifying stresses and accentuations, accelerations, decelerations and differences in fluency. She identified single elements and some combinations, recognizing rebound. Her preferences were in Effort rhythms while shape and space almost bypassed her. She said that the spatial vocabulary — directional, planar, etc. — had turned her off. She was a gifted dancer and actually quite clear in her own shapings. It was, therefore, not clear whether it was just the geometrical terminology that was alien to her. With more time, we would have tried more metaphorical approaches to the geometrical references. Her intuitive gifts had developed so creatively in the area of her experience that she could easily have learned to expand her range.

*　*　*　*　*

Dance Analysis

A dancer and Labananalyst, Ellen Goldman Shapiro, studied Effort rhythms and their content in Yemenite dances. Specific personal and cultural distinctions became clear. For example, a basic Effort phrase appeared in many variations in male dances. Although the female dances were essentially built on a similar phrase model, the difference could be seen in the women's richer use of body parts stressing successive use of limbs. Consequently, their style came out as an ornamentation of the men's theme.

The study confirmed the role of Effort organization in core differences between different cultures. Shapiro also compared the step patterns to a presentation of an Indian War Dance (Thunderbird Pow-Wow, Oakland, N.J.), where she saw steps that were very similar to the Yemenites in spatial pattern and weight shift. They differed in their relationship to the ground: The Indians constantly stressed pressing into the ground with strong Weight in contrast to the Yemenitic stress of touching the ground with light Weight, diminished Suddenness, always rebounding into Sustainment with accents off the ground. These differences reflect fundamentally different attitudes and moods.

In another study, Doris Humphrey's dance, *The Shakers*, by Suzanne Youngerman, anthropologist and Labananalyst, the relationship of dances to the cultures which create them is clearly illustrated. A clear case is made for the importance of Effort/Shape distinctions to capture the specific intent of the choreographer's interpretation of the original dance.

As Youngerman noted, "The point of recounting the history of the Shakers (in this study) was to illustrate that because the culture and the role of dance in the society differed in various periods, there can be several interpretations of *The Shakers* depending on which aspect of their life one chooses to emphasize. By controlling the Effort/Shape qualities, various dramatic moods can be created, some of which are more Shaker-like than others."

For example, there is a "relationship between various Effort patterns, especially the dialogue between the Spaceless and the Weightless drives; the predominance of certain spatial configurations, such as the use of the vertical dimension, the sagittal plane and octahedral space . . .

"In addition to [a] pattern of calm/activity/calm, and of changes of low level variations of level and back to low level, there are Effort/Shape fluctuations which follow this same general pattern. Thus, in general terms, the dance starts in Shape Flow, develops more into shaping movements including both directional movements and sculpting patterns, and then returns to a predominantly Shape Flow feeling. Furthermore, the movement starts Spaceless and Weightless, adding Weight and Space Effort elements in the middle sections, with states [Incomplete Effort actions] often turning into [Internalized] drives, ending in states based on Time and Flow. (The above analysis is based on the film; other interpretations are also discussed in the study.)

". . . The overall rhythmic quality of dance derives not just from the 'rhythm state,' [Weight/Time] although it is frequent, but also from the quality of rebound — after all, rebounding is what shaking and hopping are really about. Thus, in most cases, the states and drives mentioned above rebound into their indulging counterparts.

"The dancers, however, sometimes have difficulty in the choice of an appropriate Effort phrase which all can perform in unison. Since there is also a difference in the shaping of the shake — some, for instance, use Shape Flow, others, directional movement or shaping in the sagittal cycle — different shape phrases would also appear."

We only indicate what Youngerman spells out in detail in her study using the full Labananalysis vocabulary to describe specific movements in order to elicit the desirable emotional content. For instance, "Most of the dancers in the film begin in a state of Sustained, Bound Flow with body-oriented repetitive movements designed to mobilize the individual into either a Spaceless or Weightless drive especially Strong/Bound/Sudden or Direct/Bound/Sudden or Direct/Bound/Sustained. (Dancers in the film take both routes.) For instance, Weight and Space enter with acceleration and the change from Shape Flow to directional movement in the opening section. The Weightless drive is an appropriate one for the 'visionary' moments in the dance: for M_1 in the opening measure of the dance as he points to his vision and then melts back weightlessly into the group; for M_6 during his revelation (measure 25) and for those who stop to listen to his message; and for the Elderess during her revelation on the bench (measure 30). In the latter case, it is noted that she is in a trance . . . ; she is, in essence, not 'there' and, therefore, one of the Weightless states or drives would be appropriate. The particular dancer in this film has a great deal of natural Strength Effort, and thus does not succeed in denying her body weight. She does, however, punctuate her revelation with Bound/Sudden movements in her arms, reflecting inner vibrations. Strong/Sudden accents would reveal a more dogmatic purpose to her message. Some heaviness (going into body weight) would also be appropriate for her coming out of the trance, giving the feeling of the exhaustion of the spiritual experience."

Labananalysis has been used to describe and compare other dances, some of which are listed in the Bibliography.   *   *   *   *   *

196

Choreographing a Dance*

Although the example given below is from the journal of a young dancer of some experience, her use of Labananalysis could be applied selectively to any level of experience. It is unique as a detailed developmental record, personal and professional, of the creation of a dance directly related to the use of Labananalysis.

Carol-Lynne Moore Rose, a graduate of the Dance Notation Bureau programs in Effort/Shape aspects of Labananalysis, choreographed a dance by choosing an Effort theme as the starting point. She describes vividly in her session by session journal how she experimented with "spell" and "vision" drives which evoked a whole series of images that crystallized into a kind of magic dance she called in the end, "Fairy Tale." It is a solo but depicts the transformation from one magic figure to another one, ending in a demonic Grendl-like figure. The development of these stages is documented by notating in Effort symbols** the themes and their developments after each session. In its final version the dance was filmed and also Labanotated in motif-writing.

What is distinctive is the use of Effort as an abstract theme to stimulate images and larger themes that become integrated into a cohesive tale. It illustrates how the study of Effort can provide a tool — thinking in identifiable movement quality components — that supports and stimulates the intuitive flow of movement themes and development.

In the final crystallization of her development, there are no mimetic elements, just pure Effort/ Shape themes that carry their own poetic message in the sense of movement without exactly equivalent translatable meaning. As in music, the meaning is self-contained in the medium. Basic practice of such development takes on a distinctive character; it can never become merely mechanical and, therefore, will involve the performer's emotional, imaginative and cognitive resources with more immediate accessibility. The performer and the observer thus trained discover the inherent logic of what Laban called the grammar and syntax of Effort tension themes which can lead to transformation of the performer. Furthermore, by putting the focus on content of the movement process, the performer can extend his/her movement range. In this example, certain technical difficulties that ordinarily characterized the performer's work seemed to dissolve.

The development of a dancer must go beyond just correction of functional difficulties and should not be overburdened with endless repetitions of fragments of mechanized movement. Neither overstress on technical perfection nor the creative atmosphere of an inspiring choreographer or director alone develops the artist. What is essential is a deep familiarity with the spatial–dynamic potential of his/her own movements that should be stimulated early in a dancer's education.

---

* *Excerpts from "Fairy Tale": Journal of a Dance: Effort/Shape Certification Project. Carol-Lynne Moore Rose July 6, 1976. © Carol-Lynne Moore Rose.*
** *Verbal translation substituted below.*

197

Introduction

This dance began in my head last winter when I first started having experiences with the Spell Drive. These experiences were very important to me because they put me in touch with a certain part of myself that had been dormant — my love of fantasy, of interior romance, of castles in the air.

The real conception for the dance came from an experience in class. I chose a phrase with the Spell Drive configuration in it. Through the struggle and ultimate success with crystallizing this configuration I was transformed into a Grendl-like creature. It was a very real experience. It shook me up. And it gave me the idea for a dance called "Fairy Tale," which would be a long Effortful sequence of phrases based around the Spell Drive. I envisioned a series of transformations — the final one being Grendl.

I thought about the dance for a long time before I actually started moving in the studio. The journal that follows is a rough record of those thoughts and those working sessions.

I have placed the motif of the finished dance first. This is followed by a rough verbal outline of its sections and their nicknames — since these are the names I frequently use in the journal.

"Fairy Tale": Glossary*

1. If the body part stays the same from measure to measure, it is not notated.
2. If the body part changes, it is notated.
3. Actions of the whole body are notated in the center of the staff, without the center line dividing the staff into right and left sides.
4. General Effort qualities are notated to the far right side of each staff. If the quality is to be sustained or recreated throughout the measure it is notated with an action stroke.
5. Those measures without specific effort notations are left to the discretion of the performer. In some cases the structural information supplied lends itself to Effort, so in those measures it was unnecessary to note them specifically.
6. The floor pattern is described at the end of the score.

Preliminary Stages

Idea of transformations in a long sequence of Effort phrases crystallized around moments of spell drive, going from indulging drive to fighting drive.

Devolution. From Fairy Godmother to Grendl.

This is to be a journey, a progression through a spell to the final transformation — the transformation of the magician.

Spell drive lacks Time — there is no decision making involved. The spell casts itself. Once started there is no stopping.

---

* *See Appendix A, Documentation.*

198

Some ideas for structure:
Work on a zig-zag path:

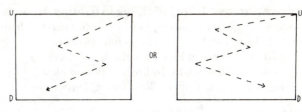

Fig. 36

Each turning point marks a transition in the weaving of the spell.
Maybe begin with gathering movements, like gathering strands together for weaving.
Working of spell might include manipulation of imaginary object.

Spell Drive Workshop with Bette Lamont 3/11/76

Fairy Godmother	EF: Light/Direct/Free Flow
Walking in your own enchanted forest	EF: Light/Indirect/Free Flow
Peter Pan	EF: Strong/Indirect/Free Flow
No definite image	EF: Strong/Direct/Free Flow
Weaving net of enchantment	EF: Light/Indirect/Free Flow
Grendl or sorcerer casting spell	EF: Strong/Indirect/Bound Flow
Walking in someone else's enchanted forest or gazing into a crystal ball	EF: Light/Direct/Bound Flow
Hypnotist	EF: Strong/Direct/Bound Flow

The above are images gathered from experiences with different crystallizations of the Spell Drive.

Accessory States to the Spell Drive 3/11/76
Images from experiences with various crystallizations of dream, stabile, and remote states:

Dream State:	EF Key: Weight/Flow
Imprisoned behind glass	EF: Light/Bound
Running in tar or luring giant	EF: Strong/Bound Flow
Mushing through clouds of whipped cream — the cliche	EF: Light/Free Flow
Overwhelming wave or hurling or fighting huge pirate in Maxfield Parrish illustration	EF: Strong/Free Flow
Stabile State:	EF Key: Weight/Space
Friendly and regal	EF: Light/Indirect
Haughty	EF: Strong/Indirect
Regal	EF: Light/Direct
Assertive	EF: Strong/Direct
Remote State:	EF Key: Flow/Space
Donovan song, wandering around on a beautiful day	EF: Free Flow/Indirect
Paranoid	EF: Bound Flow/Indirect
Wistful gaze	EF: Free Flow/Direct
Thoughtful gaze	EF: Bound Flow/Direct

Spell drive phrases* from indulging to fighting drives 3/25/76

1) Godmother gathers powers, becomes more careful, hones in
   on spell, brings all her powers carefully to bear.
   > **Effort Sequence:** Free Flow/Light/Indirect
   > to Bound Flow/Light/Indirect to Bound Flow/
   > Light/Direct to Bound Flow/Strong/Direct

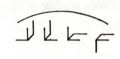

2) Godmother gathers powers, hones her attention, becomes
   more careful, all her power is concentrated.
   > **Effort Sequence:** Free Flow/Light/Indirect
   > to free Flow/Light/Direct to Bound Flow/Light/
   > Direct to Bound Flow/Strong/Direct

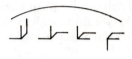

3) Godmother gathers power, concentrates power, becomes
   overwhelmed, hones in on spell.
   > **Effort Sequence:** Free Flow/Light/Indirect
   > to Free Flow/Strong/Indirect to Bound Flow/Strong/
   > Indirect to Bound Flow/Strong/Direct

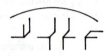

4) Godmother grooving, gains more power, hones power in, puts
   final controlling whammy on spell.
   > **Effort Sequence:** Free Flow/Light/Indirect
   > to Free Flow/Strong/Indirect to Free Flow/
   > Strong/Direct to Bound Flow/Strong/Direct

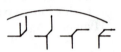

5) Godmother grooving, adds controls, gathers strength, casts
   the spell.
   > **Effort Sequence:** Free Flow/Light/Indirect to
   > Bound Flow/Light/Indirect to Bound Flow/Strong/
   > Indirect to Bound Flow/Strong/Direct

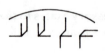

6) Godmother grooving, begins to hone in, adds power, and puts
   final degree of whammy.
   > **Effort Sequence:** Free Flow/Light/Indirect
   > to Free Flow/Light/Direct to Free Flow/Strong/
   > Direct to Bound Flow/Strong/Direct

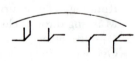

Nicknamed Sections

Measures 1–12	Opening section: turning pages reading spell, thigh slap, vision drive turn, looking through sleeves
Measures 13–19	Weaving the spell
Measure 20	Curl over, conjuring
Measures 21, 22	Spiral to ground rise, thigh slap
Measure 23	Vision drive turn
Measure 24	Shaping the ball
Measure 25	The wand

* *Labanotation has been added here as a sample. It was used throughout the original manuscript to avoid the more cumbersome verbalizations.*

Measure 26–28	Exhorting spirits, floor slap
Measure 29	Conjuring
Measure 30	Spiral to floor, rise, thigh slap
Measures 31–33	Leg extension, strong turn, thigh slap
Measures 34, 35	Pulling ball toward me
Measure 36	Vision drive turn
Measures 37, 38	Weaving (101) (deep)
Measure 39	Taking the poison (finger lick)
Measure 40–42	Effort of poison — remote
Measure 43	Arm pull with chest beating
Measure 44	Tortuous turn to almost eating apple
Measures 45–47	Fall and roll (passion)
Measure 48	Hand grab
Measures 49, 50	Eating the apple
Measures 51, 52	Ending (looking)

Choreographing the Dance

May 26, 1976: Phrases around:

1) Free Flow/Light to — might work, turning pages
   Free Flow/Light/Indirect or light slumber
2) Free Flow/Indirect to — doesn't work, remote state
   Free Flow/Light/Indirect not right for opening

Opening — dream state — turning the pages of spell book alone in tower on a summer afternoon. See spell. Sink down to read it. Like: Free Flow/Light to Sustained/Direct.

May 27: The spell needs a through line on it. Who am I casting the spell on? For what purpose?
   Might work with the idea of knots. At each bend in path a knot is tied. The final knot is me. Maybe opening phrase: Free Flow/Light to Bound Flow/Direct to Bound Flow/Sustained/Direct. Rising with leg lifted side high, let leg down, slap thigh into Sustained/Light/Indirect.

June 2: Some suggestions Susan made yesterday:
   — work for postural Light in opening.
   — connect phrases with Flow so that they don't stop at edges of kinesphere.
   — don't rise to straight vertical, but hover.
   — think up own spell — what objects do you manipulate?
      example of eating flowers from Ted Rotante dance.
   — Fairy Godmother should reappear throughout piece.
   From leg slap into Vision Drive (Bound Flow/Sudden/Direct) with peripheral tension in hands into flirtation with spirits (Free Flow/Light/Indirect) into weaving the spell (high/right to right/forward to forward/high to left/high). Step (high/right to right/forward to forward/high to left/high) into curl over jumps. Backward tilt conjuring to spiral to floor. Then spiral up into second position and back down again a couple of times.
   Through line on piece now is lazily flip pages of book, see spell, focus on spell, read spell, make decision to do spell, check to see who else is there, find the spirit I want, begin weaving spell, gather the strands together, form and crush ball.

201

June 3: Vision Drive needs different stance into Free Flow/Light/Indirect — maybe standing on one leg with the other turned in — then cross it over and take a step.

The weaving should be Bound Flow/Light/Direct.

The jumps from the spiral down should have a different Effort quality maybe.

Idea for transition into ending: Bound Flow/Strong/Direct gaze with beating arm on chest, into curling of hand into Bound Flow/Strong/Indirect.

Piece still needs through line. Structure is taking over for me and the Effort is getting lost.

After the weaving — what?

Do I want to arouse sympathy for the trapped witch? I want the end to be scary or abominable, but somewhere in the process we must feel sorry for the person — should it be moment of Passion Drive?

June 4: I got a lot of work done today.

In first part, Vision Drive is now Bound Flow/Sustained/Direct with a blues pivot turn. Then I go into crossing over the legs and looking through sleeves with Bound Flow/Light/Indirect into the web weaving part. From the conjuring in back/deep I spiral and then rise to look at up left to slap leg and jump into second with Free Flow/Light/Sudden.

From here I do another blues pivot turn accelerating with Bound Flow/Direct into Shape Flow with the crystal ball, rolling my stomach.

From here I stretch out again right/forward, grabbing the back ankle and pivoting to dive left/down/forward.

I turn and rise, lifting a little to do my curved over jumps and dive again.

This repeats, next time with the left leg in left middle, etc. Then left leg in left/high to curl over to move back/deep with conjuring. I spiral down, rise, and jump in second with slapping to spiral to other side. I rise and jump with slapping.

I think I will have to use four zig-zags instead of three. I don't have time to develop it enough in only three.

I like the structure — now I have to work on the Effort content more.

Next section needs to move into Strength and Passion Drive.

June 7: I went through the Effort organization to date roughly. The piece needs to go into Bound Flow/Strong/Direct next. Bound Flow/Strong/Direct pulling apple toward me with stamp — twice, third stamp back foot crosses over — low turn with arm extended in vision drive — scoop to down and rise as in beginning to high/right into Indirect/Light/Sustained in arms with travelling step (same stance as opening).

Quick change to relevé and Bound Flow/Light/Sudden.

Writhings in chest as arms are pulled toward stage left.

Take pivot turn in Bound Flow/Sustained/Direct to roll stomach eating the apple, almost.

Passion Drive run into beating heart — something grabs me from behind — clutch body all over with hands into Bound Flow/Strong/Indirect. Laugh, pulling face with hands. Remote ending.

June 8: This has been a day spent in a strange mind set for me. I can't exactly put my finger on what it is. I feel disconnected from things but not ill-at-ease. I am seeing things anew.

I had an experience of *deja vu* or something like it today walking through Union Square Park. I felt like a drug addict or street walker for whom the park is a familiar hanging out place. Suddenly I was in touch with the old part of me — the part that wasn't formed by these genes and this environment. I was in touch with my oldness and my darkness. Most of the time I think of myself as a child of the sun. But every once in a while I contact the dark part of me which is mostly dormant in this existence.

The new part of me is resilient and well-ordered. It keeps things neat and doesn't over-indulge.

The old sucking part is full of extremes. It is chaotic. It desires without restraint. It is rolling and seething.

One tries carefully to follow the steps of the spell — to maintain and respect the balance. But there comes a point when everything is irrevocable. There is no turning back. It has been done and will be done forever. The old takes over and the instinctual desires must be fulfilled — the dreams of dark cave nights.

— opening section should be indulgent — watch out for Bound Flow and Sustainment.
— make sure to use high/right and not forward/high on weaving.
— need to work on set of three falls and rises with leg gesture — movement and effort are not right yet — maybe I should work with left/forward/deep.
— should the extension from shaping the ball be a press?
— make second thigh slap light.
— shaping the ball travels with in and out rotation of feet?

June 9: I got the second zig-zag worked out.

Good day. Took a long time but I'm getting the rough draft done — just have to work out final part. Need to put sound with first part.

I checked the rising with the leg. The wand extends right/back/high after shaping the ball and then I slide down left/forward/deep. There are chest lifts and hovers of exhorting the spirits. I rise to slap floor and spiral to ground. Then I jump up with slapping the thighs. I extend my leg and do a strong turn to slap leg and pivot for drawing the ball toward me.

June 10: Susan saw the dance today — she liked it. Said it is definitely around Spell Drive — that I really seemed possessed at the end.

— Shaping the ball needs to be more postural.
— Arm at end should writhe and move before clutching back.
— End with arms extended — no Suddenness.
— First lick of finger must be framed better.
— No vocal sounds with first part. Maybe a sound all through piece like light chimes or gurgling water in background.
— Sound ends on final looking.
— Now I can let a few quick initiations in.

June 17: Made a small change in the dance today. I wasn't happy with the climax moment when the hand grabs me and I bite it. I added a quick turn before the bite. This also helps to get me center stage which is important in terms of lights.

June 18 — First performance: What I haven't found yet is really what doing it for an audience is. With "Few Days," which I've performed before, I had been having trouble in rehearsal recapturing the feeling I had when I first did it. But when I performed it tonight and the audience was there, it was good. I found the magic again. But since it was the first time to perform "Fairy Tale," I didn't really know what my connection with the audience was. Also the audience didn't quite know what to make of the ending.

June 19 — Second performance: Lots of people from the Bureau were here tonight. I knew that. "Fairy Tale" was very good. All the Effort combinations were clearly crystallized. Especially the transition from growling to laughing was clear. Actually from biting my hand on was very strong.

Comments tonight: Someone said that the ending is very scary and asked me how I could laugh that way. Someone else thought that I had done interesting work with the Effort/Shape material and was dealing with different, new things that dance seldom deals with.

June 20 — Third performance: I feel better about my relationship with the audience. This was an in-between performance. Though better than the first night. I felt my concentrating coming and going. The hardest place to keep concentrated is in the long weaving section. The ending transitions were good though.

I got good reviews again. Someone commented on how I kept the flow going — that is something I really learned about in doing this piece — and also on my strength, which pleased me very much.

Conclusion

My main purpose in keeping this journal was to find out something about the creative process.

The first thing I found out was that you cannot predict or plan your method of working. I had thought before I started choreographing that I would sit down and write a whole series of Effort phrases, and then I would flesh the phrases out structurally in the process of crystallizing them. It didn't work out that way.

Instead I seemed to develop a kind of dialogue between structure and Effort. Usually the structure would start the conversation in a kind of improvised outburst. Gradually Effort would modulate this outburst. Together, in fits and starts and not without arguing, the two would begin to make some kind of sense in terms of the organization and meaning of the piece as a whole.

Most of the journal entries were made after my work sessions in the studio. Unfortunately I wasn't able to record in a stream of consciousness manner what really went on. It would have been helpful if I had had a tape recorder in my head. But since I didn't, my journal entries are only an abbreviation of the actual process. The dialogue between Effort and structure, between creator, editor, and critic is lost.

There is a feeling once you have finished a piece that huge sections of it just materialized. You forget the frustrating times of working one phrase over and over, of discarding old and trying new material. I choreograph straight through, from the beginning to the end of a dance. Measure 2 was hard for me. The middle (measures 25–34) was murderous. The ending was easy. I don't know why. I don't really know how I solved problems, how I knew problems were problems, how I knew when things were okay. That's what I mean when I say that whole sections just seem to have materialized. All I know is that I went to the studio and kept trying.

The other thing I know is that when I work on a piece many seemingly unrelated things in my life begin to relate to the piece. This journal seems to me to have a dream-like quality — to be full of bits and pieces of things that I came across that eventually fed the piece in some way. I thought about the piece in a non-specific way for three months. I choreographed it in only two weeks. But it was an intense two weeks because my everyday life was feeding the piece and the piece was giving me a new way of thinking about my everyday life. Even laughter had a new sound for me.

Finally I have to say something about the relationship of the piece to Effort/Shape material. I would and could not have choreographed this piece a year ago. I didn't know about the Spell Drive then. I couldn't have had all those interesting conversations between structure and dynamics then. I wouldn't have had ideas about the spatial organization of movement then. Even though I worked intuitively (meaning my particular choices were arbitrary and spontaneous), Effort/Shape gave me a grasp on what was happening. I could be specific and objective at the same time I was being random and inspirational. Creating is so slippery — Effort/Shape makes a very good handle.

* * * * *

Walking

"From that day when the baby hauls himself up off all fours and takes his first few tottery steps till the octogenarian shuffles through his final doorway, we walk. Some walk as little as they can manage, others as much as they can find time for; but we all have that unique ability to stand erect and walk on two feet. In a very real sense, man's tenancy on this planet is a consequence of his ability to travel on foot. It has been a long, long walk.

"The really great events in mankind's history, most of them recorded only in rocks and bones, were migrations of families and tribes from one place to another, and they were all accomplished on foot. The horse and the wheel, after all, are relatively new means of travel, only a few thousand years in man's service. Before that, men walked wherever they went. And they went, almost literally, to the ends of the earth . . . .

"Is the long, long walk over? Not quite, but its pace and its objectives have changed. Having asserted his tenancy by leaving his footprints on nearly all this planet's exposed land, man now has found ways to walk the mysterious depths of the oceans and has penetrated space far enough to leave fabulous footprints on the moon . . . .

"The inner necessity persists, and the memories guide us, the race memories, though we know footprints themselves are as evanescent as dew. Wind or water or grass will wipe them out. But meanwhile, we have the peculiar privilege of mankind, the freedom to walk this earth, see its beauties, taste its sweetness, partake of its enduring strength."

Hal Borland

Walking

Walking is an excellent example for analysis because, simple as it appears, it is, in fact, a complex total body action, constantly fluctuating between mobility and stability. This "natural", "automatic" activity consists of many components subject to many variations. It is at the root of all environmental shaping activities — from utilitarian explorations and measurements to playful games and dances and to symbolic spiritual rituals. It is a clear expressive statement. Even when it has minimal Effort and shape, that too is a personal expression.

Walking is not so automated that a person's gait is unchangeable. On the contrary, changing any single factor, internal or external, can change the whole statement. The terrain to which the walker adapts, the purpose of a particular walking sequence as part of one's work or leisure activity, one's inner state that urges or impedes, individual habits developed in a particular life style, the general state of neuromuscular tone, the struggle with fatigue or physical disability — all affect the quality of one's walking gait.

Two People Walking
© Bonnie Freer.

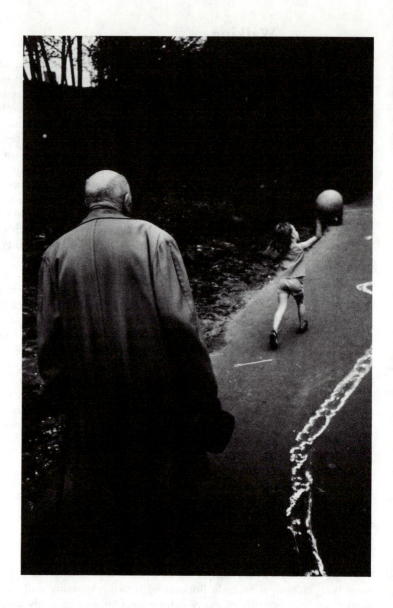

Skeletal norms or models of the structure of walking have been produced by various studies but mechanical descriptions are fragmented and incomplete. More subtle individual distinctions of qualities can be made with Labananalysis observations which include interrelationships such as limb countermovements and countertensions of the upper/lower body and their variations, the order of sequence in body parts usage, the clear distinction between the weightless phase and the graded transference of the body weight in each step. Starting from a standing position, the following factors are among those that can be observed somewhat sequentially and/or overlapping, during the walking process:

206

Breath, Effort Flow/Shape Flow.
Evenness of weight distribution.
Countertension necessary to maintain verticality.
Pelvic tilt in position of readiness.
Head–neck in position of readiness
Proximal joints in position of readiness.
Right–left weight shift involving adaptations of all above.
Beginning of asymmetry.
Rotary elements operative.
Leg freed for stepping (weightless).
Opposite arm activated.
Diagonal and its tensions.
Heel hitting floor.
Weight transfer with a spatial intent that goes beyond the actual step.
Flux more mobile in the gesture of swinging leg and more stable when the weight has been transferred.
When fluency of swing phase is very accentuated, it produces a ternary rhythm. When it becomes shorter and strongly directional, it produces a binary rhythm.
Extensive range of Effort elements and Effort combinations are possible, with Flow predominant.

A mechanical observation could define walking as a method of locomotion by the alternate use of the lower limbs in folding–unfolding patterns with transportation of the body weight in the direction of the lower limb patterns. It would describe the right–left shifts of weight and the forward–backward direction of the step. However, a spatial pattern also emerges during that process. This pattern is largely determined by the degree of fusion between the weight shift and the step direction — how much they are fused, where the emphasis is and the tensions and countertensions they produce in the body.

During the weightless phase of each step, the whole body tends toward concavity; during the weight transference phase, it goes toward a slight convexity. The degree of convex–concave change characterizes different kinds of gaits. This body shaping, occurring in the sagittal plane, is the beginning of spatial shaping.

The toddler's gait is an extreme example of a lack of fusion since it is mainly right–left weight shift. The sailor's gait is another example. In both cases, they cling to the vertical plane for stability, while pursuing and resisting the continuity pull of the sagittal plane with great caution. The spatial shaping is, consequently, minimal.

When the horizontal component — often overlooked — is incorporated into the normal walking process, shaping possibilities are extended with both grace and power. When all the factors are utilized most expansively, the activity can become running or leaping or dancing or skillful sports activities.

The 18th century ballet master, Feuillet, recognized the importance of the weight–weightless relationship as clues to the character and rhythm of dance steps and Laban incorporated those insights into his own studies.

Many skills are elaborations of walking that are adapted to special environmental conditions or to expressions of playfulness and daring, as, for example, skating and skiing, or walking on ice and snow with props. All stimulate new Effort and shape adaptations that can become dance on ice or dramatic ski jumps on mountains. Surfing is riding and walking the waves, with particular mobility–stability adaptations to the mobility of a liquid medium.

While upright walking is considered one of man's unique achievements in the animal world, man still retains the ability to use patterns that stem from his animal inheritance. He/she can still lie on the floor on his/her back and make his/her way, wriggling along either headward or footward in serpentine undulations or in various forms and levels of crawling and creeping, using all four limbs. The order in which the four limbs are used later in upright carriage is gradually established during this very important level of a child's development. How upper and lower limbs combine in a contralateral right–left relationship leads to the later fusion of right–left with forward progression in upright walking. This exploratory creeping period is also closely related to integration of vision with space awareness and body part use, also crucial to upright walking and adaptations to the environment. Thus, for example, one can creep under a low fence, squat, shrinking the whole body, amble through a low doorway or walk on one hand and hip, squeezing through a narrow opening sideways. With increasing awareness of the body's three-dimensionality in relation to the environment's multilevels and directions, patterns from all developmental stages can be selected to explore the ranges of a whole territory with walking, running, leaping in all directions and, finally, falling to the floor, continuing progression, creeping, crawling and emerging again into full height in walking and running progressions.

Stilt walking appears in many cultures, playing with an extension of the body, again with new forms of progression and balance, transforming it into a superhuman gestalt. Primitive forms of magic power are evoked as in the stilt dance of the Masai, a walking dance on very high stilts, one to a person. It is used as a preparation for the dangerous adventure of the lion hunt. The superhuman aspect of extended height still reverberates in the Greek chorus walking on stilts and the Japanese theater, where high-heeled wooden platform shoes are used, not just to enhance visibility to the audience, but to lift the action of walking to an extraordinary level. Extended height games of walking are daring, challenging balance games for children in all cultures.

Walking is ritualized in various forms of getting together, such as file or row formations for communal meetings — funerals, weddings or coronations or common allegiance to a new leader. Supported and reinforced by music, certain rhythms of walking are produced that are appropriate to the occasion. Steps are prescribed, Effort combinations are implied. The "spring" processions, for example, two steps forward, one spring back, evoke a penitential or a joyous celebratory mood, depending on the Effort combinations involved.

The level of uprightness is also significant. Lowering oneself to the level of crawling creatures may indicate the subterranean, demonic levels of men. Approaching a person of greater power or social rank with a reduced level of height conveys humility, submission.

Some processions extend the communal space by their walking progression as when images and shrines are taken from their temples and churches and carried through a city or village. Walking outside the sanctuary reaffirms the sanctity and physical shape of the territory. In ceremonies that precede the building of a sanctuary, walking in a square or circle to lay out the space defines the relation of the sanctuary to the cardinal points of the sky, where the sun rises and sets. Here, by its space–extension quality, walking becomes a measure; the length of a step is a basic unit in medieval architecture. (Even earlier, the human body was furnishing basic measure units: Elbow/forearm or a walking step.)

From such walking and trotting rituals, the beginning of dance emerged, as, for example, when two files of men would trot one behind the other with a specified number of steps, turning and repeating, establishing a rhythm, a design.

The range of everyday, "normal" walking variations seems to be infinite. For one informal study, we observed people walking in a railroad station, all of them engaged in similar sequences of activity — catching or emerging from a train, buying tickets, newspapers, refreshments, looking at time schedules, waiting around. But each person was "doing his own thing" within that framework. Their walking patterns revealed sharp glimpses into the different ways that the people organized and expressed themselves, their particular attitudes, not just toward the activity, but to themselves and others in the whole context.

Walking in a Railroad Station

Without a purpose: An elderly man walks by; his whole body seems inert, but held together by Bound Flow: both his arms are hanging down but locked in Bound Flow. He walks in an even tempo with no fluctuation. His trunk is somewhat telescoped in inertness (Neutral Flow); the legs are slightly bent with little variation throughout. There is an automaton quality about him, just going on and on, hardly any change in body form or Effort variations; his face is almost without any expression.

Somewhat fragmented: A woman, middle-aged, stands in the middle of the round ticket plaza. She makes a few small steps, stops and studies some pamphlets, walking again a few steps, pausing while continuing her bending slightly over her readings with a Bound Directness releasing into Neutrality. Her arms/hands holding the pamphlets appear separated from the rest of the body. The steps, initiated from the lower legs, also seem disconnected from the rest of the body. As she notices a porter walking with an empty carriage, she walks with a sudden start toward him. The body is still rigid while the arms move in a rowing contralateral rhythm, Free Flow, immediately Bound/Strong, which shifts the pelvis somewhat from right to left while she steps, still mainly initiating from lower leg, with the heels hitting the floor with Sudden/Bound accents.

Taking things in his stride: The porter she is addressing is a portly, middle-aged man, clearly using his body weight. In each step, the right–left shift of the weight is markedly accentuated in the pelvis–hip and the external rotation of the whole leg, with the feet everted in the process. The upper body, as he holds the cart with his hands, rotates in the opposite direction of the lower body. In each step are clear fluctuations of Free/Bound Flow with Strength accents and very fast fluctuations between Sudden and Sustained that reverberate through the whole body.

Preoccupied: A man in his fifties walks in long, straight steps in a pattern of Direct/Neutral Flow going into Sustainment/Bound Flow (Weightless Drive). His body progresses evenly. He is slightly leaning forward, his upper body and head are rigidly held, the chest hollow and the shoulders hunched up in a frozen concavity.

A clown: A young adolescent of small stature rushes toward a train gate. In a bilateral, low, spreading gesture of his arms, he keeps the upper trunk in a rigidly Bound state as he progresses — half slides — over the floor. Initiated from the lower leg, Flow spreads into the pelvic hip. In each step, he slaps the foot down with exaggerated Suddenness and some Strength — a kind of grotesque, exhibitionist performance.

Dancing together while waiting: A young couple, both tall, slim and long-legged, casually stroll back and forth in a small place before the benches. They develop a swingy rhythm, stepping towards each other and away. Though not quite in synchrony, a common rhythmical pattern forms between the two. Both initiate each step from the pelvis–hip with slight Sudden/Free Flow extending into the step while smoothly transferring body weight from stable legs to swinging legs and, immediately, when they meet, getting into Free Flow, Light/Strong variations of right–left shifts in place, the man leaning slightly toward the woman, decelerating on his last meeting step as he puts down his whole foot and slowly transfers his weight. A pause, and then they resume the game of tender, teasing reciprocal rhythm.

What is she up to? A young woman in her thirties, walking between two vigorous-looking young men. She progresses in a wide stride, long straight steps, jerkily initiating from her hip–pelvis, with the upper body rather rigid, swinging the leg forward with Free/Bound/Strength, slapping the foot down with Free/Suddenness immediately turning Bound/Strength with an additional Sudden pressure into the floor. This is accompanied by accentuated contralateral arm swing with Free/Bound/Strength/Suddenness. The face is taut, the lips pressed together, the eyes wide open in an exaggerated stare. Is it the fury of keeping up with the two men?

*   *   *   *   *

Cultural Patterns

Cultural patterns in walking have been explored in crosscultural studies of gaits. These studies are still at elementary levels of research and should be perused with caution lest they result in stereotypes. Perception of individual differences requires greater skill and refinement in observation and the many variables in age, environment, temperament, occupation, etc., have to be correlated with available materials.

One preliminary study compared gaits of four cultural groups: Caucasian-Americans, Afro-Americans, Japanese and East Indians. The subjects were observed in terms of body attitude, verticality, chest, pelvis, arms, relation to floor, initiation, gesture, touch on floor, brief moment when both feet on floor share weight, full transfer, rebound (sometimes more than one). Brief summaries of the results of detailed observation (see following chart) of these factors indicate some of the distinctions that emerged:

Japan: In general, women and men show tendency toward narrowing the upper body, subtle use of pelvic shift and rotation. Frequent peripheral use of arms–legs. Flow varies between Free and Bound with a preponderance of Bound. Effort tendencies toward Light Weight, Bound Flow and Direct Space.

India: Extremely fluent blending of phases. Serpentine/diagonal shaping in the body. Subtle changes in Effort: Small rapid fluctuations between Sudden and Sustained Time; Strong/Light Weight. Clear stress on rotation in hip/shoulder/waist. The use of the rotary element is somewhat less stressed by the men but clearly identifiable in hip and shoulder.

Afro-American: Phases are blended through the dominance of Flow with a preference for Free Flow and Shape Flow. Clear use of all articulations. Shoulders, elbows, wrists, hips, knee angles. Rotary use of upper body against lower. Main Effort combinations of Flow, Time and Weight.

Caucasian-American: Phases are frequently slurred together by abrupt Flow changes and dominance of Efforts: Strong Weight, Sudden Time and, sometimes, Direct Space. Pelvis frequently rigid.

Such studies, re-evaluated and modified by constant observation, keep one aware of the great range of human variations. In such a common activity as walking, Labananalysis can refine the observations so that rigid schemata, superficial generalizations, and cultural cliches are minimized and the variations of behavior can be viewed as rich attributes of human aliveness, expressing both extremes and subtleties of feeling.

Preliminary Crosscultural Gait Study

Notes: In details of gesture, floor touch, double support, full transfer, and rebounds, the degree of distinctions between them varies with the degree of blending that occurs during the action.

In the descriptions given below, only India shows particular male/female differences because there was a female available for the study. All the other observations were of males only.

Japan

Body Attitude Changes in Walking

Body Attitude, Verticality:	Almost always slightly inclined forward/high with chest slightly narrowed and shoulder slightly drooping. Only minor changes in body attitude
Chest:	Slightly narrowed in the upper part. Individuals vary
Pelvis:	Controlled mobility. (Moves, but with Bound Flow)
Arm/Leg Contralaterality:	Upper arms usually controlled except for very vigorous walking. Usually forearm/hand countermovements
Relation to Floor:	Scanning the floor. (Peripheral use of lower leg/foot)
Initiation:	A right step starts with a pelvic/hip shift to the left, emphasizing a slight narrowing around the front of the pelvis (pubic region), but no rotation
Gesture:	Starts around right anterior superior spine with some continued narrowing of lower abdomen; the hip is slightly flexed, spreading into knee flexion/extension, which starts the unfolding of the lower leg
Floor Touch and Double Support (of Weight) and Full Transfer:	Heel/toe come almost simultaneously down, blending into double support with Bound Flow that keeps increasing into full transfer, with no increased pressure into the floor
Rebound:	No actual rebound but immediate preparing for left step (see Initiation)

Note: In general, the steps are small and the same kind of blending of floor touch, double support, full transfer was observed in sailors and, in an even higher degree, in Noh dancing, where the pattern is seen with greater refinement.

India

Body Attitude Changes in Walking

Body Attitude, Verticality:		Vertical with some stress on contralaterality, i.e., diagonal in body
	Male:	Verticality clearly increased in weight shift
	Female:	Verticality slightly increased in weight shift, diagonal in body increased in weight shift
Chest:	Male:	Open, shoulders free
	Female:	Open with accentuated contralateral use of shoulder
Pelvis:	Male:	Mobile with controlled Free/Bound changes in Flow
	Female:	Extremely mobile with emphasis on Free Flow and successiveness in lower back/pelvis/hip
Arm/Leg Contralaterality:	Male:	Clear contralaterality of shoulder, upper chest, diminished in opposite pelvis/hip
	Female:	Marked contralaterality, spilling from shoulder into arm and into torso opposite pelvis/hip; marked use of rotation in upper and lower limb
Relation to Floor:		Serpentine adaptation to floor, somewhat more flat in the male, clearly winding in the female. Neither scanning or digging into the floor
Initiation:	Male:	Pelvis shifts laterally with some inward rotation and support from below
	Female:	Lateral shift of pelvis with marked lateral displacement of pelvis/hip spreading diagonally into the left shoulder
Gesture and Floor Touch:	Male:	Starts with hip flexion and slight knee flexion, swinging the whole leg forward into extension with increased external rotation/Free Flow which is somewhat neutralized just before touching the floor with a slightly everted foot
	Female:	Starts with successive hip/knee flexion and slight acceleration, extends through the leg, though not fully externally rotating. Shaping with Indirectness into a serpentine gesture touching the floor with marked eversion of the foot
Double Support of Weight and Full Transfer and Rebound:	Male:	With a clear acceleration and small fluctuations into Free/Bound Flow, the three phases of weight transference are completed with some reverberation in the opposite shoulder/upper chest and with graded deceleration
	Female:	Transference of weight is blended with the serpentine gesture in a very graded curved successive transference with marked emphasis on hip and upper body, shoulder contralaterality, and small graded changes in acceleration/deceleration

Afro-American

Body Attitude Changes in Walking

Body Attitude, Verticality: Clear mobile verticality, often associated with exaggerated curves of spine (sagittal)

Chest: Open, mobile, raised and sinking in rhythmical changes

Pelvis: Mobile in either sagittal or horizontal cycling. Chest/pelvis frequently in opposition: Upper horizontal, lower sagittal cycles

Arm/Leg Contralaterality: All articulations from shoulder on are used successively, shoulder initiating

Relation to Floor: Mobile use of either digging into or scanning floor

Initiation: Clear lateral shift of whole pelvis/hip to the left (for a right step), frequently also involving internal rotation of right hip

Gesture and Floor Touch and Double Support and Full Transfer and Rebound: Whole leg flexing clearly at hip/pelvis with some flexion of the knee occurring. Whole leg fluently extends — not always fully — with small fluctuations of Free Flow and some acceleration, touching with heel and immediately placing whole foot down with gradual acceleration continuing into full transference, sometimes with slight acceleration and diminished strength. At the end of this phase, Free Flow, blending into rebound with slight acceleration of knee/toe push-off from left leg to Boundness, frequently immediately starting a left pelvic shift for the preparation of the left step

Caucasian/American

Body Attitude Changes in Walking

Body Attitude, Verticality: Many variations from stiff verticality to rigid or collapsed concavity; average is neutral erect

Chest: Many variations. In general, neutral

Pelvis: Little participation, in general

Arm/Leg Contralaterality: Either little use or mild swing or active rowing (pushing/pulling)

Relation to Floor: Pressing into the floor and pushing off

Initiation: From front of pelvis, with slight narrowing around anterior superior spine/lower abdomen. (Sometimes increased tension in upper abdomen below ribs.) Lateral shifts of weight with little participation of lateral/pelvic portions

Gesture: Bending at hip and knee almost simultaneously, the leg is extended with slight acceleration

Floor Touch: Touching the floor with the heel

Double Support and Full Transfer and Rebound: Either immediately starting to press (Strength and Bound Flow) with the hip internally rotating. Increasing pressure into the floor while maintaining internal rotation of right hip. As left leg begins to externally rotate for push-off from the floor in a left step

(Variation) Rebound II, Energetic Walking: Frequently a short increase in downward pressure (Strength), followed by a Sudden/Bound push-off of the left leg as preparation for a left step

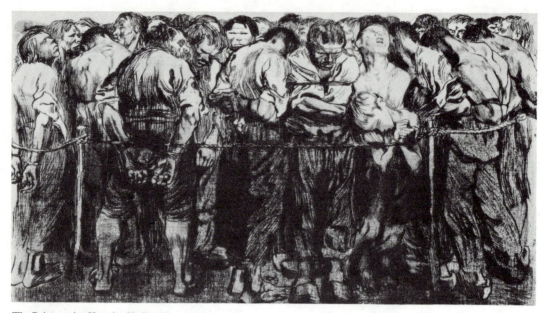

The Prisoners by Kaethe Kollwitz.

Pieter Breughel the Elder, *The Harvesters*. Courtesy of Metropolitan Museum of Art.

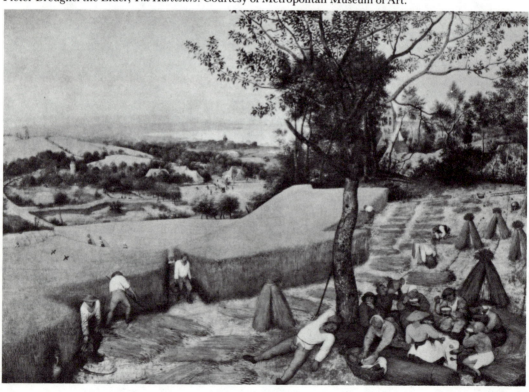

Epilogue

Rudolf Laban himself was an example of how the human body's way of translating our way of life into pure motion is reflected in the person's reasoning and behavior. When he looks at the world and speaks about it, all the petty intricacies of our usual existence drop out, the nooks and crannies are straightened, the light sweeps unhampered along generous perspectives, the eyes face a simply shaped distant goal, and the visions and thoughts and actions move to attain it.

Rudolf Arnheim

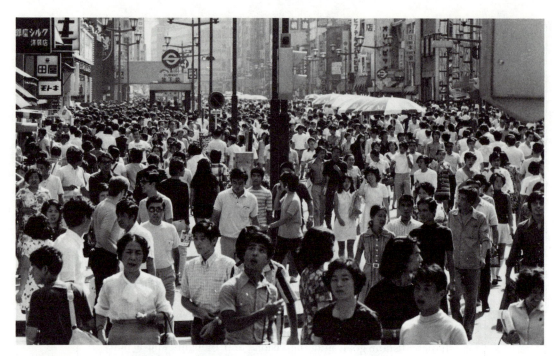

Rush Hour in Japan Courtesy of United Nations.

Brazil Pier © Bernard P. Wolff.

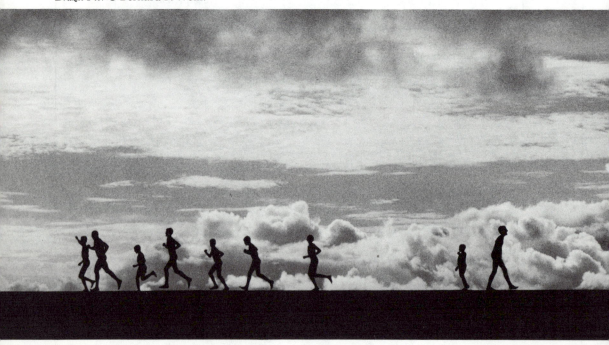

Appendix A
Documenting Observations:
Notation and Methodology

Movement events . . . can be rendered in movement notation with more exactitude than when they are described in words. A skilled reader of movement notation can not only understand what the body of the dancer does, he can (also) shudder or smile on deciphering the mental and emotional content of the symbols. Just as a skilled musician is able to hear with the inner ear the melody as he scans it in a musical score, so a skilled dancer can see with his inner eye the movements of the human body while reading the dance notation. . . .

A notation based on the combination of motion characters makes it possible to write down all styles of dance . . . Every style uses movements built up from the same motor elements. The variety of movement which can be built up from them is almost infinite, and any style with a limited number of variations, whether self-imposed or traditional, must of necessity build its movement forms out of these basic constituents of movement. . . .

One has to show in a notated dance which part of the body has been moved and its position after it has moved . . . the precise time taken for each movement has to be recorded. But all this must be done in such a way that the essential feature of a dance, namely, its flow of movement, is described in all its detail.

Rudolf Laban

Appendix A
Documentation of Observations: Notation and Methodology

From the earliest stages of Laban's work, he began to develop means of recording his perceptions in symbolic as well as verbal terms. Eventually, he and his colleagues developed a notation system that many believe surpasses verbal descriptions of movement events because the symbols immediately convey — to skilled notators — the structure and progression of the movement. The notation system records variations of body usage and as new variations continue to be observed, new ways are found to incorporate them. Choices of notation are made for use in specific research — often in combination with verbal and/or filmed documentation as well.

Albrecht Knust and, later, Ann Hutchinson, one of the founders of the Dance Notation Bureau in New York, developed and published the most comprehensive research in notation and are preparing more. Their published works are listed in the Bibliography, along with contributions by others.

Muriel Topaz, current director of the Dance Notation Bureau in New York, has, in addition to her own research and development in notation, continued to organize and develop the Bureau's collection of notated scores for some two hundred works by seventy-five choreographers. These are available to reconstructors, with the approval of the choreographer. The Bureau has also published a volume of three Doris Humphrey works scored in Labanotation.

The skills of symbolic notation require highly precise and refined observation — at its best, a reflection of extraordinary movement experience empathy. Notating movement is not simply a mechanical procedure; recording should reflect movement experience itself as in Laban's initial conception.

The symbols were not arbitrarily chosen. The genius of their simplicity is seen in the *relationship* of individual symbols which clearly expressed Laban's perception and principles of body movement. Laban considered Feuillet a master of symbolic writing because, through his symbols, one could also perceive principles. Feuillet's notation, for example, by indicating the basic trace forms of gestures of the leg, could communicate the principle of exact transference of weight in stepping.

Dramatic impact and expressive meaning of movements are sustained by the order in which the symbols appear. By contrast, word description of an event often loses the contextual framework in overcrowded enumerations of details so that, by the end, coherence is lost to apparent ambivalences.

The symbols themselves, when contextually understood, are direct representations of which part of the body does what in space and time and with what kind of dynamic stress. The skilled notator can identify the rhythms and body–spatial tensions within the movements; these are keys to the expressive content. This distinguishes Labanotation from most other movement systems that are essentially position indicators of the human figure (such as Benesh) or define movement in terms of joint angles (as in Eshkol); or choose numbers, letters or other abstractions that have no graphic or other connection to the process of movement (as in Conté); or use stick figures as a kind of memory aid to visible body–limb configurations, representing positions primarily (as in Zorn).

Labanotation can show with one symbol where the body is moving in space, what part of the body is moving, when the move is to be made and how long it takes to complete the movement. By its distribution on the staff, it will indicate the changes in weight distribution and the sequence of the movement. Additional small indicators show refinements and specificities. From a properly notated movement sequence, the skilled reader can see at one glance what is happening at any moment in every part of the body: whether limbs and trunk act in synchrony or overlap in time; or how several rhythmical–spatial events may go on at the same time in different parts of the body.

The staff consists of three basic vertical lines which represent the body's center and its left and right sides. It is read from the bottom up. The placement of a symbol shows where a specific body part is active. Its shape indicates the direction of the movement, its shading shows the level and its length, the duration of the movement.

Samples of a few individual Labanotation symbols are shown on the next pages and following that is a simple example of basic step notation and a more complex example from a notated dance.

There are hundreds of additional possibilities that provide the possibility for extraordinary expression in recording. (See Bibliography.)

Notation Primer

The Staff and Indications for Placement of Body Part Symbol

Center

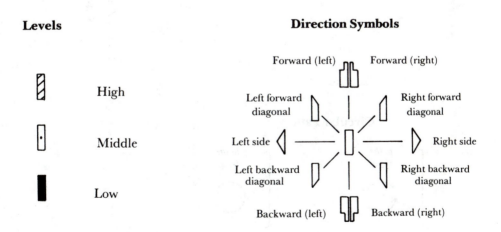

Left arm
Body
Left-leg gesture
Left support
Right support
Right-leg gesture
Body
Right arm

LEFT   RIGHT

Levels

High

Middle

Low

Direction Symbols

Forward (left)   Forward (right)

Left forward diagonal   Right forward diagonal

Left side   Right side

Left backward diagonal   Right backward diagonal

Backward (left)   Backward (right)

219

Time Duration

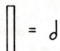

▯	= 𝅗𝅥
▯	= ♩
▯	= ♪
▯	= ♬

Measure

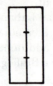

*A measure
of 3/4 time*

Turns

*Turn to right on
right foot*

*Turn to left on
left foot*

Approximately

Degree of Turn

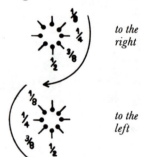

*to the
right*

*to the
left*

Circular Path

*to the
right*

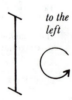

*to the
left*

The Body Signs

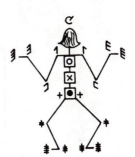

Foot Usage

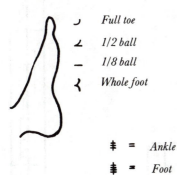

⌐	*Full toe*
⌐	*1/2 ball*
—	*1/8 ball*
⌐	*Whole foot*

‡ = *Ankle*

‡ = *Foot*

Gender

⊥ = *Man*

⊥ = *Woman*

Step Example

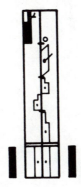

Sample: Reading up from the bottom, one sees the basic position of neutral standing with feet together, arms hanging down. Then right–forward step, middle level to a quarter note, followed by left, right forward steps, middle level as two eighth notes, followed by one-eighth turn to right, held, while left leg touches floor with the ball of the foot.

Basic Folk Dance Rhythms

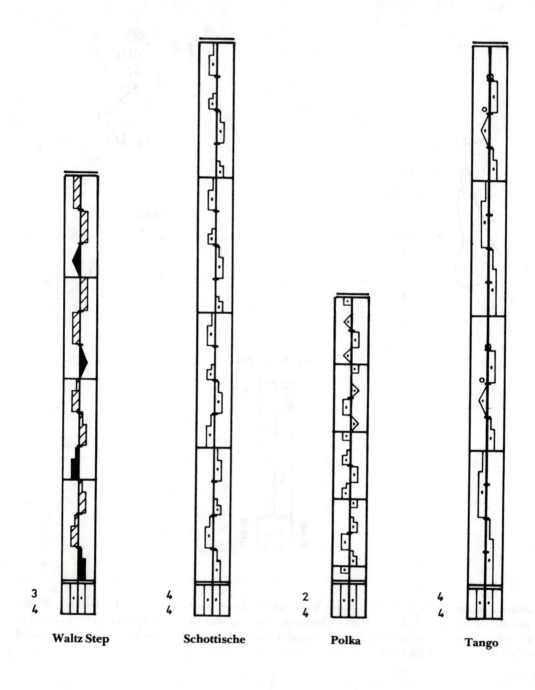

Waltz Step	Schottische	Polka	Tango
3/4	4/4	2/4	4/4

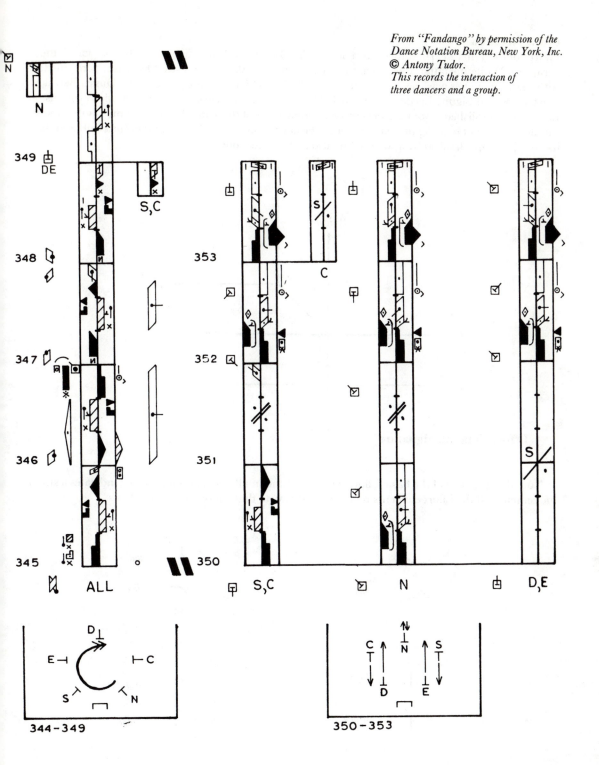

349 DE

348

347

346

345 ALL

N

S,C

353

352

351

350 S,C

C

N

D,E

344–349

350–353

223

Effort Notation

Effort notation (in its earliest theoretical form called Eukinetics) complements Labanotation (Kinetography). While the latter asks "What is the movement?" the former asks, "How is it performed?" Although Eukinetics was used as early as the 1920s by Laban and his collaborators, Dussia Bereska, Kurt Jooss and Sigurd Leeder, it was in 1947, with A.C. Lawrence, that the definitive symbols of Effort were published. From the deceptively simple basis of the symbol below, all the combinations can be rapidly notated. Again, the logic of the visualization process is captured in the symbol so that it is not just a mechanical transaction, but also a conceptual one.

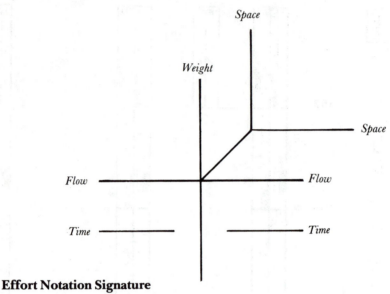

Effort Notation Signature

Note that the start of the basic Effort signature is the small diagonal sign / which indicates a stir of movement. All the Effort elements relate in some way to that stir of movement. Thus:

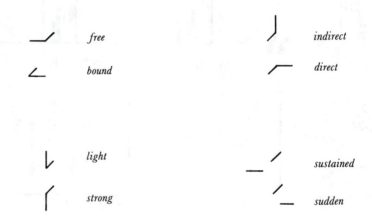

224

The addition of a line parallel to the small diagonal sign will indicate the shaping affinities. (See Warren Lamb in Bibliography.)

There is no fixed staff in Effort notation. It can be written horizontally as are letters, or it can be written outside a Labanotation score.

An overview can be perceived as shown below: Left of the diagonal — Indirect (Space), Light (Weight), Free (Flow), Sustained (Time) — are of a low intensity, spreading out, indulgent quality. Right of the diagonal — Direct (Space), Strong (Weight), Bound (Flow), Sudden (Time) — are of high intensity, condensing or fighting quality.

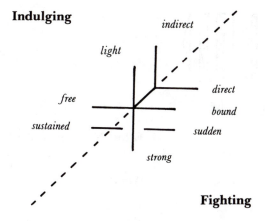

Labanotation and Effort/Shape Notation

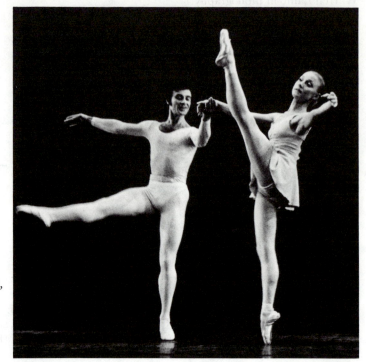

Duet from Antony Tudor's "Continuo"
© Robert Lorenz/Main Street
Photography.
The dancers are Anthony and
Sirpa Salatino of the Syracuse
Ballet Theatre.

Labanotation

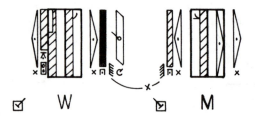

Effort Notation of the Arrested Movement

Woman   Man

Labanotation and Effort/Shape Notation

To a trained Laban notator, the Labanotation alone would include all the following information:

W (woman): she stands on her right leg on point. Her left leg is pointing forward–high.
Her trunk is tilted back high with the head slightly turned to the left.
Both arms are spread to the side at shoulder height and slightly flexed with the palm facing the floor.
Her right hand grasps the left hand of her partner from above.
M (man): he stands on his left leg raised on his forefoot.
His right leg is extended to the right at hip level.
Both arms are extended to the side at shoulder level and are slightly flexed, the left one slightly more than the right.
His trunk is straight and vertically balanced over the left leg.
His left hand touches the woman's right hand at slight diagonal angle with the palm facing up.

If Effort notation was added, as shown, the additional information about the quality of the movement would be communicated:

Woman: Light/Direct/Bound Flow
Man: Strong/Direct/Bound

The combination of Force/Space/Flow reflects the Spell Transformation Drive (Timeless) when the photograph was taken.

Methodology

The structural concepts of Labanotation and the qualitative vocabulary of Effort have stimulated new insights into movement documentation possibilities. Other selective adaptations of the notation describe more general, rather than specific aspects, such as motifs. Other kinds of symbolic recording and verbal coding sheets, rating scales and checkoff scales can be derived from notated observations.

The choice of documentation reflects the focus of the observer for a particular event. There are some differences of opinion about which selections or methods are most appropriate for different tasks and discussions continue among Laban's colleagues and followers to establish the most precise vocabulary.

It is important to acquire some speed in both observation and notation, particularly with regard to the initiation of movement, the transitions, variations in Effort and shape, fluctuations of Flow — all of which are critical to the observation of the sequence of an event. Even for the most skilled observers it is not possible to completely record in detail the speed of every event. But, they can observe the consistency with which certain combinations or transitions or initiations appear in the movement, and can then identify what is most "characteristic" of the movement.

A teacher or director can use the Laban methodology to specifically identify weak areas in a performance. The objective vocabulary frees the teacher from total dependence on his/her personal verbal and body language abilities to communicate how a body part should move, what the rhythmical accents are, and how the dynamics vary. As the behavioral scientists look more and more at body movement, they, too, are incorporating the vocabulary into their methodologies.

The Use of Film

Until recently, film was mainly used as a tool for documentation in anthropology and related disciplines for archival purposes and illustrations to record and supplement the experiences of field workers. It is increasingly used now for specific comparative research. The Choreometrics project, for example, was based entirely on existing film with all its advantages and disadvantages. When, however, focus on differentiating features of movement became more critical, the necessity arose for more specific shooting requirements, such as selection of items, length of shots, quality of light, and continuity of the event to be studied.

The special filming required for movement analysis is not always feasible within the total framework of other specific research goals. Therefore, the movement specialist is often dependent on the selections made for a study which may deal with movement in only a very marginal way. As a result, there may be concentration on just body parts instead of the whole figure: face, hands, step pattern, or the camera may shift in the middle of a movement sequence or there may be great distortion of the three-dimensionality of the movement because of light or distance. When it comes to studying choreographic sequence, it is extremely rare, even in a very good film, to have the whole event filmed in its entirety.

The state-supported folklorists in Central Europe are fortunate in being able to make films tailored to the needs of the notator who does the main work of notation and study after returning from field work. The notated script, kinetogram, and the film complement each other for the permanent record.

Helen Priest Rogers, an early American Labanotator, was the first who filmed — for the purpose of notation — a number of works by Doris Humphrey, Charles Weidman and José Limòn at the Connecticut Dance Festivals in the late forties and fifties.

Live performance has one disadvantage over film for observation purposes: The observer has only one chance to see absolutely precisely because repetitions of a sequence are never exactly the same in either a structured dance or sport sequence or a spontaneous gesture. However, since certain qualities and quality combinations reoccur in repetitive performance of a sequence, it is possible to identify single elements and combinations though transitions and combinations may vary.

Although film and video performance has the advantage of endless repetition without change, there can be distortion in the qualitative aspects — Effort — and in the three-dimensionality of movement. The distortions of Effort are the worst, especially in Weight and Flow changes. Severe distortions of the Time Effort occur especially in those films made before the 1/24 per second frame speed was established. Effort cannot be studied from film by slowing down the film. It is in the nature of Effort that it is only observable for its dynamic constellation in its natural rhythmical context at the actual speed of the event.

Appendix B
Bartenieff Fundamentals

Don't think of back bending but think 'Your head leads into backward arc towards the floor. . . .!'

. . .

Space imagination (intent) and spatial power (spatial initiation) enliven the muscle, transmit the intent to move skeletal parts . . . When we look at the expression of a pulling muscle, we see that the smallest quiver is as significant as the largest leverlike movement . . . The lifting of skeletal parts to perform a working or expressive action always makes the purpose of the muscle movement visible.

The skeleton virtually outlines in both its utilitarian and expressive movements the edges and inclinations of an invisible space crystal. This space crystal is the medium into which the tension man is built . . . The form of things speaks of the movement that created that form or has crystallized into 'intent' . . .

Only when we recognize . . . in which way the . . . realization of the . . . universal order of these crystallizations is supported and carried through will we get a glimmer of the true live idea or intent in a single movement.

Rudolf Laban

A Note About Performance of Preparatory Exercises and Bartenieff Fundamentals

Obviously, you will not absorb or experience all the exercise factors on your first attempt. Go through the motions. Each time, you will add some awareness to the experience and eventually you will not need the book guidelines or the illustrations and anatomical drawings except as a check list. Take the time to explore your experience by trying to focus on different aspects with each repetition.

We frequently observe in teaching choreutics that beginning students, who have been taught body movement mainly by imitation with emphasis on body parts and muscular tension, have difficulty with spatial exploration, that is, spatial intent. This is manifested, for instance, when they are given a task such as reaching and exploring the areas around the body with the arms, particularly in back of the body. They may go into awkward contortions of flexions, extensions, adductions, exclaiming, "I cannot get there, I am stuck." Sometimes the teacher must manipulate the rotary element and direct the arm into a new direction so the student can find a releasing action into the back area. The amazement is always great when these "new" spatial options, usually the rotary elements, are experienced after the students had tried "so hard" with only muscle–joint focus (flexion–extension) without success.

The lower unit — so crucial to weight shift and centering the whole body at any moment — always affects the upper unit and vice versa. The basic exercises, therefore, always stress the diagonal connections between lower and upper units and the changing shapes of the whole spine from base of skull to coccyx in the sequences within progressions from low on the floor to walking through the hands and up.

What is important is to reawaken your awareness of muscles and joints that are not used, used inadequately or misused so that you can extend your movement possibilities in both energy and expressiveness.

Most of the six basic exercises on the floor are simple lifting and lowering, flexing and extending of limbs or segments of limbs or trunk. Concentration is on articulation and internal physiological changes. To get the "feel" of these functional actions, they are performed with minimum Effort and space — that is, primarily Effort Flow and Shape Flow changes. However, as the exercises become more complex, Effort and spatial shaping factors begin to crystallize and become increasingly important for adequate performance of the actions.

Preparatory Exercise A
Flexion–Extension; Abduction–Adduction; Internal–External Rotation

These muscle actions all have to do with changing the angles of joints, that is, diminishing or increasing angles. They are defined for every joint in the body in its own plane range. All movements of the legs and arms are combinations of joint movements offering wide ranges of movement possibility. The exercise below will help you experience their distinctions. Flexion–extension moves in the sagittal (forward–backward) plane; abduction–adduction moves in the vertical (frontal) plane going away from or toward the vertical midline; internal–external rotation moves in the horizontal plane.

1. Stand with arms hanging down in a neutral position.
2. Raise an arm forward and swing it backward. You are flexing at the shoulder and possibly the elbow when going forward and extending when going backward. The movement is in the sagittal cycle and is controlled at the shoulder joint.
3. Swing your arm from side flat across your front to side. You are moving in the vertical cycle, again with shoulder joint control: Abducting at the side; adducting on the across.
4. From position No. 1, rotate the arm toward the body and away from the body. Watch the circle your hand is traveling in — a horizontal cycle around a vertical axis. The internal–external rotation range is the smallest of the three ranges in terms of its path in space, but not necessarily in terms of its contribution to movement at the joint.

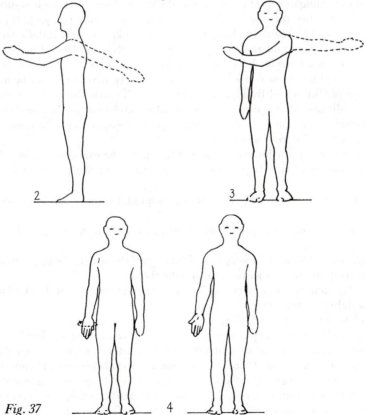

Fig. 37

231

Preparatory Exercise B
BREATH

The Use of Vowels in Control of Breath (Inner Space)

Effort and Shape Flow has been discussed as part of a growing and shrinking process which accompanies the two phases of breathing: in (full, growing) and out (empty, shrinking). This growing–shrinking process — inwardly felt and outwardly visible — also heightens awareness of the center of the body around which the process revolves.

Movement rides on the flow of the breath. Frequently, students in their overconscientiousness about breathing or negation of breath will tend to hold the breath at one part of the phase — either on the "in" or the "out." By doing this, they forego the many subtle inner shape changes in the cavities (mouth, chest, abdomen) of the body and fine gradations of changes that occur in different configurations of limbs, trunk, head. They also forego many subtleties in phrasing. "Taking a deep breath," with focus only on the goal of fullness in inhaling inhibits movement if the total body process is neglected. Depth and rate of breath adapt in rhythmic spatial patterns according to the scope and intensity of our actions, emphasizing at one time the lower cavity, at another, upper cavities, or the whole "inner" space of both which also includes mouth and nose, where the stream of air entering and leaving is further shaped.

In the "in" and "out" phases, we experience greater convexity or concavity of the torso in different degrees toward extending or rounding–flexing of the trunk. These more or less subtle changes in the inner cavities — even when they are hardly visible outwardly — play a major part in maintaining and varying uprightness; they regulate changes in the musculature, and inflationary or deflationary inside pressures in the front and along the spine between pelvis and base of the skull.

Making sounds, when lying or sitting or standing, reinforces the awareness of the stream or breath supporting the straightening or rounding of the different segments of the spine in all positions and levels. A number of Hindu and Buddhistic (particularly, Tantric Buddhism) meditation and inner concentration traditions involve inner and outer body shape changes by using definite vowels and sequences of vowels for support of different inner spaces — abdomen, chest, mouth. These sounds cause reverberations in different segments.

For example, starting at the lowest segment of the spine, the sound *oooooo*, as in "you," maintains the deepest descension of the diaphragm, reverberating into the pelvis–lower abdomen (pubic region).

The sound *oh*, extended as in "oh," reverberates around the navel and the corresponding segment of the spine.

The sound *aah*, extended as in "yoga," reverberates around and opens up the lateral portions of the lower ribs.

The sound *eeh*, extended as at the very end of "say," reverberates in the upper middle portion of the sternum and corresponding ribs without raising the shoulders.

The sound *iiih*, extended as in "meeting," reverberates at the base of the skull and in front of the throat unless a tight chin muscle prevents this.

The pitches have individual variations.

The sequence and frequency of practice of these breath vowel exercises should be varied according to the tension–relaxation state of the student. It is often desirable to start on the floor where the awareness of tension–relaxation of the lumbar spine and the abdomen can be most easily perceived. Starting with the *oooooo* and going to the *oh* and the *aah* may take quite a while and needs practice in conjunction with the lower unit exercises. You can then go to the *aah* for the lower ribs. Then practice the three sounds as a sequence *oooooo-oh-aah*, sitting on the floor in either lotus or the asymmetrical sitting position with both knees to one side, practicing on either side.

The next step is practicing — first separately, then in sequence — the sound *eeh* and the sequence *oooooo-oh-aah-eeh*. Do the same for the sound *iiih* separately and in the whole sequence *oooooo-oh-aah-eeh-iiih*.

As you experience increasing ease in maintaining uprightness, with your head "floating" on the top of the noncompressed spine, the whole practice should then switch to only practice while sitting and, instead of making these sound sequences, concentrate silently on "shaping" each sound without making it audible.

Several other factors that should guide graded practice of these sequences are:

1. Initiating the sound: When first practicing the sound *oooooo*, try to avoid localizing the production of the sound in your mouth and throat. That localization often arises from tensions in the upper neck, throat muscles, upper shoulders and, especially, the chin "pushing" downward. Instead of forcing the initiation of the sound from such localized areas, start with a gentle humming of "m-m-m-m" and gradually let it slide into a *oooooo*, evoking the image of the inside of a bell.

2. Maintaining the sound: Here, again, do not force. With the *oooooo*, imagine your whole inner space as the inside of a resounding bell, letting the sound travel from the bottom of the spine upward — unhindered and unforced — as a process of flowing, shaping of the lowest, deepest part of your inner space. Essentially, you open yourself to the flow of sound–breath through that image of inner shaping of the inside of a bell, allowing this shape to spread in all three dimensions. You can then spread the sound sequence from *oooooo* to *oooooo-oh* and from *oooooo-oh* to *aah*. Do not force the prolongation of the sound by any input of Effort, such as Strength or Bound Flow which actually "chokes" the sound.

3. In group sound: Feel supported by the sounds of others rather than give in to the temptation of outdoing others by intensity (yelling) or, forceful choking prolongation. By allowing yourself to be carried by the sounds of others you will give in to the flowing nature of breath–sound and share a feeling of communication.

* * * * *

Preparatory Exercise C
ROCK AND ROLL

Purpose

To introduce with a rhythmic foot movement (up and down flexion and extension from the ankle), the connections to the tilting forward and backward of the pelvis*: a) the connection of the pelvic area to the heel (grounding), and b) the connection of the two main muscles regulating flexion and extension actions (the iliopsoas in flexion from the groin, and the hamstrings in extension from the sit bones, ischium).

Action

Lie flat on the floor, legs and arms extended, the arms resting at the side of the body.

Bend your feet downward toward the floor initiating from the ankle, which retracts the heels and tilts the pelvis slightly forward (iliopsoas action).

Reverse the action from the ankle to bring the feet up. This stretches the heels and tilts the pelvis slightly backward (hamstring action).

Repeat the two foot actions which reverberate into the pelvic area and produce a rhythmical rocking of pelvis and feet.

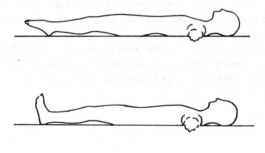

Fig. 38

Experience

It is important that the foot movement is always initiated from the ankle, not the toes, and that no tension occurs in lumbar extensor muscles and surface abdominals, particularly the rectus abdominis. Otherwise the connection between heel and pelvic floor cannot be experienced.

The hamstrings and iliopsoas actions are always relating to each other. As one is active, the other becomes passive and vice versa. It is as if they play with each other.

Function

The complex interaction of these areas in all lower unit movements will be clarified through the description of the six basic exercises and is involved at some level in all movements.

$$* \quad * \quad * \quad * \quad *$$

---

* *Tilt forward has the lower pelvic floor forward; tilt backward has the lower pelvic floor back.*

Exercise No. 1A
THIGH LIFT: Pre-Lift

Purpose

To raise the thigh with maximum efficiency, i.e., using iliopsoas muscle, without using extraneous
  muscles. The iliopsoas is the key to pure hip movement.

To become aware of "pure" joint and segmental movement.

Action

Lie on your back, legs extended, arms to the side and palms on the floor.

Breathe. On the exhalation, let the abdomen become empty and hollow as you simultaneously slide
  the heel to bring the knee up. Heel aims exactly towards the ischium. Whole foot is now in contact
  with the floor.

Rest.

Leading with heel, slide the leg out to the starting position.

Repeat with other leg. Then alternate.

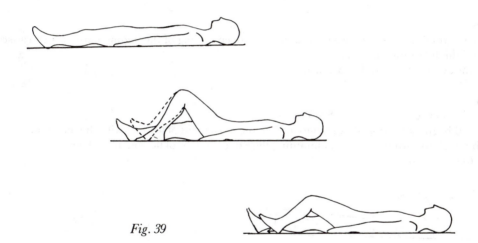

Fig. 39

Experience

From start of action, feel continuous folding of inguinal area in front.

Feel continuous lengthening of lower back by relaxing lumbar muscles, so lower back sinks into floor.

Continuous heel to ischium to sacrum–coccyx connection.

On return, feel ischium to heel connection by activating hamstrings from the ischium, not from the
  knee–lower leg.

Effort and Space

The two phases of pulling up the knee with heel contact and lowering it toward the floor require no
  more than folding–unfolding Shape Flow and fluctuations in Free/Bound Effort Flow. In the
  pulling up, Free Flow Effort increases slightly toward Bound; in lowering, the Flow increases
  toward Free and ends Neutral. No stress on Time or Weight or Space Effort elements.

Notes

Avoid tension around the sternum (chest bone) and inside of thighs. If you have tension on inside of thigh, it is because you are tending to adduct (pulling leg toward midline of body) and have thus lost the straight aim of the heel toward ischium.

As you slide leg up, don't bulge the abdomen (i.e., keep abdomen hollow). If you are bulging the abdomen, it is because you are overusing the superficial abdominals.

Don't shorten the lower back by contracting or "holding" the lumbar muscles in contraction.

Function

Initiation for walking and leg raising.

* * * * *

Exercise No. 1B
THIGH LIFT: Lift

Purpose

To raise the thigh through iliopsoas initiation and deep folding of the inguinal area which causes a "pure" thigh flexion movement.

To become aware of the graded pelvic tilt.

Action

Lie back in "knees-up" position. (See Pre-Lift.)

Exhale and begin hollowing abdomen to initiate the movement of leading with the top of the knee to lift the thigh toward the chest, maintaining the same amount of flexion in the knee.

Return to starting position.

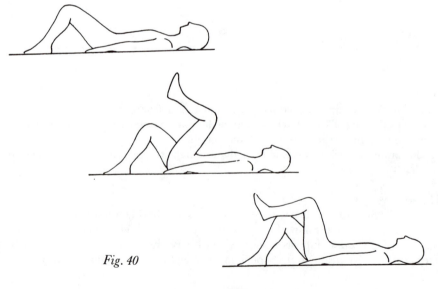

Fig. 40

Experience

As pelvis starts moving with the anterior superior spine going into a backward arc, a deep fold occurs in the inguinal area. Lumbar extensor muscles begin to lengthen (i.e., tension diminishes in them). The gluteal extensor muscles (buttock muscles) gradually relax so the whole sacrum settles on floor. This allows the iliopsoas to function. This whole process will be experienced as changing tensions around the big trochanters.

On return, feel the action initiating from around the ischium (by the hamstrings), and the reversal of the angle of the inguinal region — both supported by coccyx and lower sacrum.

Anchoring the rest of the body occurs in the opposite leg from ischium to heel and in the utmost width across the back and front of the chest.

Weight of upper body is cradled by the scapula.

Effort and Space

The same is true in 1B as in 1A: Essentially slight Shape Flow, Effort Flow changes occur in the hip-knee segment to the chest in phase one. In phase two, lowering the thigh and bringing the foot to the exact place on the floor introduces a short-lived use of Space Effort, slightly Bound Flow with Directness.

Notes

Avoid bulging your abdomen (excess superficial abdominal tension).

Avoid pulling your knees toward each other (adductor leg tension).

Avoid tension in back of knees.

Avoid any tension increase in chin, neck–shoulder in this and following exercises.

With the first shock of experiencing the weight of the leg, there is a tendency to brace it by contraction of the hamstrings flexing the lower leg, and of contracting the lumbar muscles. To avoid this and maintain the angle at the knee, it may be necessary to think of the lower part of the leg slightly lifting. This leads to the proper feeling of weightlessness of the leg.

On the return, the initiation in the hamstrings is particularly important to maintain the weightless feeling on the way back, while the heel aims at the original starting place.

Function

For creeping, walking, running and marching, and climbing stairs.

* * * * *

Exercise No. 2
PELVIC FORWARD SHIFT

Purpose
To mobilize the weight by means of pelvic shift and use of the pelvic floor.
To prepare for forward and backward weight transference and level change.

Action
Lie on back in "knees up" position, hands and arms comfortably at sides.
Exhale and hollow abdomen to initiate following action.
Preparatory rock and roll.
Raise pelvis and shift the center of weight forward toward the feet and up in the air, so that you seem
    to be standing on your feet.
Reverse the movement.

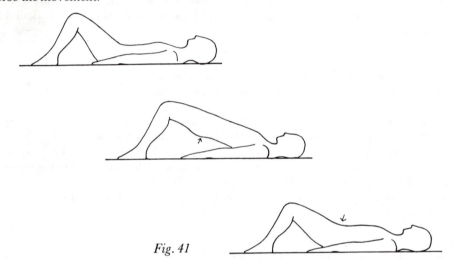

Fig. 41

Experience
Feel the front of the hip area opening (inguinal area flattens) by pressing into heels and supporting
    the movement from the coccyx and hamstrings. The space between the anterior superior spine and
    about an inch below the inguinal area (into the thigh) should be straight throughout the lift.
On reversal, sink into the groin, lengthening the lower back, supported by the coccyx.
Feel the connection between the feet and the pelvis.
Feel the support of the coccyx through the predominant use of the pelvic floor.

Effort and Space
Preparatory rock and roll of pelvis by pointing the foot down (plantar flexion) and alternating it with
    raising the foot by a stretch from the heel (dorsiflexion) is accompanied by Effort Flow changes:
    Free to Bound in both cases.
Raising the pelvis and opening the inguinal area elicits spatial intent: aiming forward and up in the
    raising and some Weight Effort (reduced Strength) and some Time Effort (reduced Suddenness).
The lowering of the pelvis in the second phase is done with Shape Flow (folding) and Free Effort Flow
    going into Neutral (near passivity) in reaching the floor.

Notes

Avoid using arms and hands as support.

Avoid overuse of buttock muscles. It is an indication of insufficient coccyx support and bypassing of pelvic floor muscle use.

Function

To prepare for standing from sitting or lying.

*　*　*　*　*

<h1 style="text-align:center">Exercise No. 3
PELVIC LATERAL SHIFT</h1>

Purpose

To shift the weight laterally without any twist, by using the area of lowest components of the pelvic–hip action. The latter is known as the "pelvic floor" (roughly between pubic bones, ischium and coccyx).

To establish the predominance of the pelvic floor muscles in lateral weight shifts and the fusion of the pelvic floor muscles with extensors of the hip in forward weight shifts in forward progression.

To establish the predominance of the pelvic floor muscles as rotators (internal and external) of the thigh–legs with abduction and adduction of the thigh–legs.

Action

Lie on back in "knees up" position.

Exhale and hollow abdomen to initiate the following action.

After preparatory rock and roll, let it take you into slightly lifting the pelvis, initiating with support from coccyx.

Shift pelvis to right on an absolutely straight path and gently lower into floor.

Rest a moment.

Lift pelvis again initiating with support from the coccyx.

Shift it back to midline and lower into sacrum onto floor which brings you back to starting position.

Repeat to the other side.

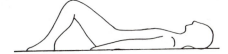 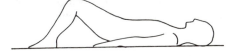

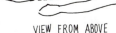

VIEW FROM ABOVE

Fig. 42

239

Experience

The exhalation will carry you through the whole movement until the rest, when you inhale.

On lift, lead with coccyx while lengthening back.

On the shift, experience the shifting tensions from above and below the trochanters on a straight right–left axis, that is, without hiking the hip up. The big trochanters are the axes for the shift.

Maintain the support from the coccyx and ischium (hamstrings).

What is experienced as movement of the pelvic floor is probably a complex interplay of abductor and adductor muscles with the hamstrings, parts of iliopsoas, and the posterior external rotators. This experience cannot be finely detailed in the use of individual muscles. Even electromyography has not yet made explicit differentiations. Therefore, it is especially important to localize the bony landmarks as guides to the activity.

Effort and Space

Just a Shape Flow, Effort Flow action with slight folding–unfolding of the pelvis through flexion of the feet in both directions with fluctuations of either Free or Bound Flow.

The slight lift of the pelvis is a Shape Flow unfolding lifting of the pelvis with no spatial intent.

In the shift from side to side, clear spatial intent causes the directional, one-dimensional displacement of the pelvis initiated from the greater trochanter. This is accompanied by Effort Flow fluctuations and reduced Strength. Lowering the pelvis at the side is a Shape Flow folding action with Effort Flow going from Free/Bound to Neutral Flow with readiness for change.

Lifting again and shifting as earlier with the corresponding directional path has the same accompanying Effort Flow changes.

Notes

The horizontal axis should only be felt through the greater trochanters. If the axis is felt above the upper rim of the pelvis, you are bypassing the pelvic floor muscles and the hip abductors.

Avoid initiating the movement from anything above the pelvic rim. The most common error is hiking the hip (with the quadratus lumborum, a pelvic abductor), which causes a slight twist at the waist as a substitute for the pure lateral shift along the horizontal axis of the greater trochanters.

Avoid all unnecessary upper body and leg tension.

Function

In normal walking: for the fusion of lateral weight shift and forward progression, and for steering it by the rotary element of the legs.

In side stepping: lateral weight shift.

*   *   *   *   *

Exercise No. 4
BODY HALF (VERTICAL)

Purpose

To become aware of the vertical midline of the body which separates right and left sides.
Simultaneous use of right (or left) arm and leg in vertical plane.
Preparation for right–left asymmetry.
Preparation for alternating use of right and left sides of whole body.

Action

Lie on back in "X" position.
Exhale as you lead simultaneously with the right elbow and right knee drawing toward each other on
    the floor, shortening right side of trunk as in a side bend. Head tilts to side.
Reverse the action by retracing the original path, leading with the fingers and toes.
Repeat exercise on the left.

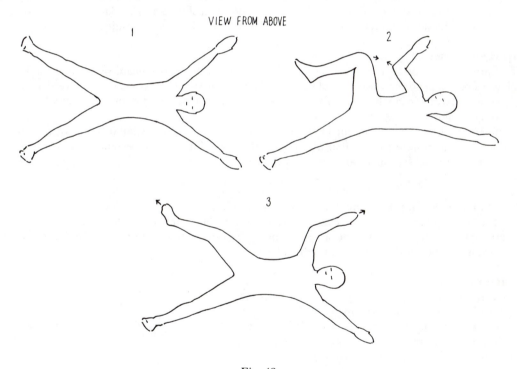

VIEW FROM ABOVE

Fig. 43

241

Experience

Feel vertical midline of the body.

Stay as flat as possible, in the vertical plane with minimal twisting. The flatness is more important than the degree of the side bend. The flatter you are the more you activate the pure side movement without deviating forward or back.

Upper body and lower body activate simultaneously as they swing to the side to facilitate getting elbow and knee together with maximal lateral flatness.

Opposite side is anchored by slightly rotating the proximal joints (hip) outward (external).

Reversal feels like opening the space as the upper and lower parts of body go away from each other, spreading and lengthening.

When the effort is made to confine a movement so absolutely strictly to one plane, the movement expresses an unnatural quality because it is inherent in human body movement to function in two or three dimensions, not one.

People easily distinguish upper and lower initiation. However, they have much less awareness of the midline division of the body separating one side from the other. Therefore, they cannot easily distinguish right (upper–lower) initiation from left (upper–lower) initiation.

In this exercise, it is not so important that you fulfill each part to its utmost as that you have a clear sense, during the process, about which side of your body is operating. For example, although you may have trouble staying altogether flat on the floor, you should stay as flat as possible so your focus is on the side contraction which will prevent your getting into the sagittal plane.

Effort and Space

The flatness of the body and the precision of the simultaneous use of head, right upper and right lower body depends on the clarity of the spatial intent with which elbow goes downward and knee goes upward alongside the body in an Effort Flow pattern of increased Boundness (avoiding use of Strength Effort).

In the reversal, the spatial intent of the fingers is upward and the spatial intent of the foot is downward to restore the original position on the floor. Effort Flow becomes increasingly Free ending in almost Neutral as body reassumes starting position.

Notes

Do not initiate by central contraction; initiation is simultaneous from elbows and knees.

Avoid letting either the arm or leg lead. Upper and lower should move together.

Be sure to keep in the vertical plane; avoid letting the leg deviate toward forward or backward. Try to maintain contact with the floor in thigh and leg.

Function

Preparation for:

First walking patterns of the young child.

Vertical turning, as in ballet.

Chain turns or barrel turns in acrobatics or log rolling.

Passé and side bending dance movements.

*   *   *   *   *

Exercise No. 5A
KNEE DROP

Purpose

To establish a clear twist of the lower unit against the upper unit.

To establish the predominance (unilateral use) of pelvic floor (rotators) with abduction and adduction.

To establish heel to coccyx connection.

Action

Lie on back in "knees up" position, arms out to side, palms down, with feet in full contact with floor. Feet are in line with ischia.

Feet tilt to right side, changing support to outer rim of right foot and heel and inner rim of left foot and heel as knees lower to same side.

Rest a moment.

Exhale, hollowing the abdomen. Leading with coccyx, return knees to starting position, and regain stance of the feet.

Feel drop of knees as a passive movement. Feel return as an active movement.

Practice leading with the coccyx — lower pelvic floor — with and without surface abdominal tension so you really understand the difference. This movement should always be without abdominal tension.

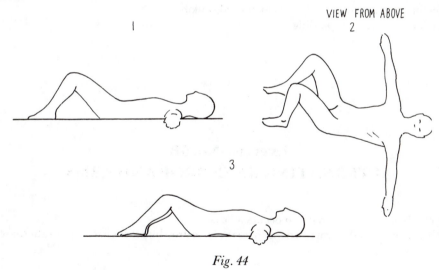

VIEW FROM ABOVE

Fig. 44

Experience

Changes in foot area of support.

The continuing connection from knees to ischium during the knee drop.

During rest, feel diagonal pull of the right hip and the left shoulder.

During exhalation–hollowing, feel the activation of coccyx–trochanter–heel connection to prepare for reversal of action.

Returning, feel the whole back lengthening with coccyx–sacrum as you sink into groin (inguinal region).

243

Effort and Space

The dropping of the thighs–lower legs, initiated from the knees, is essentially a Shape Flow action in which the right thigh unfolds (out) and the left folds (in). Effort Flow becomes increasingly Free and finally Neutral as the weight of the thighs becomes "heavy."

Reversal of action: The thighs reverse their Shape Flow action, returning to starting position. Effort Free Flow initiates going into Neutral when it reaches end position. Spatial intent and other Effort elements are minimized because the main attention is on the succession of body parts.

The diagonal pull between right hip and left shoulder described here is at first experienced more in its contralateral body limb relationship than as a spatial pull, though it prepares for more complex spatial and Effort combinations.

Notes

Avoid abdominal tension.

Avoid increased tension in tensor fascia lata and front of thigh, i.e., around anterior superior spine.

In the reversal of the action, the initiation from sacrum–coccyx is crucial. Initiation from knee and front of thigh (right rectus femoris and sartorius) prevents the proper function of the iliopsoas and the interplay of right and left greater trochanters and of right and left hamstrings from the ischia. With such *improper* input, there would be a disturbance of walking patterns; for instance, the lower leg would initiate thrust forward, leading the walk.

When feet return to starting position, be sure it is a result of pelvic–heel action.

Function

Preparation for contralateral use of limbs in normal walking.

Preparation for twisting and spiraling.

*　　*　　*　　*　　*

Exercise No. 5B
ALTERNATING KNEE DROP AND ARMS

Purpose

To further emphasize the diagonal that occurs in 5A.

To establish awareness of the arm relationship to the knee drop by practicing drops to alternate sides.

Action

Lie on back in "knees up" position with feet in full contact with the floor as in Exercise 5A. The arms are spread horizontally with palms down and with full support on both scapulae.

On the first knee drop to the right, allow its effect to spread into the left shoulder, extending arm up overhead and to the left, as a diagonal counterpull to the right lower body. The right arm stays straight spread to the right.

As you start changing the knee drop to the left, first pull the knees up to center with support from sacrum–coccyx as you simultaneously begin to move the left arm toward the straight side–left and the right arm toward the diagonal high–right, leading with the finger tips.

244

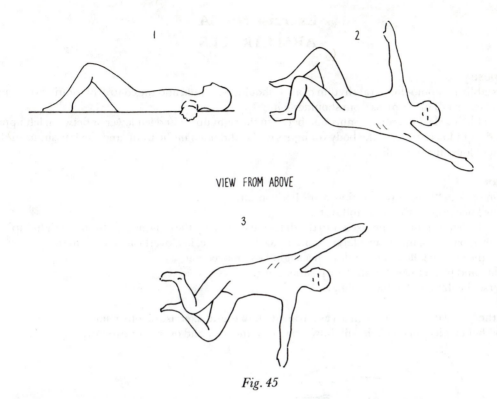

VIEW FROM ABOVE

Fig. 45

Experience

The experience of Exercise 5A is further refined by the synchronized counteraction of the two arms shifting from diagonal to directional spatial tension.

Adjusting the opposite arm into a diagonal countertension left and overhead introduces awareness of the whole diagonal tension developing between left arm and right lower abdomen and pelvic frontal area. The same tension develops when the movement is performed on the other side, producing the opposite diagonal.

When synchrony of upper–lower is fully achieved, the whole movement will be performed with great smoothness and graded flow changes.

Effort and Space

Essentially Shape Flow (one through folding, the other unfolding) in lower body with fluctuations of Effort Flow. Effort Flow increasingly Free to Neutral, while weight of thighs becomes heavy.

A peripheral spatial tension from the arm movement balances the Effort Flow and heaviness of body weight. There is minimal use of other Effort elements.

Function

See Exercise No. 5A.

* * * * *

Exercise No. 6A
ARM CIRCLES

Purpose
To establish scapulo–humeral rhythm of arm–shoulder–scapula and the control of rotation (internal and external) in the arms from shoulder joint.

To establish a clear diagonal connection between the right upper and left lower or between left upper and right lower parts of the body (obliques of the abdomen in the front, and the latissimus in the back) for contralaterality.

Action
Lie on back in "knees up" position, arms horizontally spread.

Do the knee drop to the right and rest.

Allow the left arm to extend itself into the diagonal caused by the oblique pull from the right hip.

Left arm, palm up, moves in a large counter-clockwise circle, i.e., overhead and around.

Allow the eyes to follow the hand, with a slight head movement.

When hand has returned to starting position, rest.

Reverse the direction of the circling.

Rest.

Use the "knee drop" exercise in 5B as a transition to repeat exercise on other side.

If you hold a piece of chalk, it will draw a circle on the floor and over your two hips.

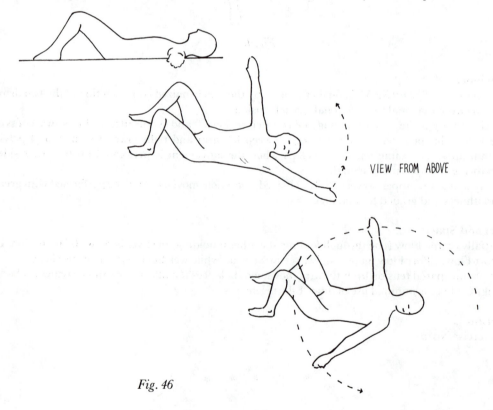

VIEW FROM ABOVE

Fig. 46

Experience

As soon as you begin to circle, you are moving with a gradual outward rotation of the arm.

Feel that the arm has two changes in rotation during the circle: at the top and the bottom. The palm faces the ceiling at the top of the circle and the floor at the bottom, although the rotation occurs gradually.

The pelvis is anchored as you allow the upper body to twist against it as the arm reaches to its opposite side.

The arm movement should be as smooth and easy as possible.

Effort and Space

Dropping the knee to the right side is a near passive movement with minimal spatial intent and Effort Flow fluctuations which end in Neutral Flow.

The tracing with the third finger of a complete, planar circle is directed by the spatial intent of going across, down, side and up. This shaping of the circle is dependent on constantly shifting spatial diagonals. This clear spatial shaping is accompanied by Effort Flow/Time changes that reach a maximum Bound at the top of the head and maximal Free at the bottom below the pubic region.

The smoothness and full roundedness of the circle depends on clear two-dimensional shaping. This evokes not only Effort Flow changes but also definable Effort element changes.

Starting from diagonally overhead moving to directly overhead, there is an increase in lightness and Bound Flow.

Starting from directly overhead moving to across and down to the hips, there is an increase in Bound Flow and Sustainment.

In the left arm's movement across the body to left out and back up and moving back to the starting position, there is an increase in Free Flow, some diminished Suddenness, and increasing Light/Sustainment in the last quarter of the cycle.

Notes

To avoid a jerky or sudden rotation, make sure to grade the rotation in the arm.

Do not lock the elbow.

Do not let the circle be lopsided or otherwise irregular.

Do not confine your attention to the shoulder-joint body action at the expense of the spatial shaping.

Function

Preparation for large circular movements of the arms and upper body for shaping motions in work, manipulation of tools or in expressive movement.

*   *   *   *   *

Exercise No. 6B
DIAGONAL SITUP

Purpose

Same purpose as 6A plus its extension into using the momentum of 6A lift into a situp, taking the
body weight into space.

To initiate from upper body with support from lower.

Action

Lie on back in "knees up" position, arms horizontally spread, palms down.

Do the knee drop to the right and rest.

Allow the left arm to extend itself into the diagonal caused by the oblique pull from the right hip.

Left arm, palm facing the ceiling, moves in a large counter-clockwise circle, i.e., overhead and
around.

Allow the eyes to follow the hand, with a slight head movement.

When hand has returned to starting position, rest.

Reverse the direction of the circling.

Rest.

Use the "knee drop" exercise as a transition to repeat exercise on other side, starting with right arm
which will have to go clockwise to go overhead and around.

Repeat circle, with gradual energy increase in reaching toward left knee until it gets you into a full
sweeping trunk–arm circle that brings you into a twisted sitting position with the right hip slightly
off the floor to follow right arm beyond left knee.

Continue circle, never interrupting the arm movement as you sink diagonally back into the left
groin–pelvis and finish the cycle by placing your scapula–shoulder–arm–hand back into the
diagonal knee drop position on the floor with weight distributed over both left and right pelvis.

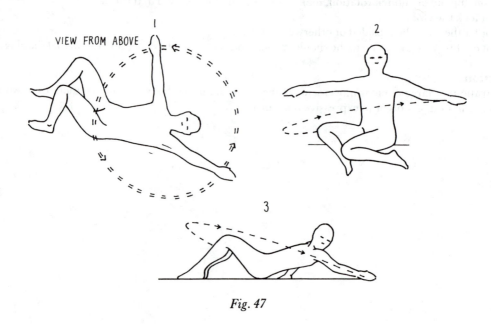

Fig. 47

Experience

As in Exercise No. 6A, watch carefully the changes in arm rotation which occur at top and bottom of circle.

Grade it carefully.

Watch the sweep of your circle, letting your head accompany the eye motion.

Experience the increasing drive of the circular arm sweeping, causing a shift of the weight in the lower body from right to left, which actually gets you up into sitting.

Finishing the circle lying down is again experienced as a smooth shift of weight in the lower body from left to right, spreading into the pelvis–lower back–thoracic spine–scapular arm.

Effort and Space

See previous exercise.

As you increase the sweep of the circle by enlarging the range of the spatial form including the whole upper body, Strength and Suddenness appear as accents: maximum Strength/Suddenness appearing when the arm–body sweeps across and when the arm is overhead reaching its maximum openness. When you do the whole circle, you will sit up at the maximal point of acrossness and lie down as you open into widening. Lying down is then accompanied by decrease in Effort accents and increase in Free/Bound Flow fluctuations.

Notes

The continuous maintenance of the upper–lower connection is the key to the performance. The pelvis actually performs a circular shifting of the lower body weight.

Both the pelvic weight shift and the scapular-arm movement must be continued simultaneously without interrupting the spatial drive of the shaping movement making a large circle.

Function

To prepare for the performance of large spatial shapes in dance and work, as in using an ax to fell a tree.

This closes the cycle of the six basic exercises which moved from initiation of movement in lower part of body to initiation of movement in upper part of body. The exercises that follow are examples of some of the additional Bartenieff Fundamentals. They incorporate the six basic exercises into other actions.

*   *   *   *   *

Exercise No. 7
THE SEESAW, A PARTNER EXERCISE

Purpose

To experience initiation of movement from lower unit with upper unit following.

To experience the interrelationship of breath and body weight.

To experience the active and passive aspects of body weight.

To interrelate the breath and weight rhythm between two people.

Action

Partner I lies on floor with knees flexed and feet together in full contact with floor.

Partner II, standing, faces Partner I. His feet enclose the feet of his partner.

They reach for each other with straight arms, grasping each other's hands.

Partner II sits down with flexed knees and lies on his back, keeping the knees flexed while slowly letting his breath go out, with a tendency to give in to his passive weight.

This process raises Partner I from the floor into standing while breathing in, filling himself with air. He becomes lighter, buoyant, more active.

The arms stay extended all through this and there is no active pulling or pushing from either partner in the upper body.

This process is repeated with Partner I sitting–lying down and Partner II being raised into standing.

Continuing that process through a number of repetitions, with concentration on the rhythmical change between the passive, heavy phase and the active one in the lower body makes the breathing regulate its rhythm automatically.

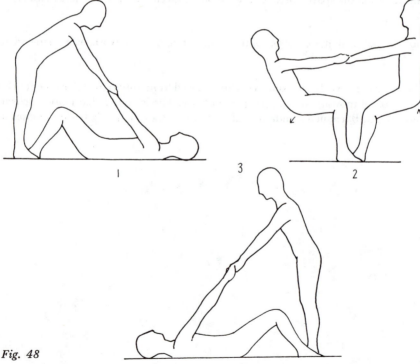

Fig. 48

Experience

Be aware of breath, passive body weight changes and the changes between concave and convex body shape: passive body weight in the process of going from standing to lying while letting the breath out; active support of weight from the incoming breath in the process of going from lying to standing. In both phases, there should be no active pulling or pushing with the arms.

Effort and Space

This exercise deals with a gradual, graded tuning in to a partner's sitting and standing through the synchronized use of breath and body weight. Till this tuning in is finally achieved, one can observe jerky, arhythmical Effort and Shape Flow changes, extremes of muscular tensions in either the upper body or other parts of the trunk. With concentration on the heavy (breath out) passive body weight and the full (breath in) active weight, gradually the Shape Flow of folding and unfolding regulates itself together with rhythmical changes in the Effort Flow. In this exercise there is no spatial intent.

Notes

Avoid any pushing and pulling in the arms

Avoid any talking or laughing during the repetitions; give yourself over to the rhythm developing between the partners.

Function

This interaction of breath and passive–active alternations serves as a recuperative experience and should be tried also in states of fatigue after major exertions.

*   *   *   *   *

Exercise No. 8
PREPARATORY EXERCISE FOR CREEPING TO STANDING
(EX. 9 & 10)

Purpose

To become aware of the importance of initiation from groin, trochanters, and lower sacrum–coccyx in any level changes.

Action

Start from lying on back on floor, legs together, arms at side.

Initiating from the groin–lower sacrum–trochanter, roll over to the side while flexing the whole body into a ball.

Initiating from trochanter–groin–lower sacrum, roll back to starting position.

Repeat several times.

Then, condense the sideward roll suddenly into a total shift of the body onto the knees and elbows. The head faces the floor.

Straighten the arms directly underneath your shoulders to lift the pelvis. You are now ready to creep or crawl. Face should be facing forward.

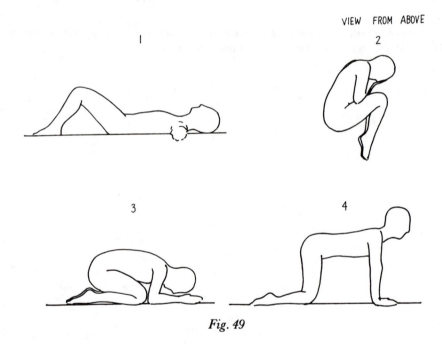

Fig. 49

Experience

Feel the fusion of the roll with the flexion. They should be occurring simultaneously.

Awareness of the trochanter involvement strengthens the lateral component of the roll because of the lateral axis between the trochanters.

On the condensation, the simultaneity is crucial.

When the arms straighten, keep the neck and shoulders free of extraneous tension.

252

Effort and Space
The condensed rounding and rolling evokes extreme Flow changes between Free and Bound along
   with Sudden Time and Strong Weight.
In the unrolling, these are smaller Flow fluctuations with more Sustainment and Neutral Weight.

Function
To prepare for changes of level from lying to creeping.

* * * * *

Exercise No. 9
LOWER UNIT SEQUENCE
WALKING THROUGH HANDS FROM QUADRUPED POSITION

Purpose
To establish the use of the lowest part of the pelvis–hip in lower level locomotion (squat, creep). To
   intensify training of iliopsoas and the rotators of the hip.

Action
Start from creeping position with straight arms underneath shoulder and full lower leg–knee support.
Hands are stationary as knees walk toward them. Lower back muscles lengthen while the inguinal
   fold steadily increases.
Head gradually inclines forward facing the floor. It is part of the total rounding of the back from the
   base of the skull to the lowest part of pelvis–coccyx.
Knee–walk through hands and beyond until you are forced, by whatever means are available to you,
   without stopping forward motion, to land on your feet and walk your feet so the legs unfold and you
   sit down with straight legs.
Lower part of body stays as low as possible and upper part (neck, chin, shoulders) as mobile as
   possible as feet walk through the hands.

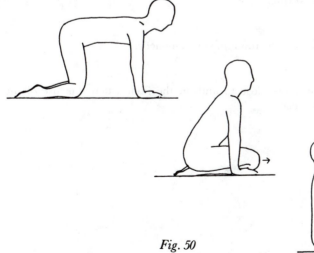

Fig. 50

253

Reversal

With arms–hands slightly in back of body for support on hands (fingers facing forward), pull up the knees, bringing the feet toward the ischium as closely as possible, and with that momentum, continue to lift the lower body immediately in a slightly forward–upward arc from the ischium–coccyx which causes the upper body to tilt slightly forward while you walk your feet back through your hands in a very deep squat.

Continuing backward, you will get on your knees again, in the original creeping position, with the back neither rounded nor hyperextended.

Experience

As soon as you begin to walk, feel the lengthening in the lower back, curling the lowest part of the sacrum–coccyx increasingly under you without tension.

This feeling of lengthening and rounding of the whole torso increases until you are through the hands, maintaining a low squat.

As you continue to progress forward, offer no resistance in either head or shoulders or ankles–feet; you wriggle through.

In the reversal, feel the backward pull of the pelvis initiated by a slight lift of the ischia and coccyx. This is possible only through pelvic floor participation.

Effort and Space

Walking on the knees toward the hands is clearly spatially directed forward, the spatial intent being renewed in each alternation of right and left. Allow the small fluctuations between Free Flow and slight Bound to spread into the whole body so Bound Flow countertensions would not develop around shoulder–neck. This is particularly crucial when you pass through the two hands and keep renewing the spatial intent forward until you sit with straight legs.

In the reversal toward backward, it is crucial to lift the lowest part of the pelvis slightly from the ischium back, which shifts head–neck somewhat forward–down. This allows the Flow fluctuations to develop in pelvis–leg and pull the thighs back and under to start the knee creeping backward, gradually straightening the whole body shape. These spatial adjustments are supported mainly by Effort Flow fluctuations and only minimally by other Effort elements. You experience here how the spatial intent of the forward or backward creeping produces changes in the shape of the trunk–neck toward growing and shrinking.

Notes

Avoid any neck tension fighting against the rounding of torso–neck.

Function

Prepares for the very low weight shifts close to and on the floor where the use of the pelvis, particularly the pelvic floor, is crucial.

*   *   *   *   *

254

Exercise No. 10
CONDENSING TO SITTING FROM LYING

This relates to sequences of getting up from the floor (Exercise No. 6B and sequences 11A, 11B, 12). The difference is that this exercise is not a sequence but is instead, one condensed shaping action.

Purpose
To sit up from lying in one concerted action using straight and oblique muscles in front together with full hip flexion (iliopsoas) and immediate full contact with heel–ischium–coccyx.
To get quickly to readiness for upper unit action.

Action
Lie on back on floor with arms and legs spread into a large X, palms facing ceiling.
Exhale and condense your whole body–head–limbs forward into an all around folding to the center of the body; heels never leaving the floor.

VIEW FROM ABOVE

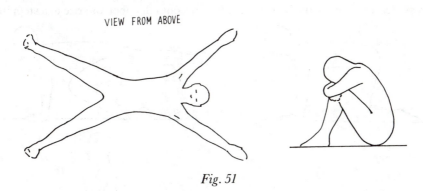

Fig. 51

Experience
Feel the flexion in the sagittal plane as shortening between chest and pelvis.
Feel the body–limbs narrowing toward the vertical midline. Experience the whole as one action: a highly intensive concerted action of folding and narrowing reinforced by the iliopsoas, oblique abdominals, hamstrings.

Effort and Space
This exercise illustrates the concerted participation of spatial intent up and clear Effort elements. Its performance commands an immediate readiness for simultaneous use of upper–lower body and Effort elements of Strength and Suddenness.

Note
This exercise involves two opposite diagonal tensions (as experienced in Exercise 6B) neutralizing each other.

Function
To rise quickly from lying to sitting.

* * * * *

Exercise No. 11A
CREEPING TO STANDING LEVEL FOR LOCOMOTION

Purpose

To establish the use of the lowest part of pelvis in the transfer of body weight forward and up to move from creeping (flexion) level to standing–walking (extension) level.

Action

Start from creeping position with straight arms underneath shoulders and full support from knee–lower leg.

Initiating from groin, swing right leg forward with knee bent and initiating from sit bone, swing back into extension.

Repeat the swing forward and place right foot on the floor between both hands.

Swing leg going back to starting position.

After several repetitions of this sequence, alter the forward swing midway by releasing the right hand from the floor and replacing it with the right foot. Without stopping, with continuing support from the coccyx–sacrum, transfer the body weight forward onto that foot and rise to a stepping stance.

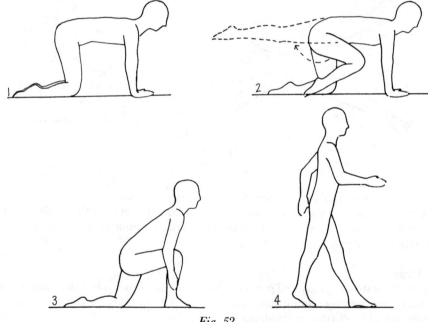

Fig. 52

Experience

In the creeping position there is no added tension in either the neck or the lumbar muscles.

In the swinging action of the leg forward (flexion) and backward (extension) allow the pelvic–femoral rhythm to develop fully.

The placing of the foot between the hands causes a slight increase in the total rounding of the back from the base of skull to the coccyx. Do not fight or force the action but try to slip the foot smoothly into place.

In replacing the right hand with the right foot use the momentum of the forward–up swing to the fullest, continuing smoothly into the stepping stance that leads into the rising up and forward (sagittal plane) never losing the coccyx–sacrum connection.

Effort and Space
The easy swinging of the leg forward and backward with Shape Flow changes is followed by placing the foot forward with spatial intent as well as Effort Flow fluctuations with fleeting Suddennesses.

Function
To increase the ease of getting up from the floor with readiness to go immediately into locomotion.

*   *   *   *   *

<h1 align="center">Exercise No. 11B</h1>
<h1 align="center">CREEPING TO STABLE STANDING</h1>

Purpose
To use lower sacrum–coccyx support for getting from the floor to vertical stable standing by transferring the body weight up and slightly forward.

Action
Start on knees and forearms, hands with palms flat on the floor and elbows touching the knees. Head bent deeply forward with forehead resting on floor between the hands.
Lift right leg backward.
Straighten arms underneath shoulders to lift chest and head vertically up from the floor.
Releasing right hand place right foot where hand had been. Transfer weight minimally forward and maximally up into standing as you straighten the body.

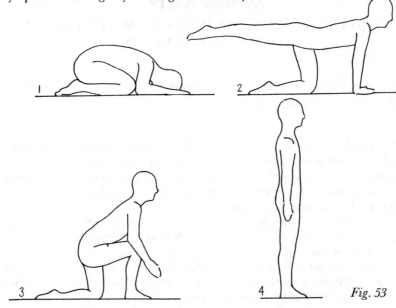

Fig. 53

Experience

The starting position brings upper and lower unit much closer together than in 11A, condensing it into an almost ball-like shape. In the unfolding, there is a greater emphasis on the vertical direction up than on transporting the body forward in the sagittal plane. Therefore, there is no readiness to locomote. You are simply standing.

Effort and Space

From folded body shape your spatial intents shift with accompanying Effort shifts. Right leg is lifted backward with Bound/Free Flow fluctuation, accompanied by some diminished Strength with clear backward spatial intent.

Straightening of arms heightens spatial intent of pressing into the floor with Free Flow becoming Direct with some diminished Strength.

Flow fluctuations accompany the release of the hands and the placement of the right foot. The spatial intent of the foot is forward and is accompanied by Effort fluctuations of Free/Bound with Sudden Neutral Time.

Transfer of weight forward with Bound Flow; the vertical lift adds increasing Strength.

Note:

It is recommended that the two exercises, 11A and 11B, be done alternately for comparison.

Function:

To arrive at stable standing position with appropriate support.

*   *   *   *   *

Exercise No. 12
SITTING TO STANDING TO WALKING
PROPULSION SEQUENCE

Purpose

To use the forward–upward shift of the pelvis, as taught in Exercise No. 2, to get up from the floor through the use of the lower pelvis support.

Action

Start sitting with straight legs slightly spread on the floor. The arms are straight and slightly spread, placed in back of the pelvis with palms down and finger tips facing back.

Pull both knees up while exhaling with a maximum hollowing of the abdomen (to allow the iliopsoas to function) until the feet are flat on the floor. This rounds the back from the base of the skull to the coccyx and lets the lumbar muscles lengthen.

Initiating from the lower pelvis (with maximal support from the sacrum coccyx, and flattening the inguinal region) transfer the weight forward and slightly up on to the feet and continue advancing on to the knees. Release the hands as you get upright on your knees.

Place right foot (with knee bent) forward on the floor. Transfer weight forward and up, rising into stepping forward, fully flattening the inguinal region and continually supporting from the lowest part of the pelvis as the body-leg straightens toward and up.

Fig. 54

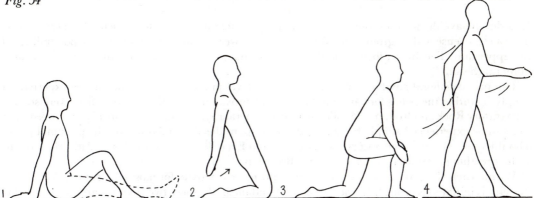

Experience

The preparation for the shift — using hollowed abdomen and releasing the lumbar muscles — is crucial for the transference of weight onto the feet forward and up. This fully straightens the inguinal region.

The spatial intent forward and up, initiated from the lower pelvis, is maintained throughout all the phases in order to make full use of the momentum which gets you off the floor.

As you get onto the knees when the arms are released, the body is for a moment slightly tilted forward. It is therefore important that the stepping with the right foot is immediately started and that the forward–up tension is spread into the upper body and head. This makes for the propulsion.

Effort and Space

The pulling up of both knees is performed with Flow fluctuations and causes a slight rounding of the back (Shape Flow condensing).

The transfer of weight forward is accompanied by Free Flow/Suddenness/Directness, which becomes slightly Bound Flow and diminished Sustainment, as you land on your knees. Simultaneously the arms are released from the floor with Free Flow/Lightness/Suddenness. Immediately, as the body straightens, the right foot with bent knee is placed forward with the Free Flow/Suddenness and the weight immediately transferred into a forward step (Bound/Sudden), straightening the body with Bound Strength/diminished Suddenness into a stable uprightness. This produces a propulsive lift of the body weight forward and up from the floor of Strength/Suddenness, Sustainment and Directness.

Note

If the full transference of body weight onto the knees presents difficulties, use the support of your hands on the floor as a support for the back, walking them forward as you aim to get on the knees so that you gently and gradually place the full body weight forward–up. This straightens the torso–head into upright kneeling without strain on your back.

Function

This is the basis also for all getting up from sitting on chairs or any elevated plane. It reinforces the immediate straightening of the hips and strengthens the connection from hip (sit bones) into the floor. It should replace the heaviness so often seen in rising, characterized by bending over and lifting the body by holding on to the thighs.

Summary Notes on Exercises and Anatomical Illustrations

In order to have the widest ranges of Effort and spatial shaping available to the mover, he/she must have a clear sense of the "grounding" function in the lower unit and the manipulative possibilities of the upper unit. The former focuses on the "pelvic–femoral rhythm" and the latter on the "scapulo–humeral rhythm."

The pelvic–femoral rhythm is activated at some level in all movement and can be experienced simply by tilting the pelvis forward and back on the proximal joints (hip joints). (See Exercise "C" Preparatory Rock and Roll, p. 234.) The scapulo-humeral rhythm is activated in all arm movements and can be experienced simply by raising the arm up, to the side and down on the proximal joints (shoulder joints). (See Preparatory Exercise "A" and Exercise 6A, Arm Circles, p. 246.) Both relate to the breathing process. (See Exercise "B," Breath, p. 232.)

Within each rhythm, there is a symbiotic multi-muscle activity for most efficient use. Where the activity is initiated is crucial. In the Bartenieff Fundamentals, these two rhythms are emphasized to point out often neglected components and show why it is important that they be restored to their appropriate participation.

Pelvic–Femoral Rhythm

The pelvic–femoral rhythm is created in the sequence of interplay of pelvic–hip and pelvic–thigh movement. The interaction is between three distinguishable muscle groups (see illustration, p. 271 ff):

1. above the pelvis–lower trunk (suprapelvic)
2. the sacrum and hip joint level (pelvis–hip joint)
3. the lowest level of sacrum–coccyx–ischium–pubic region (the "pelvic floor")*

This interaction is present in all movement involving the full potential of the ball and socket joints of the hip in all ranges and combinations of flexion–extension, abduction–adduction, and internal and external rotation.

There are three critical factors in the interaction of these three groups. One is initiation, the second is rotation and the third is the participation of the lowest component, the pelvic floor.

In the pelvic–femoral rhythm, the pelvic tilt and the femur work in finely graded collaboration. In order for this to happen, the posterior external rotators have to actively participate in conjunction with the iliopsoas and the hamstrings.

Of the six posterior external rotators, which are distributed over the whole lowest part of the back of the pelvis, some accompany the forward tilt initiated by the iliopsoas, which shortens causing the hamstrings to stretch in passive response. Other rotators accompany the backward tilt initiated at the ischia by the hamstrings which shorten, causing the iliopsoas to stretch in passive response.

When the iliopsoas is not used appropriately in the pelvic tilt, including thigh lifting (flexion), then the rectus abdominis and rectus femoris are over-used and the rhythm cannot be established.**

When the hamstrings are not appropriately incorporated into the pelvic–femoral rhythm by the activity of the rotators, their usefulness is reduced to that of simple extensors of the knees.

---

* *Use of the term "pelvic floor" differs in the literature. It is here defined as the area bounded on the lower part by the sacrum and coccyx, the ischia, and the obturator foramen, and bounded in front by the pubic junction.*

** *In appropriate use, the rectus abdominis is used in trunk flexion, but always in balance with other abdominal muscles, such as the external oblique and internal oblique and the iliopsoas in its role as trunk flexor. The rectus femoris is used appropriately in thigh lift but as an accessory to the iliopsoas in its role as hip flexor.*

Scapulo–Humeral Rhythm

The bone structure supporting the scapulo–humeral rhythm is less solid than the structure supporting the pelvic–femoral rhythm. Therefore, the muscle interaction in the scapulo–humeral rhythm is more complex. There is constant involvement and interaction of all three muscle groups: flexor/extensor, abductor/adductor, and internal/external rotators.

Three main muscle groups control the movements of the scapulo–humeral rhythm. All three should be involved in any shoulder–arm movement, although not to the same degree. See illustrations, pp. 266 to 269.

1. The upper trapezius (surface muscles) and some neck muscles are dominant in vertical–horizontal movements of the arm.
2. The middle trapezius (surface back); the rhomboids (deep) and the pectoralis major (surface front) commonly referred to as chest muscles, are dominant in horizontal–sagittal movements.
3. The lower trapezius (surface back); serratus anterior (surface); latissimus dorsi (surface back) are dominant in sagittal–vertical movements.

Internal and external rotator groups of the scapulo–humeral rhythm are distributed over outer and inner surfaces of scapula. Here again, as in the pelvic–femoral rhythm, there is finely graded collaboration among the components. All participate but with shifting degrees of accommodations to the dominance of one at any given time.

Whether we interpret the many lower back and neck problems in our time as a still incomplete use of our verticality, or see them as deterioration through urban life and reduced physical activity, they are undoubtedly related to incomplete use of the scapulo–humeral and the pelvic–femoral interplay so widespread throughout the population, even among trained dancers and athletes.

The outstanding feature of that incomplete use of the scapular and shoulder joint potential is the weak use of the serratus anterior and lower trapezius, the lowest angle and lateral border of the scapula. As a result, one finds overuse of the upper component, causing neck–shoulder tension. This weakened use of the lower scapula component influences full uprightness, full use of neck–head, and full use of the reach space around. It also prevents making full use of the connections through the large muscle groups that connect the shoulder girdle with the lumbar–sacral region. Lack of these connections cuts off the supportive and balancing forces of body weight in upper unit activity.

The Rotary Factor

Anatomically, the structure of the spine — as central axis of the body and vertical axis of uprightness — has a built-in potential for each vertebrae to move clearly sagitally and laterally and, also, to rotate slightly. The spine extends from the base of the skull to the end of the coccyx.

The rotary possibilities of the spinal vertebrae tremendously increase the range and variety of trunk–limb movements in space. The proximal ball and socket joints at the shoulder and hip are the rotary links between trunk and limbs and give them the mobility for three-dimensional spatial shaping.

The rotary possibilities of the head are controlled by two joints that link the top of the spine to the base of the skull. The rotation of the head itself is a very small movement which can be increased only by including additional vertebrae of the neck.

The upper unit has a majority of internal rotators; the lower unit has a majority of external rotators. Internal rotators are more stabilizing and external more mobilizing. Thus, the bony structure the shoulder girdle is given stability by a preponderance of internal rotators and the more solid bony structure of the pelvis area is given more mobility by a preponderance of external rotators.

261

The rotary muscle groups — along with the flexion–extension and abductor–adductor groups — make diagonal spatial pathways possible and changes in rotation can therefore affect not only the function but also the expressive content of an action.

It is particularly in relation to the rotary element that spatial and anatomical aspects of movement enhance each other. All notions of "simple," straight directions or "simple" vectors are dispelled as the mover becomes sensitized to the rotary role.

Overstress on the sagittal or vertical cycles usually happens at the expense of the horizontal cycle. That is usually directly related to under-use of the rotary element and creates two-dimensional movement even when three-dimensional movement would be preferable. A turning, twisting quality is unavailable without the rotary–horizontal input. Some cultures — in India, Southeast Asia, China, Japan, the Pacific and Africa — seem to incorporate the horizontal with its rotary factor to a greater extent than many western cultures.

Bony Landmarks and Muscles
It would be helpful during the preparation and/or performance of the exercises to refer to the anatomical drawings and find the bony landmarks that can be ascertained by touch and visibly traced. Surrounding areas in relation to the most important muscle groups can be identified in such a way that muscle tensions can be felt or checked. Both the pelvic–femoral rhythm and the scapulo–humeral rhythm activate many more muscles than the major ones described here. In normal activity, muscles never operate in isolation. Selections have been emphasized in this book to make particular points; it is not possible here to include the total picture. A future volume will deal with these in greater depth and will include many more upper body exercises and variations on the basic themes of the Bartenieff Fundamentals. It will also include discussion of and exercises for particular movement problems and elaborations on the basic factors which are only generally discussed here.

*   *   *   *   *

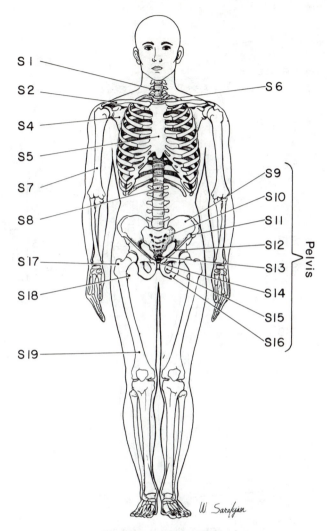

Skeleton: Front View

S1	Neck (cervical spine)	S11	Anterior superior spine
S2	Clavicle	S12	Inguinal ligament
S4	Scapula	S13	Coccyx
S5	Sternum	S14	Junction of pubic bone
S6	First thoracic vertebra (begins thoracic spine)	S15	Obturator foramen
S7	Humerus	S16	Ischium
S8	First lumbar vertebra (begins lumbar spine)	S17	Greater trochanter
S9	Ilium	S18	Lesser trochanter
S10	Sacrum	S19	Femur

263

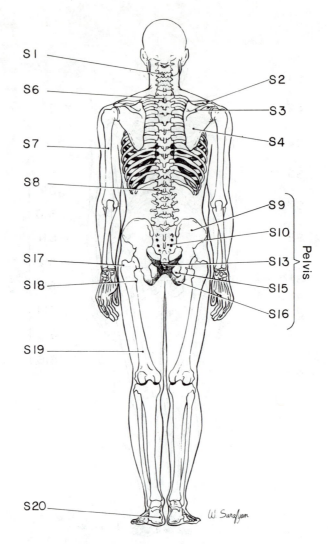

Skeleton: Back View

S1	Neck (cervical spine)	S10	Sacrum
S2	Clavicle	S13	Coccyx
S3	Spine of scapula	S15	Obturator foramen
S4	Scapula	S16	Ischium
S6	First thoracic vertebra (begins thoracic spine)	S17	Greater trochanter
S7	Humerus	S18	Lesser trochanter
S8	First lumbar vertebra (begins lumbar spine)	S19	Femur
S9	Ilium	S20	Heel

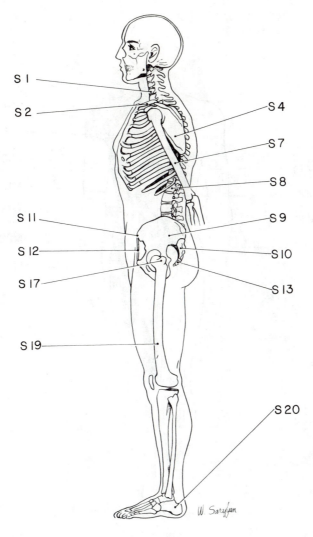

Skeleton: Side View

S1	Neck (cervical spine)	S11	Anterior superior spine
S2	Clavicle	S12	Inguinal ligament
S4	Scapula	S13	Coccyx
S7	Humerus	S17	Greater trochanter
S8	First lumbar vertebra (begins lumbar spine)	S19	Femur
S9	Ilium	S20	Heel
S10	Sacrum		

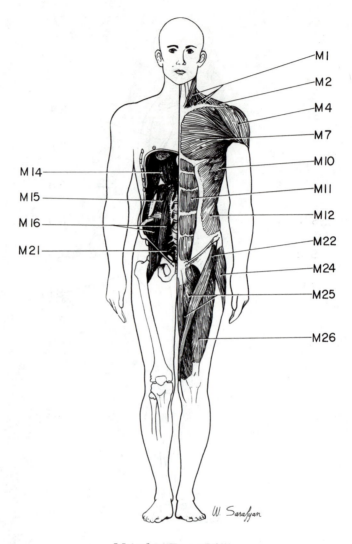

Muscles: Front View

M1	Neck muscles	M15	Quadratus lumborum
M2	Upper trapezius	M16	Iliopsoas (deep)
M4	Deltoid	M21	Posterior rotator group
M7	Pectoralis major	M22	Sartorius
M10	Serratus anterior	M24	Tensor fascia lata
M11	Rectus abdominis	M25	Adductor group
M12	External oblique	M26	Rectus femoris
M14	Diaphragm		

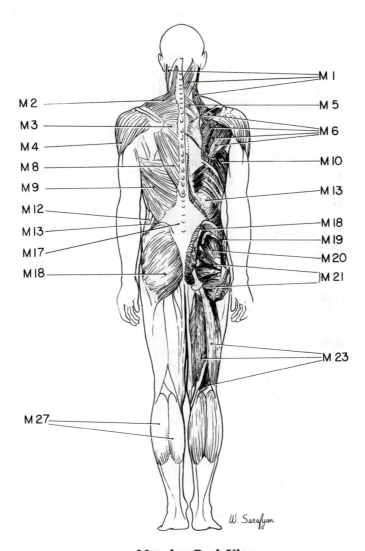

M1
M2
M3
M4
M8
M9
M12
M13
M17
M18

M1
M5
M6
M10
M13
M18
M19
M20
M21
M23
M27

W. Sarafian

Muscles: Back View

M1	Neck muscles	M12	External oblique
M2	Upper trapezius	M13	Internal oblique (deep)
M3	Middle trapezius	M17	Area covering lumbar extensor
M4	Deltoid		muscle group
M5	Rhomboids (deep)	M18	Gluteus maximus
M6	External rotator group of scapulo–humerus*	M19	Gluteus medius
M8	Lower trapezius	M20	Gluteus minimus
M9	Latissimus dorsi	M21	Posterior rotator group
M10	Serratus anterior	M23	Hamstrings
		M27	Calf muscles

* *The external rotator group and the internal rotator group (not shown) of the scapulo–humerus are distributed over the outer and inner surfaces of the scapula.*

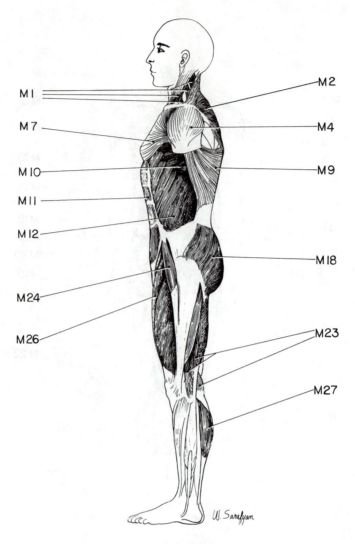

M1

M2

M7

M4

M10

M9

M11

M12

M18

M24

M26

M23

M27

W. Sarafyan

Muscles: Side View

M1	Neck muscles	M12	External oblique
M2	Upper trapezius	M18	Gluteus maximus
M4	Deltoid	M23	Hamstrings
M7	Pectoralis major	M24	Tensor fascia lata
M9	Latissimus dorsi	M26	Rectus femoris
M10	Serratus anterior	M27	Calf muscles
M11	Rectus abdominis		

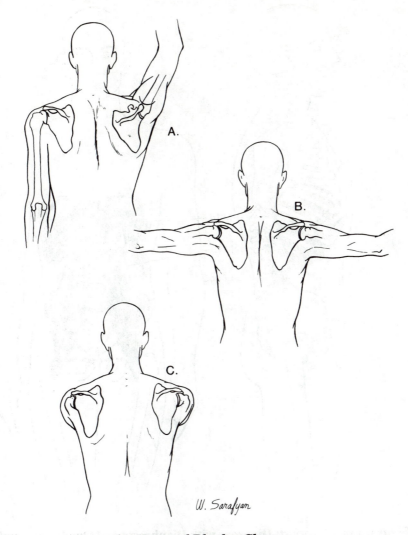

W. Sarafyan

Scapulo–Humeral Rhythm Changes
A. Vertical–Horizontal Movement
B. Horizontal–Sagittal Movement
C. Sagittal–Vertical Movement

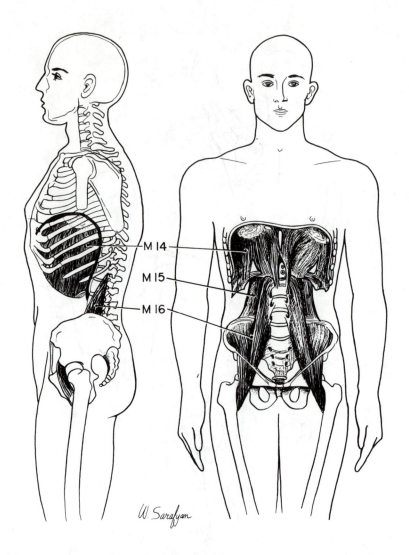

M 14

M 15

M 16

W. Sarafyan

Central Inner Support: Iliopsoas with Diaphragm and Quadratus Lumborum

Side view: Diaphragm (M14) and Iliopsoas (M16)
Front view: Diaphragm, Quadratus Lumborum (M15) and Iliopsoas

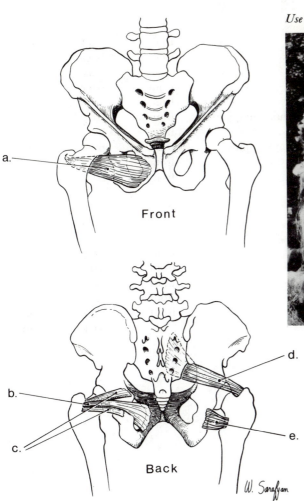

Front

Back

W. Sarafian

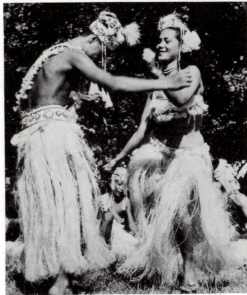

Courtesy of UTA French Airlines.

Neglected Factor in Pelvic–Femoral Rhythm Support: Posterior External Rotators*

Front view
a.   obturator externus
Back view
b.   obturator internus (left)
c.   gemelli (left)
d.   piriformis (right)
e.   quadratus femoris (right)

* *Five of the six rotators are shown. The sixth, coccygeus, is hidden by the others. One set of six is on each side of the body but, for clarity, only one set is illustrated.*

271

Anatomical Labels: Skeletal

S1	Neck (cervical spine)	front	back	side
S2	Clavicle	front	back	side
S3	Spine of scapula		back	
S4	Scapula	front	back	side
S5	Sternum	front		
S6	First thoracic vertebra (begins thoracic spine)	front	back	
S7	Humerus	front	back	side
S8	First lumbar vertebra (begins lumbar spine)	front	back	side
S9	Ilium	front	back	side
S10	Sacrum	front	back	side
S11	Anterior superior spine	front		side
S12	Inguinal ligament	front		side
S13	Coccyx	front	back	side
S14	Junction of pubic bone	front		
S15	Obturator foramen	front	back	
S16	Ischium	front	back	
S17	Greater trochanter	front	back	side
S18	Lesser trochanter	front	back	
S19	Femur	front	back	side
S20	Heel		back	side

Pelvis [bracket spanning S9–S16]

272

Anatomical Labels: Muscular

M1	Neck muscles	front	back	side
M2	Upper trapezius	front	back	side
M3	Middle trapezius		back	
M4	Deltoid	front	back	side
M5	Rhomboids (deep)		back	
M6	External rotator group of scapulo–humerus*		back	
M7	Pectoralis major	front		side
M8	Lower trapezius		back	
M9	Latissimus dorsi		back	side
M10	Serratus anterior	front	back	side
M11	Rectus abdominis	front		side
M12	External oblique	front	back	side
M13	Internal oblique (deep)		back	

Sectional view
M14	Diaphragm	front		
M15	Quadratus lumborum	front		
M16	Iliopsoas (deep)	front		

M17	Area covering lumbar extensor muscle group		back	
M18	Gluteus maximus		back	side
M19	Gluteus medius		back	
M20	Gluteus minimus		back	
M21	Posterior rotator group	front	back	

Sectional view
- a. obturator externus
- b. obturator internus
- c. gemelli
- d. piriformis
- e. quadratus femoris
- f. coccygeus (not shown)

M22	Sartorius	front		
M23	Hamstrings		back	side
M24	Tensor fascia lata	front		side
M25	Adductor group	front		
M26	Rectus femoris	front		side
M27	Calf muscles		back	side

---

* *The external rotator group and the internal rotator group (not shown) of the scapulo–humerus are distributed over the outer and inner surfaces of the scapula.*

273

Sources of the Quotations

(see also Bibliography)

Laban, *Gymnastik und Tenz*, p. 46
Laban, *Choreutics*, pp. 111–112
Laban, *Choreutics*, p. 25
Laban, *Choreutics*, p. 45
Laban, *Choreutics*, p. 4
Laban, *The Mastery of Movement* (2nd edition), p. v
Laban, *Choreutics*, p. 112
Laban, *Gymnastik und Tenz*, p. 35
Laban, *Choreutics*, p. 46
Rose, "Mathematics Offers Key to Choreutics," Laban Institute
  Newsletter, January, 1979
Laban, *Gymnastik und Tenz*, p. 69
Laban, *Choreutics*, p. 94
Laban, *Choreutics*, p. 5
Laban, *Choreutics*, p. 112
Laban, *Choreographie*, p. 80
Kestenberg, *Children and Parents*, p. 236
Cousins, "Litany for Modern Man," *Saturday Review*, August 8,
  1953
Schnitt, "Duet in Canon: Problems of Conformity," Dance
  Notation Bureau Student Project (unpublished)
Laban, *Gymnastik und Tenz*, pp. 9, 132
Laban, *Gymnastik und Tenz*, p. 131
Laban, *Gymnastik und Tenz*, p. 133
Schoop, *Won't You Join the Dance?*, p. 45
"What is Dance Therapy, Really?," Proceedings of the 7th
  Annual Conference ADTA, October 19–23, 1972, first page
Laban, *The Mastery of Movement*, pp. 88–89
Lomax, *Folk Song Style and Culture*
Bartenieff and Paulay, "Cross-Cultural Example" from *Dance —
  An Art in Academe*
Laban, *Choreutics*, p. 48
Laban, *Gymnastik und Tenz*, pp. 8–9
Laban, *Gymnastik und Tenz*, p. 73
Youngerman, "Translation of a Culture into Choreography:
  A Study of Doris Humphrey's *The Shakers* Based on
  Labananalysis," Woodruff, ed., *Essays in Dance Research*
Rose, "Fairy Tale," Dance Notation Bureau Student Project
Borland, *The Gentle Art of Walking*, pp. v, x
Arnheim, Laban Centennial Address, Laban Institute of
  Movement Studies, New York, June 8–10, 1979
Laban, *Principles of Dance and Movement Notation*, pp. 17, 15, 13
Laban, *Gymnastik und Tenz*, pp. 114–115

Bibliography

Works by Rudolf Laban*

Die Welt des Tänzers: fünf Gedankenreigen. Stuttgart: W. Seifert, 1920. 264 pp.
Choreographie. Jena, Germany: Eugen Diederichs, 1926. 103 pp.
Des Kindes Gymnastik und Tanz. Oldenburg, Germany: G. Stalling, 1926. 134 pp.
Schrifttanz. Wien, Leipzig: Universal Edition, c1928. 1 v.
Ein Leben für den Tanz: Erinnerungen. Dresden: C. Reissner, 1935. 228 pp.; Reprint ed., *A Life for Dance: Reminiscences.* Translated and annotated by Lisa Ullmann. London: Macdonald & Evans, 1975; New York: Theatre Art Books, 1975. 193 pp.
Choreutics. Annotated and edited by Lisa Ullmann. London: Macdonald & Evans, 1966; 1st American ed., *The Language of Movement: A Guidebook to Choreutics.* Annotated and edited by Lisa Ullmann. Boston: Plays, Inc., 1974, c1966. 214 pp.
Effort. With F.C. Lawrence. London: Macdonald & Evans, 1947. 88 pp.; 2nd ed., *Effort: Economy in Body Movement.* Boston: Plays, Inc., 1974. 98 pp.
Modern Educational Dance. 3rd ed., revised with additions by Lisa Ullmann. London: Macdonald & Evans, 1975. 114 pp.
The Mastery of Movement on the Stage. London: Macdonald & Evans, 1950. 190 pp.; 2nd ed., *The Mastery of Movement.* Rev. & enl. by Lisa Ullmann. London: Macdonald & Evans, 1960; Boston: Plays, Inc., 1972. 186 pp.
Principles of Dance and Movement Notation. London: Macdonald & Evans, 1956. 56 pp.; 2nd ed., *Laban's Principles of Dance and Movement Notation.* Revised and annotated by Roderyk Lange. Boston: Plays, Inc., 1975. 61 pp.
Rudolf Laban Speaks About Movement and Dance. Lectures and articles selected and edited by Lisa Ullmann. Woburn Hill, Addlestone, Surrey, England: Laban Art of Movement Centre, 1971. 68 pp.

Works by Irmgard Bartenieff*

(Irma Dombois-Bartenieff) with Irma Otte-Betz. "Elementary Studies in Laban Notation," *Dance Notation Record*, Dec. 1944.
With Ann Hutchinson. "A Tribute to Rudolf Laban by Irmgard Bartenieff and Ann Hutchinson," *Dance Observer* (Dec. 1949), pp. 145–146.
"Functional Approach to the Early Treatment of Poliomyelitis," *Physical Therapy Review*, 35 (Dec. 1955).
"Feuillet's l'Art d'écrire la Danse: A Modern Notator Takes a Look at a System of the Past," *Dance Notation Record*, 7 (1956), pp. 2–9.
Effort Observation and Effort Assessment in Rehabilitation. New York: Dance Notation Bureau, 1962.
With Lucy Venable. "A Presentation of Movement Notation." Unpublished paper presented at the Center for Cognitive Studies, Harvard University, April 1962.
"Contributions of Effort/Shape to Technique and Style in Dance." *Proceedings of the Ninth Annual Conference on Creative Teaching of Dance.* New York: 1965.
With Lucy Venable. "Training the Teacher's Eye." *Proceedings of the Tenth Annual Conference on Creative Teaching of Dance.* New York: 1966.
With Martha Davis. "Effort/Shape Analysis of Movement: The Unity of Expression and Function." Unpublished monograph, Albert Einstein College of Medicine, New York: 1965; Reprinted in *Research Approaches to Movement and Personality.* New York: Arno Press, 1973.
With Forrestine Paulay. "Research in Anthropology: A Study of Dance Styles in Primitive Cultures." *Research in Dance: Problems and Possibilities.* New York: Committee on Research in Dance (CORD), 1967.
With Martha Davis. "An Analysis of the Movement Behavior within a Group Psychotherapy Session." Unpublished paper presented at the Conference of the American Group Psychotherapy Association, Jan. 1968.
With Forrestine Paulay. "Choreometrics Profiles," in Alan Lomax, ed., *Folk Song Style and Culture.* Washington, D.C.: American Association for the Advancement of Science, Publication no. 88, 1968.

* *In chronological order.*

"Laban's Space Harmony in Relation to Anatomical and Neurophysiological Concepts," in Bartenieff, Martha Davis and Forrestine Paulay, *Four Adaptations of Effort Theory in Research and Teaching*. New York: Dance Notation Bureau, 1970.

With Carol Boggs. "Laban's Space Harmony in Relation to Dance." Unpublished paper presented at the Department of Art, Harvard University, Spring 1971.

Notes on a Course in Correctives. New York: Dance Notation Bureau, 1970

"The Roots of Laban Theory: aesthetics and beyond," in Bartenieff, Martha Davis and Forrestine Paulay, *Four Adaptations of Effort Theory in Research and Teaching*. New York: Dance Notation Bureau, 1970.

With Forrestine Paulay. "Cross-Cultural Study of Dance: Description and implication," in Bartenieff, Martha Davis and Forrestine Paulay, *Four Adaptations of Effort Theory in Research and Teaching*. New York: Dance Notation Bureau, 1970.

With Forrestine Paulay. "Dance as Cultural Expression," in M. Haberman and T.G. Meisel, eds., *Dance; An Art in Academe*. New York: Teachers College Press, Columbia University, 1970.

"Dance Therapy: A New Profession or a Rediscovery of an Ancient Role of the Dance?" *Dance Scope*, 7 (1972–3), pp. 6–18.

"Effort/Shape in Teaching Ethnic Dance," in *New Dimensions in Dance research: Anthropology and Dance. I. The American Indian*. Proceedings of the Third Conference of Research in Dance, 1972. Edited by Tamara Comstock. New York: Committee on Research in Dance (CORD), 1974.

With Alan Lomax and Forrestine Paulay. "Choreometrics: A Method for the Study of Cross Cultural Pattern in Film," in *New Dimensions in Dance Research: Anthropology and Dance. I. The American Indian*. Proceedings of the Third Conference on Research in Dance, 1972. Edited by Tamara Comstock. New York: Committee on research in Dance (CORD), 1974.

"Effort/Shape, A Tool in Dance Therapy," in *Proceedings of the American Dance Therapy Association Conference*. New York: 1973.

"Space, Effort and the Brain," *Main Currents in Modern Thought*, 31 (1974), pp. 37–40.

Laban Theory and Applications

Anthropological Perspectives of Movement. New York: Arno Press, 1975.

Cassirer, Ernst. *The Philosophy of Symbolic Forms*. Translated from the French by Ralph Manheim. Preface and introduction by Charles W. Hendel. New Haven, Conn.: Yale Univ. Pr., 1953–57.

Chilkovsky, Nadia. *Three R's for Dancing*. Illustrated by Nicholas Nahumck. New York: M. Witmark, c1955–56. 3 V.

——————. *A Comprehensive Curriculum in Dance for Secondary Schools*. Philadelphia: Univ. of Pennsylvania, 1970. 238 pp.

Cohen, Lynn Renee. "An Inquiry into the Use of Effort/Shape Analysis in the Exploration of Leadership in Small Groups: A Systems View." Unpublished Ph.D. dissertation, Columbia University, 1975.

Dauer, Alfons M. *Der Jazz, Seine Ursprünge und Seine Entwicklung*. Kassel, Germany: E. Roth-Verlag, 1958. 284 pp.

Daubenmire, Jean et al. *Synchronics: A Notation System for the Quantitative and Qualitative Description of Presenting Behaviors*. Columbus, Ohio: Ohio State University Research Foundation, 1977. 217 pp.

Davis, Flora. *Inside Intuition: what we know about nonverbal communication*. New York: McGraw-Hill, 1973. 245 pp.

Davis, Martha. "Effort/Shape Analysis: Evaluation of Its Logic and Consistency and Its Systematic Use in Research," in Irmgard Bartenieff, Martha Davis and Forrestine Paulay, *Four Adaptations of Effort Theory in Research and Teaching*. New York: Dance Notation Bureau, 1970.

——————. "Movement Characteristics of Hospitalized Psychiatric Patients." Proceedings of the American Dance Therapy Association, 1970.

——————. "Movement as Patterns of Process," *Main Currents in Modern Thought*, 31 (1974), pp. 18–22.

——————. "The Potential of Nonverbal Communication Research for Research in Dance," *Committee on Research in Dance (CORD) News*, 6 (1973), pp. 10–28.

——————. *Towards Understanding the Intrinsic in Body Movement*. New York: Arno Pr., 1975, c1973. 132 pp.

——————. *Understanding Body Movement. An Annotated Bibliography*. New York: Arno Pr., 1972. 190 pp.

——————, and Shirley Weitz. "Sex Differences in Nonverbal Communication: A Laban Analysis." Presented at the American Psychological Association Meetings, Toronto, 1978.

Dell, Cecily. "A Language for Movement," *Music Journal*, XXIV (1966), pp. 50, 56–57.

——————. *A Primer for Movement Description: Using Effort/Shape and Supplementary Concepts*. New York: Dance

Notation Bureau, 1970. 123 pp.

——————. *Space Harmony: Basic Terms*. Revised by Aileen Crow. New York: Dance Notation Bureau, c1970. 12pp.

Eisenberg, Philip. *Expressive Movements Related to Feeling of Dominance*. Archives of Psychology, no. 211. 1937. Reprinted in *Research Approaches to Movement and Personality*. Edited by Martha Davis. New York: Arno Pr., 1973. 73 pp.

Gellerman, Jill. "The *Mayim* Pattern as an Indicator of Cultural Attitudes in Three American Hasidic Communities: A Comparative Approach Based on Labananalysis." Unpublished student project. Effort/Shape Certification Program, Dance Notation Bureau, New York, 1977.

Goodridge, Janet. *Creative Drama and Improvised Movement for Children*. Boston: Plays, Inc., 1972, c1970. 158 pp. (First published in 1970 under title: *Drama in the Primary School*. London: Heinemann Educational Books.)

Hutchinson, Ann. *Labanotation; or, Kinetography Laban; The System for Recording Movement*. Rev. and exp. ed. Illustrated by Doug Anderson. New York: Theatre Arts Books, 1970. 508 pp.

Jablonko, Allison Peters. "Dance and Daily Activities among the Maring People of New Guinea: A Cinematographic Analysis of Body Movement Style." Unpublished Ph.D. dissertation, Columbia University, 1968.

Jooss, Kurt. "Rudolf von Laban on His 60th Birthday," *The Dancing Times*, Dec. 1939, pp. 129–131.

Kalish, Beth Isaacs. "Body Movement Scale for Autistic and Other Atypical Children: An Exploratory Study Using a Normal Group and an Atypical Group." Unpublished Ph.D. dissertation, Bryn Mawr College, 1976.

Kestenberg, Judith S. *Children and Parents: psychoanalytic studies in development*. New York: Aronson, 1975. 496 pp.

——————. "The Role of Movement Patterns in Development: I. Rhythms of Movement," *Psychoanalytical Quarterly*, 34 (1965), pp. 1–36.

——————. "The Role of Movement Patterns in Development: II. Flow of Tension and Effort," *Psychoanalytical Quarterly*, 34 (1965), pp. 517–563.

——————. "The Role of Movement Patterns in Development: III. The Control of Shape," *Psychoanalytical Quarterly*, 36 (1967), pp. 356–409.

Kleinman, Seymour. "Effort–Shape for Physical Educators," *Journal of Health, Physical Education and Recreation*, September 1974.

Knust, Albrecht. "Dictionary of Kinetographie Laban." Unpublished manuscript, 1954. Copies available from Roderyk Lange.

——————. *Handbook of Kinetography Laban*. Hamburg, Germany: Verlag Das Tanzarchiv, 1958. 2 V.

——————. and Kurt Peters. *Kinetographisches Lexikon der Klassischen Tanztechnik* (Kinetographic Dictionary of Classical Ballet Technique). Hamburg, Germany: Verlag Das Tanzarchiv, 1965. 16 l.

Lamb, Warren. *Posture and Gesture: An Introduction to the Study of Physical Behaviour*. London: Duckworth & Co., 1965. 189 pp.

——————, and David Turner. *Management Behaviour*. New York: International Universities Pr., 1969. 177 pp.

Lange, Roderyk. "Every Man a Dancer," in *Studio 25, Anniversary Issue*, Addlestone, Surrey, England: The Art of Movement Studio, 1971, pp. 26–32.

——————. *The Nature of Dance: An Anthropological Perspective*. London: Macdonald & Evans, 1975. 142 pp.

Miles, Allan. *Labanotation Workbook*, Rev. ed. New York: Dance Notation Bureau, c1962. 26 pp.

North, Marion. *Body Movement for Children; an introduction to movement study and teaching*. Boston: Plays, Inc., 1972, c1971. 104 pp. (London ed. published under title: Introduction to Movement Study and Teaching.)

——————. *Personality Assessment through Movement*. Boston: Plays, Inc., 1975, c1972. 300 pp.

——————. *A Simple Guide to Movement Teaching; movement in every day life and examples of this experience in developing art of movement teaching in schools*. 4th ed. London: by the author, 1964. 85 pp.

——————. *Movement Education: Child Development through Body Motion*. New York: E.P. Dutton & Co., 1973.

Otte-Betz, Irma. "The Work of Rudolf von Laban," *Dance Observer*. Pt. 1, Dec. 1938, pp. 147; Pt. 2, Jan. 1939, pp. 161–162; Pt. 3, Mar. 1939, pp. 189–190.

Paulay, Forrestine with Alan Lomax. Films: "Step Style," "Palm Play," "Dance and Human History." Berkeley, Ca.: Extension Media Center, University of California, 1974.

——————, Choreometric Findings (untitled work in progress).

Pforsich, Janis. "Effort/Shape Theory Curriculum." Unpublished student project. Effort/Shape Certification Program, Dance Notation Bureau, New York.

Preston-Dunlop, Valerie Monthland. *A Handbook for Modern Educational Dance*. London: Macdonald & Evans, 1963. 187 pp.

277

———— . "A Notation System for Recording Observable Motion," *International Journal of Man–Machine Studies*, 1 (1969), pp. 361—386.

———— . *Practical Kinetography Laban*. London: Macdonald & Evans, 1969; Reprint ed., Brooklyn: Dance Horizons, 1973. 216 pp.

———— . *Readers in Kinetography Laban*, series A. London: Macdonald & Evans, 1966. 3 V.

———— . *Readers in Kinetography Laban*, series B: motif writing for dance. London: Macdonald & Evans, 1967. 4 V.

Ramsden, Pamela. *Top Team Planning: a study of the power of individual motivation in management*. London: Associated Business Programmes; distr. by Cassell, 1973. 262 pp.

Redfern, Betty. *Introducing Laban Art of Movement*. London: Macdonald & Evans, 1965. (2nd ed. of "The Art of Movement in Education, Work and Recreation"), 32 pp.

Redfern, H.B. "Rudolf Laban and the Aesthetics of Dance," *British Journal of Aesthetics*, 16: 61–67, 1976.

Rose, Carol Lynne Moore, "Fairy Tale: Journal of a Dance." Unpublished student project. Effort/Shape Certification Program, Dance Notation Bureau, New York, 1976.

Russell, Joan. *Creative Dance in the Primary School*. London: Macdonald & Evans, 1968. 68 pp.

———— . *Creative Dance in the Secondary School*. London: Macdonald & Evans, 1969. 102 pp.

———— . *Modern Dance in Education*. London: Macdonald & Evans, 1966. 99 pp.

Schmais, Claire and Elissa Q. White. "Movement Analysis: A Must for Dance Therapists," in *Proceedings of the American Dance Therapy Association*, 4th Annual Conference, New York, 1969.

Siegel, Marcia B. *At the Vanishing Point; a critic looks at dance*. New York: Saturday Review Pr., 1972. 320 pp.

———— . "Effort–Shape and the Therapeutic Community." *Dance Magazine*, XLII (1968), pp. 57–59, 71–73.

———— . "Gesture as Language," *Ballet Review*, 3 (1971), pp. 55–63.

———— . "Training an Audience for Dance," *Arts in Society*, Summer (1967), pp. 435–440.

———— . *The Shapes of Change: Images of American Dance*. Boston: Houghton Mifflin Co., 1979. 386 pp.

Thornton, Samuel. *Laban's Theory of Movement; a new perspective*. Boston: Plays, Inc., 1971. 134 pp. (First published in Great Britain under the title: *A Movement Perspective of Rudolf Laban*.)

Ullmann, Lisa. "Movement Education," *The Laban Art of Movement Guild Magazine*, March 1960, pp. 19–28.

Venable, Lucy. "1976 Labananalysis Workshop." Columbus, Ohio: Ohio State University, 1976. (Coding Sheets and Glossary.)

White, Elissa Q. "Effort–Shape: Its Importance to Dance Therapy and Movement Research," *Focus on Dance*, VII: 33–38, 1974.

Whyte, Lancelot Law, ed. *Aspects of Form: a Symposium on Form in Nature and Art*. Bloomington, Ind.: Indiana Univ. Pr., 1961, c1951. 249 pp.

Winearls, Jane. *Modern Dance: The Jooss–Leeder Method*. Foreword by Rudolf Laban, preface by A.V. Coton, with 275 drawings by Peter Krummins. London: Black, 1968. 168 pp.

Wolff, Peter H. "Observations on Newborn Infants," *Psychosomatic Medicine*, 21 (1959), pp. 110–118.

Woodruff, Diane L., ed. *Essays in Dance Research from the Fifth CORD Conference*, Dance Research Annual IX. New York: Committee on Research in Dance, 1978.

Youngerman, Suzanne. "Translation of a Culture into Choreography: A Study of Doris Humphrey's *The Shakers* Based on Labananalysis," in Diane L. Woodruff, ed., *Essays in Dance Research*. Dance Research Annual IX. New York: Committee on Research in Dance, 1978.

Zacharias, Jody. "The Kestenberg Movement Assessment Profile: One Profile, An Explanation and Movement Interpretations." M.A. dissertation, New York University, 1973.

Zalk, Kayla Kazahn and Naima Prevots. *The Laban Factor (A Contextual Biography)*. (In preparation.)

Works on Related Subjects*

Argyle, Michael. *Bodily Communication*. New York: International Universities Press, Inc., 1975. 403 pp.

Allport, Gordon and Philip E. Vernon. *Studies in Expressive Movement*. New York: Hafner, 1967. 269 pp. (Reprint of 1933 edition.)

Arnheim, Rudolf. *Art and Visual Perception: a psychology of the creative eye*. New version, exp. and rev. ed. Berkeley: Univ. of California Pr., 1974. 508 pp.

* *Includes works referred to in text.*

—————. "The Gestalt Theory of Expression," *Psychological Review*, 56 (1949), pp. 165–171.

Basmajian, John V. *Primary Anatomy*. 6th ed. Baltimore: Williams & Wilkins, 1970. 404 pp.

Bateson, Gregory and Claire Holt. "Form and Function of Dance in Traditional Balinese Culture," in Jane Belo, ed., *Traditional Balinese Culture*. New York: Columbia Univ. Pr., c1967.

Birdwhistell, Ray L. "Kinesic Level in the Investigation of the Emotions," in Peter H. Knapp, ed., *Expression of the Emotions in Man*. New York: International Universities Pr., 1963.

—————. "Kinesics and Communication," in Edmund Carpenter and Marshall McLuhan, eds., *Explorations in Communication*. Boston: Beacon Pr., c1960.

—————. *Kinesics and Context; essays on body motion*. University of Pennsylvania Publications in Conduct and Communication, no. 2. Philadelphia: University of Pennsylvania Pr., 1970. 338 pp.

Blair, Lawrence. *Rhythms of Visions; the changing patterns of belief*. Foreword by Lyall Watson. New York: Warner Books, 1977. 234 pp.

Bloomer, Kent C. and Charles W. Moore. *Body, Memory, and Architecture*. New Haven, Conn.: Yale University Press, 1977.

The Body as a Medium of Expression: essays based on a course of lectures given at the Institute of Contemporary Arts, London, edited by Jonathan Benthall and Theodore Polhemus. New York: E.P. Dutton, 1975. 339 pp.

Bosmajian, Haig A., comp. *The Rhetoric of Nonverbal Communication; readings*. Glenview, Ill.: Scott, Foresman, 1971. 180 pp.

Boston Women's Health Book Collective. *Our Bodies Ourselves*. Rev. 2nd ed. New York: Simon and Schuster, 1976.

Brain and Human Behavior, edited by A.G. Karczmar and J.C. Eccles. Berlin: Springer–Verlag, 1972. 475 pp.

Brooks, Charles Van Wyck. *Sensory Awareness; the rediscovery of experiencing*. New York: Viking, 1974. 244 pp.

Bull, Nina. *The Body and Its Mind; an introduction to attitude psychology*. New York: Las Americas, 1962. 99 pp.

Chace, Marian. *Marian Chace her papers*. Edited by Harris Chaiklin. Kensington, Md.: American Dance Therapy Assn., c1975. 261 pp.

Chaiklin, Sharon. "Dance Therapy," in *American Handbook of Psychiatry*. 2nd ed., vol. 5. New York: Basic Books, 1975.

Cheng Man-ch'ing, and Robert W. Smith. *T'ai Chi; the "supreme ultimate" exercise for health, sport, and self-defense*. Rutland, Vt.: Tuttle, c1966. 112 pp.

Cho Won-Kyung. *Dances of Korea*. New York: Dance Notation Bureau, 1962. 38 pp.

Cirlot, Juan Edwardo. *A Dictionary of Symbols*. Translated from the Spanish by Jack Sage. Foreword by Herbert Read. London: Routledge & Kegan Paul, 1962. 400 pp.

Clynes, Manfred. *Sentics: The Touch of Emotions*. Garden City, N.Y.: Anchor Press/Doubleday, 1977. 249 pp.

Conté, Pierre. *La Danse & ses lois; expression par gestes & locomotion, les arts dynamiques*. Paris: Arts et Mouvement, 1952. 239 pp.

Costonis, Maureen Needham. *Therapy in Motion*. Urbana, Ill.: University of Illinois Press, 1978. 278 pp.

Critchlow, Keith. *Order in Space; a design source book*. New York: Viking Pr., 1976. 120 pp.

Crouch, James E. *Functional Human Anatomy*. 3rd ed. Philadelphia: Lea & Febiger, 1978.

Dance in Africa, Asia, and the Pacific: selected readings. Edited by Judy Van Zile. New York: MSS Information Corp., c1976. 177 pp.

Darwin, Charles Robert. *The Expression of the Emotions in Man and Animals*. With a preface by Margaret Mead. New York: Philosophical Library, 1955. 372 pp.

De Mille, Agnes. *The Book of the Dance*. New York: Golden Pr., 1963. 252 pp.

Denby, Edwin. *Dancers, Buildings and People in the Streets*. With an introduction by Frank O'Hara. New York: Horizon Pr., 1965. 287 pp.

Deutsch, Felix. "Analytic Posturology," *Psychoanalytic Quarterly*, 21 (1952), pp. 196–214.

—————. "Analytic Posturology and Synesthesiology: some important theoretical and clinical aspects," *Psychoanalytic Review*, 50 (1963), pp. 40–67.

Dittman, A.T. "Kinesic Research and Therapeutic Process," in Peter H. Knapp, ed., *Symposium on Expression of the Emotions in Man*, 1960. New York: International Universities Pr., 1963.

Draeger, Donn F. and Robert W. Smith. *Asian Fighting Arts*. Palo Alto, Calif.: Kodansha International, 1969. 207 pp.

Duncan, Starkey and Donald W. Fiske. *Face-to-Face Interaction: Research, Methods and Theory*. Hillsdale, N.J.: Lawrence Erlbaum Associates, Publishers, 1977. 361 pp.

Efron, David. *Gesture and Environment*. New York: Kings Crown, 1941. 226 pp.

Eibl-Eibesfeldt, Irenäus. "Similarities and Differences Between Cultures in Expressive Movements," in Robert A. Hinde, ed., *Non-Verbal Communication*. London: Cambridge Univ. Pr., 1972.

Ekman, Paul. "Body Position, Facial Expression and Verbal Behavior during Interviews," *Journal of Abnormal and Social Psychology*, 68 (1964), pp. 295–301.

——————. "Communication through Nonverbal Behavior: a source of information about an interpersonal relationship," in S.S. Tompkins and C.E. Izard, eds., *Affect, Cognition and Personality*. New York: Springer, 1965.

——————. "Universals of Cultural Differences in Facial Expressions of Emotion," in James K. Cole and Donald D. Jensen, eds., *Nebraska Symposium on Motivation*. Lincoln, Neb.: Univ. of Nebraska Pr., 1972.

——————, ed. *Darwin and Facial Expression*. New York: Academic Press, 1973. 273 pp.

——————. *Unmasking the Face; a guide to recognizing emotions from facial clues*. Englewood Cliffs, N.J.: Prentice-Hall, 1975. 212 pp.

——————, and Wallace V. Friesen. "Constants Across Cultures in the Face and Emotions," *Journal of Personality and Social Psychology*, 17 (1971), pp. 124–129.

——————, ——————. "Head and Body Cues in the Judgment of Emotion: a Reformulation," *Perceptual and Motor Skills*, 24 (1967), pp. 711–724.

——————, ——————. "The Repertoire of Nonverbal Behavior: Categories, Origins, Usage and Coding," *Semiotica*, 1 (1969), pp. 49–98.

——————, ——————, and Phoebe Ellsworth. *Emotion in the Human Face*. New York: Pergamon Pr., 1972. 191 pp.

——————, ——————, and E.R. Sorenson. "Pan-Culture Elements in Facial Displays of Emotion," *Science*, 164 (1969), pp. 86–88.

Espenak, Liljan. *Body Dynamics and Dance in Individual Psychotherapy*. Monograph no. 2, pp. 111–127. Columbia, Md.: American Dance Therapy Assn., 1972.

Ferber, Andrew and Adam Kendon. "A Description of Some Human Greetings," in R.P. Michael and J.H. Crook, eds., *Comparative Ecology and Behaviour of Primates:* proceedings of a conference held at the Zoological Society, London, 1971. London: Academic Pr., 1973.

Freedman, Norbert and Stanley Grand, eds. *Communicative Structures and Psychic Structures*. New York: Plenum Press, 1977. 465 pp.

Fries, Margaret E. "Longitudinal Study: Prenatal Period to Parenthood," *Psychoanalytic Association Journal*, 1 (1977), pp. 115-132.

——————, with Beatrice Lewi. "Interrelated Factors in Development: A Study of Pregnancy, Labor, Delivery, Lying-in Period, and Childhood." *American Journal for Orthopsychiatry*, vol. XIII, no. 4, October 1938. pp. 726-752.

Fuller, Richard Buckminster. *Ideas and Integrities*; a spontaneous autobiographical disclosure. Edited by Robert W. Marks. Englewood Cliffs, NJ: Prentice-Hall, 1963. 318 pp.

——————*Synergetics: Explorations in the Geometry of Thinking*. Preface and contribution by Arthur L. Loeb. New York: Macmillan, 1975. 876 pp.

Goffman, Erving. *Behavior in Public Places*; notes on the social organization of gatherings. New York: Free Press of Glencoe, 1963. 248 pp.

——————*Interaction Ritual: Essays on Face-to-Face Behavior*. Garden City, NY: Doubleday, c1967.

——————. *The Presentation of Self in Everyday Life*. Garden City, NY: Doubleday, 1959. 255 pp.

Goodman, Nelson. *Languages of Art*; an approach to a theory of symbols. Indianapolis: Bobbs-Merrill, 1968. 277 pp.

Hall, Edward T. "The Anthropology of Manner," *Scientific American*, 192 (1955), pp. 85–89.

——————. *The Hidden Dimension*. Garden City, N.Y.: Doubleday, 1969. 217 pp.

——————. "The Language of Space," *A.I.A. Journal*, Feb. 1961.

——————. *The Silent Language*. Garden City, N.Y.: Doubleday, 1959. 240 pp.

——————. "A System for the Notation of Proxemic Behavior," *American Anthropologist*, 65 (1963), pp. 1003–1026.

Hayes, F. "Gestures: A Working Bibliography," *Southern Folklore Quarterly*, 21 (1957), pp. 218–317.

H'Doubler, Margaret Newell. *Dance: A Creative Art Experience*. With dance sketches by Wayne Lm. Claxton. 2nd ed. Madison, Wisc.: The Univ. of Wisconsin Pr., 1957. 167 pp.

——————. *The Art of Making Dances*. Madison, Wisc.: Univ. of Wisconsin Pr., 1966.

Henley, Nancy M. *Body Politics: Power, Sex and Nonverbal Communication*. Englewood Cliffs, N.J.: Prentice-Hall, 1977. 214 pp.

Hewes, Gordon W. "The Anthropology of Posture," *Scientific American*, 196 (1957), pp. 123–132.

——————. "World Distribution of Certain Postural Habits," *American Anthropologist*, 57 (1957), pp. 231–244.

Hollingshead, William Henry. *Functional Anatomy of the Limbs and Back: a text for students of physical therapy and others interested in the locomotor apparatus.* 3rd ed. Philadelphia: W.B. Saunders, 1969. 420 pp.

Hood, Mantle. *The Ethnomusicologist.* New York: McGraw-Hill, 1971. 386 pp.

Human Relations Area File (HRAF). Yale University, 1963. (Founded 1949: collects data on world's cultures.)

Huang, Al Chung-liang. *Embrace Tiger. Return to Mountain: the essence of t'ai chi.* Moab, Utah: Real people Pr., c1973. 188 pp.

Jablonko, Allison. "Physical Movement and Ethnographic Film (The Maring of New Guinea)." Unpublished paper presented at the 65th annual meeting of the American Anthropological Association, 1966.

Jacob, Stanley W. and Clarice Ashworth Freancone. *Structure and Function in Man.* 2nd ed. Philadelphia: W.B. Saunders, 1970. 591 pp.

Jacobson, Edmund. *Biology of Emotions; New Understanding Derived from Biological Multidisciplinary Investigation; First Electrophysiological Measurements.* Springfield, Ill.: Thomas, 1967. 211 pp.

Jammer, Max. *Concepts of Force; a study in the foundations of dynamics.* Cambridge, Mass.: Harvard Univ. Pr., 1957. 269 pp.

—————. *Concepts of Space: the history of theories in physics.* Foreword by Albert Einstein. Cambridge, Mass.: Harvard Univ. Pr., 1954. 196 pp.

Jankovic, Ljubica S. *Problem and Theory of Individual Arrhythmy in the Rhythm of the Whole of Performance of Folk Dance and Folk Melody.* Serbian Ethnographic Anthology, 82. Belgrad, Yugoslavia: Serbian Academy of Arts and Sciences, 1968.

Jaques-Dalcroze, Emile. *Rhythm, Music and Education.* Translated from the French by Harold F. Rubinstein. New York: G.P. Putnam's Sons, 1921. 334 pp. London: Dalcroze Society, 1967. 200 pp.

Kaeppler, Adrienne Lois. "The Structure of Tongan Dance." Unpublished Ph.D. dissertation. University of Hawaii, 1967.

Kealiinohomoku, Joanne. "Theory and Methods for an Anthropological Study of Dance." Ph.D. disseration, Indiana University, 1976. (Available through Ann Arbor Referencing System.)

Kendon, Adam. "Some Functions of Gaze–Direction in Social Interaction," *Acta Psychologica*, 26 (1967), pp. 22–63.

—————, Richard M. Harris and Mary Ritchie Key, eds. *Organization of Behavior in Face-to-Face Interaction.* The Hague and Paris: Mouton Publishers, 1975. 509 pp.

Kepes, Gyorgy, ed., Vision + Value Series: *The Nature of Art and Motion; Education of Vision; Structure in Art and Science.* New York: Braziller, 1965. 195 pp.; 233 pp.; 189 pp.

Key, Mary Ritchie. *Nonverbal Communication: A Research Guide and Bibliography.* Metuchen, N.J.: Scarecrow Pr., 1977. 439 pp.

—————. *Paralanguage and Kinesics.* (Nonverbal communication), with a bibliography. Metuchen, N.J.: Scarecrow Pr., 1975. 246 pp.

Knapp, Mark. *Nonverbal Communication in Human Interaction.* New York: Holt, Rinehart and Winston, 1978. 213 pp.

Kostrubala, Thaddeus. *The Joy of Running.* Philadelphia: J.B. Lippincott, c1976. 158 pp.

Krout, Maurice Haim. *Autistic Gestures: an experimental study in symbolic movement.* (Psychological Monographs, vol. 46, no. 208.) Columbus, Ohio: Psychological Review, 1935. 126 pp.

—————. "An Experimental Attempt to Produce Unconscious Manual Symbolic Movements," *Journal of General Psychology*, 51 (1954), pp. 93–120.

Kurath, Gertrude P. "Panorama of Dance Ethnology," *Current Anthropology*, 1 (1960), pp. 233–254.

La Barre, Weston. "The Cultural Basis of Emotions and Gestures," *Journal of Personality and Social Psychology*, 16 (1947), pp. 49–68.

—————. "Paralinguistics, Kinesics and Cultural Anthropology," in Thomas A. Sebeok, Alfred S. Hayes and Mary Catherine Bateson, eds., *Approaches to Semiotics.* The Hague: Mouton, c1964. 294 pp.

LaFrance, Marianne and Clara Mayo. *Moving Bodies: Nonverbal Communication in Social Relationships.* Monterey, Ca.: Brooks/Cole, 1978. 225 pp.

Lange, Roderyk. *The Nature of Dance: An Anthropological Perspective.* London: Macdonald & Evans, 1975. 142 pp.

Langer, Susanne Katherina. *Feeling and Form; a theory of art.* New York: Scribner, 1953. 431 pp.

—————. *Philosophy in a New Key; a study in the symbolism of reason, rite, and art.* 2nd ed. New York: New American Library, c1951. 256 pp.

The Language of Pattern; an enquiry inspired by Islamic decoration. New York: Harper & Row, 1974. 112 pp.

Lasswell, Harold et al. *The Comparative Study of Symbols.* Stanford, Ca.: Stanford University Press, 1952. 87 pp.

Lerner, Ira and Tex Yukiso Yamamoto. *Diary of the Way, three paths to enlightenment.* New York: A. & W. Publs., 1977. 160 pp.

Lettvin, Maggie. *Maggie Lettvin and Her Famous Television Exercise Program, the Beautiful Machine.* New York: Knopf, 1972. 1 case.

Lockhart, Robert D. *Living Anatomy: a photographic atlas of muscles in action and surface contours.* 6th ed. London: Faber, 1970. 91 pp.

Lomax, Alan. *Folk Song Style and Culture.* With contributions by the Cantometrics staff and with the editorial assistance of Edwin E. Erickson. New Brunswick, N.J.: Transaction Books. Repr. of 1968 ed. publ. by American Association for the Advancement of Science, Washington, D.C., publ. no. 88. 363 pp.

Lott, Dale F. and Robert Sommer. "Seating Arrangements and Status," *Journal of Personality and Social Psychology,* 7 (1967), pp. 90–95.

Lowen, Alexander. *The Betrayal of the Body.* New York: Macmillan, 1967. 307 pp.

———. *Bioenergetics.* New York: Penguin, 1976, c1975. (Reprint of ed. published by Coward, McCann & Geoghegan.)

———. *The Language of the Body.* New York: Collier Books, 1971. 400 pp. (Originally published as "Physical Dynamics of Character Structure.")

Lu Hui-ching. *T'ai Chi Ch'uan; a manual of instruction.* New York: St. Martin's Pr., c1973. 166 pp.

Machotka, Paul. "Defensive Style and Esthetic Distortion," *Journal of Personality and Social Psychology,* 35 (1967), pp. 600–622.

Maisel, Edward. *Tai Chi for Health.* New York: Holt, Rinehart and Winston, 1972. 212 pp.

Marey, Etienne Jules. *Movement.* Translated from the French by Eric Pritchard. New York: International Scientific Series, Vol. 73, 1895. Reprint ed. New York: Arno Pr., 1972. 323 pp.

Mead, Margaret and Frances Cooke Macgregor. *Growth and Culture: A Photographic Study of Balinese Childhood.* Based upon photos by Gregory Bateson, analyzed in Gesell categories. New York: Putnam, 1951. 223 pp.

Mehrabian, Albert. "Significance of Posture and Position in the Communication of Attitude and Status Relationships," *Psychological Bulletin,* 71 (1969), pp 359-372.

Merleau-Ponty, Maurice. *The Structure of Behavior.* Translated by Alden L. Fisher. Boston: Beacon Pr., 1963. 256 pp.

Morris, Charles William. "Signs, Language, Behavior," in his *Writings on the General Theory of Signs.* The Hague: Mouton, 1971.

Munro, Thomas. *Form and Style in the Arts:* an introduction to aesthetic morphology. Published in collaboration with the Cleveland Museum of Art. Cleveland, Ohio: Press of Case Western Reserve University, 1970. 467 pp.

Murdock, George Peter and Timothy J. O'Leary *Ethnographic Bibliography of North America.* 4th ed. New Haven: Human Relations Area Files, 1975. 5 v.

Parsons, T.E. et al. "Some Fundamental Categories of the Theory of Action: A General Statement," in Parsons and E. Shils, eds., *Towards a General Theory of Action.* Cambridge, Mass.: Harvard Univ. Pr., 1951.

Polhemus, Ted, ed., *The Body Reader: Social Aspects of the Human Body.* New York: Pantheon, 1978. 336 pp.

Pollenz, Philippa. "Methods for the Comparative Study of the Dance," *American Anthropologist,* 51, (1938), pp 428-435.

Reich, Wilhelm. *Character-analysis.* 3d. enl. ed., translated by Theodore P. Wolfe. New York: Farrar, Straus and Giroux (The Noonday Press), 1949. 516 pp.

———. *The Function of the Orgasm; sex-economic problems of biological energy.* Translated from the German manuscript by Theodore P. Wolfe. New York: Noonday Press, 1961. 368 pp.

Reichard, Gladys Amanda. *Navaho Religion, a Study in Symbolism.* 2d ed. New York: Bollingen Foundation; distr. by Pantheon Books, 1963. 804 pp.

Renneker, R.E. "Some Methodological Considerations Regarding Kinesic Research," in Peter H. Knapp, ed., *Expression of the Emotions in Man.* New York: International Universities Prs., 1963.

Research Approaches to Movement and Personality. New York: Arno Press, 1972. (Reprint of 3 publications.) 73 pp. 71 pp. 130 pp.

Risner, Vicky J. "Dance Ethnography Data Inventory Project." Dept. of Dance, Univ. of California, Los Angeles, Calif., 1973.

Royce, Anya Peterson. *The Anthropology of Dance.* Bloomington, Ind.: Indiana Univ. Pr., 1977. 238 pp.

Rush, Anne Kent. *Getting Clear: body work for women.* New York: Random House, 1973. 290 pp.

Saitz, Robert L. and Edward J. Cervenka. "Handbook of Gestures," *Semiotica,* 31 (1972), pp.

Sasamori, Junzo and Gordon Warner. *This is Kendo: the Art of Japanese Fencing.* Rutland, Vt.: Charles E. Tuttle, 1964. 159 pp.

Saunders, Ernest Dale. *Mudra;* a study of symbolic gestures in Japanese Buddhist sculpture. New York: Pantheon Books, 1960. 296 pp.

Scheflen, Albert E. *How Behavior Means*. New York: Gordon and Breach, 1973. 167 pp.

——————— with Alice Scheflen. *Body Language and the Social Order*. Englewood Cliffs, N.J.: Prentice-Hall, Inc., 1972. 208 pp.

Schilder, Paul. *The Image and Appearance of the Human Body:* studies in the constructive energies of the psyche. New York: International Universities Pr., 1950. 353 pp.

Schoop, Trudi, with Peggy Mitchell. *Won't You Join the Dance?* A dancer's essay into the treatment of psychosis. Palo Alto, Calif.: National Pr. Books, 1974. 194 pp.

Selye, Hans. *The Stress of Life*. New York: McGraw-Hill, 1956. 324 pp.

Shawn, Ted. *Every Little Movement;* A book about Francois Delsarte . . . 2d ed. Pittsfleld, Mass.: Eagle Print and Binding, 1963; Reprint ed., Brooklyn, Dance Horizons, 1968. 127 pp.

Sheehan, George, *Dr. George Sheehan's Medical Advice for Runners*. Mountain View, Ca.: World Publications, Inc., 1978. 303 pp.

Shore, Herb. "Cultural Innovation in Advanced Technological Societies." Unpublished report for the US National Commission for UNESCO. Spring 1977.

Siegman, Aron W. and Stanley Feldstein. *Nonverbal Behavior and Communication*. Hillsdale, N.J.: Lawrence Erlbaum Associates, Publishers. 1978. 400 pp.

Soo, Clifford Chee. *The Chinese Art of T'ai Chi Ch'uan*. London: Gordon & Cremonesi, 1976. 206 pp.

Sorell, Walter. "Marginal Notes," *Dance Scope*, Fall/Winter (1973–74).

Spiegel, John Paul and Paul Machotka. *Messages of the Body*. New York: Free Press, 1974. 440 pp.

Stebbins, Genevieve. *Delsarte System of Expression*, with 32 illustrations from Greek art. Rev. New York: S. Werner, 1902. 507 pp.

Stevens, Peter S. *Patterns in Nature*. Boston: Little, Brown, 1974. 240 pp.

Szasz, Suzanne. *The Body Language of Children*. New York: W.W. Norton and Co., 1978. 159 pp.

Tegner, Bruce. *Kung Fu & Tai Chi: Chinese Karate & Classical Exercises*. Rev. Ventura, Calif.: Thor, 1973. 127 pp.

Thompson, D'Arcy Wentworth. *On Growth and Form*. An abridged ed., edited by John Tyler Bonner. Cambridge, England: Cambridge Pr., 1961. 345 pp. (An unabridged ed., 2nd ed., reprinted by Cambridge Univ. Pr., 1959, 2 V.)

Thompson, Robert Farris. *African Art in Motion; icon and art in the collection of Katherine Coryton White*. Catalog of an exhibition. National Gallery of Art, Washington, D.C.; Frederick S. Wight Art Gallery, University of California Press, 1974. 275 pp.

Van Zile, Judy. *Dance in India*. An annotated guide to source materials. Providence, R.I.: Asian Music publs., 1973. 129 pp.

Vatsyayan, Kapila. *Classical Indian Dance in Literature and the Arts*. New Delhi, India: Sangeet Natak Akademi, 1968. 431 pp.

Waxer, Peter H. *Nonverbal Aspects of Psychotherapy*. New York: Praeger Publishers, 1978. 119 pp.

Wentinck, Charles. *The Human Figure in Art from Prehistoric Times to the Present Day*. Translated from the French by Eva Cooper. Wynnewood, Pa.: Livingston, 1971. 160 pp.

Whitehouse, Mary. "The Transference in Dance Therapy," *American Journal for Dance Therapy*, Spring 1977.

——————— . "Reflections on the Metamorphosis," *Impulse*, 1969–70.

——————— . "Creative Expression in Physical Movement Is Language Without Words." Unpublished talk to the Psychoanalytic Club, Los Angeles, 1963.

——————— . "Physical Movement and Personality." Unpublished talk given at the Psychoanalytic Club, Los Angeles, 1963.

——————— . "The Tao of the Body." Unpublished talk given at the Psychoanalytic Club, Los Angeles, 1958.

Wigman, Mary. *The Language of Dance*. Translated from the German by Walter Sorrell. Middletown, Conn.: Wesleyan Univ. Pr., 1966. 118 pp.

Wilson, Jim. *Illustrated Guide to the Art of Oriental Self Defense*. London: Cavendish, 1975. 88 pp.

Wolz, Carl. "Dance in the Noh Theatre," *The World of Music*, 3 (1961), pp. 26–32.

Wosien, Maria Gabriele. *Sacred Dance*. Encounter with the gods. London: Thames & Hudson, 1974. 128 pp.

Wundt, Willhelm. *The Language of Gestures*. With an introduction by Arthur L. Blumenthal and additional essays by George Herbert Mead and Karl Bühler. The Hague: Mouton, 1973. 149 pp.

Documentation and Notation

Brown, Maxine Diane. "A Graphic Editor for Labanotation." Masters Thesis, Department of Computer Science, The Moore School of Electrical Engineering, University of Pennsylvania, Aug. 1976.

Benesh, Rudolf and Joan Benesh. *An Introduction to Benesh Notation*. With a foreword by Arnold L. Haskell. London: A. and C. Black, 1956. 48 pp.

Eshkol, Noa and Abraham Wachmann. *Movement Notation*. London: Weidenfeld & Nicholson, 1958. 203 pp.

György, Martin. *Magyar Tánctipusok és Táncdialektusok*. (Dance-types and Dance Dialects from Hungary. One text vol. and I, II, III notation vols.) Notated by A. Lanyi. Budapest: Nepmuvelesi Propaganda Iroda, 1970–1972.

Feuillet, Raoul Auger. *Choreographie, ou l'Art d'écrire la dance par caracteres, figures, et signes démonstratifs, avec lesquels on apprend facilement de soy-même toutes sortes de dances*. Paris: l'auteur, 1700. 106, 84, 72 pp.

Hutchinson, Ann. "A Survey of Systems of Dance Notation." Unpublished manuscript, illustrated with slides. Available from Dance Notation Bureau, New York. Includes Benesh, Feuillet, Jay, Morris, Stepanov, Sullivan, Sutton, and Zorn notations.

Kurath, Gertrude P. "A New Method of Choreographic Notation," *American Anthropologist*, 52 (1950), pp. 120–123.

Laban, Juana de. "Introduction to Dance Notation," *Dance Index*, V (April–May, 1946), pp. 89–129.

"Labanotated Dances." A list available from the Dance Notation Bureau, 505 Eighth Avenue, New York, N.Y. 10018.

Lange, Roderyk. "Kinetography Laban and the Folk Dance Research in Poland." *Lud*, PTL (Polish Ethnological Society), 50 (Warsaw), 1966, pp. 378–391. 5 kinetograms. Summary of lectures given at the International Congress of Anthropological and Ethnological Sciences, University of Moscow, Moscow, 1964.

—————. "On Differences Between the Rural and the Urban: Traditional Polish Peasant Dancing." *1974 Yearbook of the International Folk Music Council*, Ontario, Canada: n.p., 1975. pp. 44–51.

—————. "The Traditional Dances of Poland." *Viltis* 29 (1) (Denver, Colorado), May, 1970, pp. 4–41. 20 illustrations, 6 kinetograms, 1 map, music, 1 synoptic table, list of selected books.

Mahoney, Billie. *Body-tone-ology in Modern Jazz*. New York: Dance Notation Bureau, 1961. Labanotated examples.

Morris, Margaret. *The Notation of Movement, Psyche Miniatures*. Text, drawings and diagrams by Margaret Morris; with an introduction by H. Levy. London: K. Paul, Trench, Trubner, 1928. 103 pp.

Topaz, Muriel, ed. *Catalog of Dance Reconstruction in Labanotation*. New York: Dance Notation Bureau, 1973.

Zorn, Friedrich Albert. *Grammar of the Art of Dancing, Theoretical and Practical*. Lessons in the arts of dancing and dance writing (choreography) with drawings, musical examples, choreographic symbols, and special music scores. Translated from the German by Benjamin P. Coates. Edited by Alfonso Josephs Sheafe. Boston: The Ileintzemann Pr., 1905. 302 pp.

Fundamentals

Alexander, Frederick Matthias. *The Resurrection of the Body*. The Writings of F. Matthias Alexander. Selected and introduced by Edward Maisel. With a preface by Raymond A. Dart. New York: University Books, 1969. 204 pp.

Alexander, Gerda. *L'Eutonie*. Munich: Koesel Verlag, 1976.

Arnheim, Daniel D., with Joan Schlaich. *Dance Injuries, Their Prevention and Care*. With 125 illustrations. Drawings by Helene Arnheim. St. Louis, Mo.: C.V. Mosby, 1975. 183 pp.

Ayres, Anna Jean. *Sensory Integration and Learning Disorders*. Los Angeles: Western Psychological Services, c1972. 294 pp.

Basmajian, John V. *Muscles Alive: their functions revealed by electromyography*. 3rd ed. Baltimore, Md.: Williams & Wilkins, 1974. 525 pp.

Benjamin, Ben E. *Sports Without Pain*. New York: Summit Books; 1979. 247 pp.

Brunnstrom, Signe. *Clinical Kinesiology*. Philadelphia: F.A. Davis, 1962. 339 pp.

Daniels, Lucille, Marian Williams and Catherine Worthingham. *Muscle Testing: Techniques of Manual Examination*. Format and text illustrated by Harold Black. Anatomical drawings by Lorene Sigal. 2nd ed. Philadelphia: W.B. Saunders, 1956. 176 pp.

Duchenne, Guillaume Benjamin Armand. *Physiology of Motion Demonstrated by Means of Electrical Stimulation . . .* Translated and edited by Emanuel B. Kaplan. Philadelphia: W.B. Saunders, 1959. 612 pp.

Feldenkrais, Moshé. *Awareness Through Movement: health exercises for personal growth.* New York: Harper & Row, 1972. 173 pp.

Finneson, Bernard E., with Arthur S. Freese. *Dr. Finneson on Low Back Pain.* New York: Putnam, 1975. 254 pp.

Fiorentino, Mary R. *Reflex Testing Methods for Evaluation of Central Nervous System Development.* With foreword by Burr H. Curtis. American Lectures in Orthopaedic Surgery, no. 543. Springfield, Ill.: Thomas, 1963, 58 pp.

Gelabert, Raoul. *Gelabert's Anatomy for the Dancer.* With exercises to improve technique and prevent injuries. Edited by William Como. Photographs by Jack Mitchell. New York: *Dance Magazine,* c1964–66. 2 V. (First published as a series in *Dance Magazine,* V. 37, no. 1, Jan. 1963, to July 1966, under the title: *Anatomy for the Ballet Teacher.*)

Glaser, Volkmar. *Integrale Tonus Regulation*: das Wirkungsprincip der Psychotaktilen Therapie nach Glaser-Veldman. Zeitschrift für allgemeine und spezielle Medizin: Physikalische Medizin und Rehabilitation. Vol. 11, no. 5, Mai 1970.

——————. Krankengymnastische Behandlung von Haltungsschaden. Zeitschrift für allgemeine und spezielle Medizin: Physikalische Medizin und Rehabilitation. Vol. 8, no. 5, November 1967.

——————. *Das Menschenbild der westlichen Welt im Meridiansystem der oestlichen Welt.* Unpublished material.

Goodgold, Joseph. *Anatomical Correlates of Clinical Electromyography.* Baltimore, Md.: William & Wilkins, 1974. 153 pp.

Granit, Ragnar. *Receptors and Sensory Perception.* A discussion of aims, means, and results of electrophysiological research into the process of reception. New Haven, Conn.: Yale Univ. Pr., 1955. 369 pp.

Gray, Henry. *Anatomy, descriptive and surgical.* Edited by T. Pickering Pick and Robert Howden. Philadelphia: Running Press, c1974. 1257 pp. (Facsimile reprint of 1901 ed.) Also, Philadelphia: Lea and Febiger, 1973 (29th ed.).

Hecox, Bernadette, Ellen Levine and Diana Scott. "Dance in Physical Rehabilitation," *Physical Therapy,* 56 (1976), pp. 919–924.

Hollingshead, William Henry. *Functional Anatomy of the Limbs and Back: A Text for Students of Physical Therapy and Others Interested in the Locomotor Apparatus.* 3rd ed. Philadelphia: W.B. Saunders, 1969. 420 pp.

Inman, Verne T. "Function of the Adductor Muscle," *Journal of Bone and Joint Surgery,* 29 (1949), pp. 607–615.

——————. "Some Observations of the Function of the Shoulder Joint," *Journal of Bone and Joint Surgery,* 26 (1944), pp. 1–36.

Jacobson, Edmund. *Biology of Emotions: New Understanding Derived from Biological Multidisciplinary Investigation; First Electrophysiological Measurements.* Springfield, Ill.: Thomas, 1967. 211 pp.

——————. *Progressive Relaxation.* A physiological and clinical investigation of muscular states and their significance in psychology and medical practice. 2nd ed. Chicago: Univ. of Chicago Pr., 1938. 493 pp.

——————. comp. *Tension in Medicine.* Springfield, Ill.: Thomas, 1967. 148 pp.

Jones, Frank Pierce. *Body Awareness in Action: A Study of the Alexander Technique.* New York: Schocken Books, Inc., 1976. 176 pp.

Kabat, H. et al. "Relaxation of Spasticity by Physiological Techniques," *Archives of Physical Medicine and Rehabilitation,* 35 (1944), pp. 214–223.

Kahn, Fritz. *The Human Body.* New York: Random House, 1965. 288 pp.

Kendall, Henry Otis and Florence Peterson Kendall. *Muscles, Testing and Function.* Baltimore, Md.: Williams & Wilkins, 1949. 278 pp.

——————, ——————, and G.E. Wadsworth. *Muscles: Testing and Functioning.* Baltimore, Md.: Williams & Wilkins Co., 1971 (2nd ed.). 284 pp.

Kent, Barbara E. Functional Anatomy of the Shoulder Complex. *Physical Therapy Review,* vol. 51, no. 5, August, 1971.

Knott, Margaret and Dorothy E. Voss. *Proprioceptive Neuromuscular Facilitation: Patterns and Techniques.* 2nd ed. With illustrations by Helen Drew Hipshman and James B. Buckley. Foreword by Sedgwick Mead. New York: Hoeber Medical Division, Harper & Row, 1968. 225 pp.

Lagerwerff, Ellen B. and Karen A. Perlroth. *Mensendieck: your posture and your pains.* Line drawings by Ellen B. Lagerwerff. Anatomy drawings by Karen A. Perlroth. Garden City, Anchor Pr., 1973. 263 pp.

Latchaw, Marjorie and Glen Egstrom. *Human Movement.* With concepts applied to children's movement activities. Englewood Cliffs, N.J.: Prentice-Hall, 1969. 337 pp.

Leonard, George Burr. *The Ultimate Athlete: re-visioning sports, physical education and the body.* New York: Viking Pr., 1975. 273 pp.

285

Liebowitz, Judith. "For the Victims of Our Culture: The Alexander Technique," *Dance Scope*, Fall/Winter (1967–8), pp. 32–3.

MacConaill, Michael Aloysius and John V. Basmajian. *Muscles and Movements: A Basis for Human Kinesiology.* New rev. ed. Huntington, N.Y.: Krieger, 1977. 400 pp.

McGraw, Myrtle Byram. *The Neuromuscular Maturation of the Human Infant.* Reprint edition with new introduction and updated bibliography. New York: Hafner, 1963, c1949. 140 pp.

Mensendieck, Bess M. *Körperkultur der Frau: praktisch hygienische und praktisch ästhetische Winke.* Munich: F. Bruckmann, 1919. 200 pp.

Michele, Arthur Albert. *Iliopsoas: Development of Anomalies in Man,* Springfield, Ill.: Thomas, 1962. 550 pp.

————— . *Orthotherapy.* Illustrations by Rosemary Torre. New York: Evans, 1971. 223 pp.

Mollier, Siegfried A.E. *Plastische Anatomie: die konstruktive form des meschlichen körpers.* With illustrations by Hermann Sachs. Munich: J.F. Bergmann, 1924. 296 pp.

Muybridge, Eadweard. *The Human Figure in Motion.* Introduction by Robert Taft. New York: Dover, 1955. 195 pp.

Nuvga, Vincent C. *Manipulation of the Spine.* Baltimore: Williams & Wilkins, 1976.

Rathbone, Josephine Langworthy. *Corrective Physical Education.* Philadelphia: W.B. Saunders, 1934. 292 pp.

Schmidt, Richard A. *Motor Skills.* New York: Harper & Row, 1975. 158 pp.

Schmitt, Johannes Ludwig, in collaboration with Frederike Richter. *Atemheilkunst.* Munich: Müller, 1956. 619 pp.

Sparger, Celia. *Anatomy and Ballet.* A handbook for teachers of ballet. Foreword by S.L. Higgs. Introduction by Dame Ninette de Valois. 2nd ed. London: A. and C. Black, 1952. 79 pp.

Steindler, Arthur. *Kinesiology of the Human Body.* Under normal and pathological conditions. Springfield, Ill.: Thomas, 1955. 706 pp.

Stough, Carl and Reece Stough. *Dr. Breath: The Story of Breathing Co-ordination.* New York: Wm. Morrow & Co,. Inc., 1970. 255 pp.

Sweigard, Lulu E. *Human Movement Potential: Its Ideokinetic Facilitation.* New York: Dodd, Mead, 1974. 320 pp.

Todd, Mabel Elsworth. *The Thinking Body.* A study of balancing forces of dynamic man. Foreword by E.G. Brackett. Brooklyn, Dance Horizons, 1968, c1959. 314 pp.

Whitfield, D. "Human Skill as a Determinant of Allocation of Function," in W.T. Singleton, R.S. Easterby and D.C. Whitfield, eds., *Proceedings of the Conference on the Human Operator in Complex Systems.* London: Taylor & Francis, 1967.

Yesudian, Selva Raja. *Sport and Yoga.* Thielle, Switzerland: Edouard Frankhauser, 1949. 282 pp.

Young, J.Z. *Programs of the Brain.* Oxford: Oxford University Press, 1978. 325 pp.

Index

Actions, 73
  phrasing in, 73-74, 76-78
    multi-phasic, 73, 74, 77
    two-phasic, 73-74, 76, 78
Affinities, of body, space and Effort, 85-100
  cube diagonals and basic Effort, 91-92
  examples of, 94-100
Albert Einstein Medical College, 9
Alexander technique, 147
American Dance Guild, 167
American Dance Therapy Association
    (ADTA), 143
Arnheim, Rudolf, 215
Authentic response, 138-39

Balkan dances, 74
Bartenieff, Irmgard, 112, 169
Bartenieff, Michail, 118-19
Bartenieff Fundamentals, 5, 15, 87, 159
  exercises according to, 19, 20-22, 230-62
    additional, 250-59
    basic, 235-49
    how to use, 230
    preparatory, 231-34
    summary notes on, 260-62
  role of, in dance therapy, 145-46, 162
Basic Effort Actions, 57, 58-59, 61, 63
  Drives, 91-92
Basic exercises, 20, 21
  bodily awareness, 20-21
See also Exercises, according to Bartenieff
    Fundamentals
Bateson, Gregory, 167
Bellevue Hospital, 6
Bereska, Dussia, 224
Berger, Lynn Flexner, 155
Birdwhistell, Raymond, 112, 167
Bishop Museum (Honolulu), 168
Blythedale Hospital (Valhalla, N.Y.), 6-9,
    154
Boas, Franziska, 143
Body architecture:
  connectedness, 21
  joints, 19, 26
  muscles, 19-20
  segments, 19, 26
  spine, 19
Body attitude, 109, 110-11
Body tensions, 71
  tension flows, 71, 85
Borland, Hall, 205
Brainard, Susan, 162
Bronz State Hospital, 15, 162, 163
Budapest Opera House, 168
Bugaku, Japanese, 168

Chace, marian, 139, 143, 146-47
Child Development Research Center for
    Parents and Children, 85
Chilkovsky, Nadja, 167
Choreometrics, 111, 169-73, 178, 228
Choreutics, 99-100, 103
Columbia University, 169
Connectedness, 21-22
Connecticut Dance Festivals, 228

CORD (Committee on Research in
    Dance), 167
"Core" qualities, 160-61, 170, 178
Counterbalance (tension), law of, 101
Countershaping. See Tensions and
    countertensions
Countertension. See Tensions and
    countertensions

Dance:
  as an art, Laban's definition of, 191
  choreographer, functions of, 192
  Effort combinations in, 192-93
  growth in activity, 194
  Labananalysis: as aid in training and
      communication, 194-95
    for analysis, 195-96
    for choreographing, 197-204
  movement in, Laban on, 193
  tensions in, 192
  walking as beginning of, 208
Dance Ethnology Inventory, 167
Dance Notation Bureau, 167, 171, 197, 203,
    218
Dance therapy, 9-10, 11-15, 143-63
  definition of, 143
  examples: with the aged, 163
    core qualities to show child
        development, 160-61
    with mentally retarded, 162
    movement analysis of hospitalized
        patients, 157-58
    movement therapy with individual
        patients, 152-54, 155
    phrasing, use of, 154
    post-partum psychosis, release from,
        156-67
    props, working with, 154-55
    shared with art therapy, 154, 155
    visual limitation and mobility, 158-59
  by groups, 11-12, 139
    movement choirs, 139-40
    movement analysis and, 143, 144-45,
        149, 150
  other techniques and disciplines,
      incorporating, 146-48
  resources: Bartenieff Fundamentals, role
      of, 145-46, 162
    dance, role of, 144-45
    Labananalysis as key, 144, 145, 148-
        50, 162
  values of, 151
    integration with other therapies, 151
Dauer, Alphons, 79
Davis, Martha, 9-10, 14, 112, 137n
Day Hospital Unit, Jacobi Hospital
    (Bronx, N.Y.), 9-15
de Mille, Agnes, 79
  "Oklahoma," 79
Deaver, George, 3, 6
Degree of flux, law of, 101
Dynamic space, 101

Effort, 51-68
  affinities of body, space and, 85-93

  examples of, 94-100
  combinations of, 56, 57
    basic Effort Actions, 57, 58-59
    in dance, 192-93
    examples, 64-68
    Full Efforts (Complete Drives), 58, 63
    Incomplete Efforts (Inner Attitudes or
        States), 58, 59-60, 62, 63
    Transformation Drives, 57, 61-63
    in walking, 208
  Effort elements continuum, 51-56
    Flow Effort, 53-55, 61
      predilections of, 53
    Space Effort, 55
    Time Effort, 56
    Weight Effort, 55-56
  gestural, 111
  observations of, 56-57
    identifying distinctions among, 56-57
  postural, 111
    as style-defining factor, 176
Effort Flow. See Flow Effort
Efron, David, 167
Engert, E.M., 118
Erdman, Jean, 178
Espenak, Lilyan, 143
Eukinetics, 224
Exercises, according to Bartenieff
        Fundamentals, 19, 20-22, 230-
        62
  additional: condensing to sitting from
      lying (10), 255
    creeping to stable standing (11B), 257-
        58
    creeping to standing level for
        locomotion (11A), 256-57
    preparatory for creeping to standing
        (8), 252-53
    seesaw (with partner; 7), 145-46, 250-
        51
    sitting to standing to walking
        (propulsion sequence; 12), 258-
        59
    walking through hands from
        quadruped position (9), 253-54
  basic: alternating knee drop and arms
      (5B), 244-45
    arm circles (6A), 246-47
    body half (vertical; 4), 241-42
    diagonal situp (6B), 248-49
    knee drop (5A), 243-44
    pelvic forward shift (2), 238-39
    pelvic lateral shift (3), 239-40
    thigh lift (lift; 1B), 236-37
    thigh lift (pre-lift; 1A), 235-36
  preparatory: angles of joints, changing
      (A), 231
    breath, proper use of (B), 232-33
    rock and roll (C), 234
  summary notes on, 260-62
    bony landmarks and muscles, 262
    pelvic-femoral rhythm, 260
    rotary factor, 261-62
    scapulo-humeral rhythm, 261
Exertion/recuperation, 71-74, 75, 78, 90,
    136

287

"Fairy Tale," 197-204
Ferber, Andrew, 134
Feuillet (ballet master), 207, 218
Fidler, Jay, 137
Film for documentation, use of, 228
Flow, 51-55, 57, 59-60, 63
Flow Effort, 61, 85-87, 132
  Bound, 53, 55
  Free, 53-55
Folkwangschule (Essen-Werden), 168
Force. See Weight
Freedom, 144
Fries, Margaret, 160-61
Full Efforts (Complete Drives), 58, 63, 92

Gestural Effort, 111
Gesture, 109, 110, 111, 112
  Laban on, 110, 193
Gleisner, Martin, 139
Graham, Martha, 79
Group interaction, 129-40
  examples: authentic response in group
    session, 138-39
  dance confrontations, 135
  dance duet in canon, 136-37
  family hierarchy configuration, 135
  group Effort rhythms, 136
  groups on subway station, 136
  interrelation in actors' training class,
    137
  movement behavior in group therapy
    session, 137-38
  movement choirs, 139-40
  spatial configurations and
    confrontations, 130-34
    circles, 132
    files, 131
    greeting behaviour, 134
    group dances, 133-34
    other groupings, 133
    rows, 131
    spontaneous movements and
      improvisations, 133-34
Gurewitsch, David, 6
Guzman, Paschal, 116
Gymnastics, Laban on, 191
Gymnastik und Tanz, 139, 140
Gyoergy, Martin, 168

Hall, Edward, 167
Hawaii, University of, Department of
  Theatre and Drama, 168
Hawkins, Alma, 143
H'Doubler, Margaret, 169
Hood, Mantle, 167
Huang, Al Chung-liang, 147
Hubbard tanks, 5, 6
Humphrey, Doris, 79, 218, 228
  The Shakers, 196
  "Water Study," 79
Hutchinson, Ann, 218

Icosahedron, 33-35, 38, 40
  "A" and "B" scales on, 34-35, 38-40, 44,
    193
  other scales: axis, 34, 43, 44
    girdle, 45
    peripheral, 34, 43, 44
    primary, 34, 44

transverse or peripheral rings, 43
scale sequences derived from, 80-82
Incomplete Efforts. See Inner States
Inner States (Inner Attitudes; Incomplete
  Efforts), 58, 59-60, 62, 63
Institute for Nonverbal Communication
  Research, 9, 171

Jankovic, Ljubica, 79
Jooss, Kurt, 168, 224

Kaeppler, Adrienne, 168
Kealiinohomoku, Joann W., 168
Kendo, 189-90
  Kata, 189
  Labananalysis observations on, 190
  suburi, 189
Kendon, Adam, 134
Kenny, Sister, 4
Kestenberg, Judith, 53, 71, 85, 87, 111, 112
Kinesphere, 25, 32, 34, 105, 107, 148, 154,
  159, 160, 161, 185
Kinetography Laban. See Labanotation
Knust, Albrecht, 139, 168, 218
Kurath, Gertrude, 167

Laban, Rudolf, 29, 30, 33, 44, 46, 71, 85,
  100, 103, 105, 111, 112, 146, 167,
  207, 215
  body in movement, focus on, 3
  on dance: as an art, 191
    movement, 193
  on gesture, 110, 193
  on gymnastics, 191
  Gymnastik und Tanz, 139, 140
  motion factors identified by, 51
    Effort, 51-68
  shadow-movements (-forms), 109
  movement choirs, development of, 139,
    194
  on movement notation, 217
Oriental martial arts, study of, 188
  and posture, 110
Laban Institute of Movement Studies, 171
Labananalysis, 3, 6, 7, 9-10, 12-13, 14, 16,
  20, 21, 29, 57, 90, 111, 138-39,
  146, 154, 158, 160, 167, 178, 187
  aid in dance training and
    communication, 194-96
  of animal movements, 184-85
  in choreographing a dance, 197-204
  and choreometrics, 111, 169-71
  dance therapy, contributions to, 144,
    145, 148-50, 162, 163
  and group interaction studies, 129,
    137
  Kendo: description of, 189
    observations on, 190
  misuse of yoga according to, 147-48
  and movement choirs, 139
  preparing pizza, 95-96
  walking, observations of, 206-07
Labanotation, 99, 167, 168, 197, 200
  beginnings of, 218
  choice of symbols, 218-19
    Effort notation, 224-25
    Effort/Shape notation, 226-27
    primer, 219-23
  kinetograms, 168

methodology, 227
Lamb, Warren, 111
Lamont, Bette, 199
Lange, Roderyk, 168
Lanyi, I., 168
Lawrence, A.C., 224
Leeder, Sigurd, 224
Limòn, José, 228
Locomotion, 26
  walking as, 207
Lomax, Alan, Choreometrics project, 111
  169-73, 228
Lugosy, Emma, 168

Masai stilt dance, 208
Mead, Margaret, 167
Motivation of physically handicapped, 7-9
Movement:
  actions in, 73
  analysis of, in animals, 183-85
    mare and foal, 183
    mountain lion and wild boar, 184-85
    using Labananalysis, 184-85
  body, study of, 167-79, 186-90
    choreometrics, 169-71
    ethnic aspects, 167-71
    Japanese Kendo, 188-90
    two musicians contrasted, 187
    walking, rehabilitation of, 186
  in dance, Laban on, 193
  ethnic studies of, examples from, 172-79
    American Indian (Yaqui)
      intracultural comparison, 174-
      75
    choreometric profile, 172
    cross-cultural comparison, 173
    Effort as style-defining factor, 176
    ethnic dances, teaching, 178-79
    inter-cultural comparison of same
      task, 179
    intra-cultural analysis (Blackfoot
      Indians), 176
    Japanese Kabuki dancer and Western
      ballet, 177
  inner impulses toward, 51
  organization of, 51-68
  rehabilitation of, 4-8
  rhythms in, 74-75
  as total spatial shapes, 108-09
  See also Space harmony scales
Movement analysis, 143, 144-45, 149, 150,
  157-58, 167
Movement choirs, 133, 139-40, 194
  Labananalysis and, 139
Movement impulse, 9
Movement notation, 217
  beginnings of, 218
  systems of, 218
  See also Labanotation
Movement therapy, 152-54, 155, 162
Muscles, stretching, 5

New York University:
  Institute of Rehabilitation, 3
  Performing Arts School, 178
Noh dancing, 211

Octahedron, 30-31
Ohio University, 171

288

One-dimensional and diagonal grounding,
    fusing of, 47

Parkinson's Disease, 105-07
Passion Drive. *See* Transformation Drives:
    Spaceless
Paulay, Forrestine, 169
Phrasing, 73-74, 76-78
    multi-phasic, 73, 74, 77
    two-phasic, 73-74, 76, 78
Physical therapy, 3-6
    patients' fears during, 5
Polio, treatment for, 4-6, 7
Postural Effort, 111
Posture, 109, 110, 111, 112
Preston-Dunlop, Valerie, 99-100
Primus, pearl, 110
Progressions, spatial, 29
    space harmony scales, 29-46
Props, use of, 150, 154-55, 163

Reich, Wilhelm, 143
Rhythm, 71-82
    in dance, 79, 193
    industrialization and, 75
    patterns of, 71-82
        exertion/recuperation, 71-74, 75, 78,
            90
        phrasing, 71, 73-74, 76-78
        preparatory action/main action, 73
        scale sequences in, 74, 80-82
        symmetrical and asymmetrical, 74, 79
        in work, 78
Rituals, 149-50
Robbins, Jerome, 79
    "West Side Story," 79
Rogers, Helen Priest, 228
Rolf, Ida, technique, 147
Rose, Carol-Lynne Moore, 197-204
Rotantge, Ted, 201
Rusk, Howard, 3

St. Elizabeth's Hospital (Washington,
    D.C.), 146
Scheflen, Albert, 112
Schmais, Claire, 14
Schmitt, Diana, 136*n*, 136-37
Schoop, Trudi, 143
Seeger, Pete, 78
"Seesaw" exercise, 145-46, 250-51
Segments, body, 19, 26
Shadow-movements (-forms), 109
Shankar, Udar, 192
Shape Flow, 85-87, 107
Shapiro, Ellen Goldman, 195
Simultaneity, 173
Space, 51-53, 57, 58, 59-60, 63
Space Effort, 55, 89, 90
    Direct, 55
    Indirect, 55
Space harmony scales, 29-46
    one-dimensional or defense, 29-30, 36,
        89-90
    cross of axes, 29
    three-dimensional 32-35, 91

"A" and "B" scale sequences, 34-35,
    38-40, 44, 92, 193
    diagonal cross of axes, 32-33
    icosahedron, 33-35, 38, 40-46, 92
    modified diagonals, 33, 193
    other scales, 34-35, 43-46
    two-dimensional, 30-32, 90-91
        octahedron cycles, 30-31
        three planes available, 31-32, 36-38
Spatial intent, 5, 21, 108, 148, 159, 229, 230
Spatial paths, 107
Spatial shaping, 103, 107, 108-09, 207
    and spatial intent, 108
Spatial zones of action, 26
    directions of movement, 27-28
Spell Drive. *See* Transformation Drives:
    Timeless
Steeples, 35
Stilts, use of, 208
Sudan Dogons Ritual Dance for the Dead,
    118
Szentpal, Maria, 168

Tagore, Rabindranath, 192
T'ai Chi Ch'uan training, 47, 143, 147, 169
Takemoto, Y., 162
Tension Flow, 71, 85
Tensions and Countertensions, 103-25,
    145, 148
    center of initiation, 108
    countertensions, 103-07, 108, 114, 115,
        116, 118
        mini-countertensions, 105-07
    dance, tensions in, 192
    examples: chordic tensions, 116-17
        comparison of tensions, sequence for,
            113
        countershaping and Effort, 118
        countertension, 114
        peripheral and transversal sequences
            in animal and human actions,
            121-22
        renewing countertension, 114
        same movement activity by many
            people, 124-25
        spiral shape, tensions of, 115
        three Commedia dell'Arte figurines,
            120-21
        two musicians, contrast between, 187
        utmost mobility: dance Michail
            Bartenieff, 118-19
        walking, rehabilitation of, 186
        work action: two construction workers
            compared, 122-23
    spatial tensions, 103, 107
        paths of, 107
        and spatial intent, 108, 114
Tetrahedral tensions, 97-99
Tetrahedron, 46-47
Therapy:
    art, 154, 155
    dance, 9-10, 11-15, 139-40, 143-63
    family, 14
    group, 14
    mental, 3

movement, 152-54, 155, 162
    occupational, 162
    patients' images of therapists, 4-5
    physical, 3-6, 162
    total, 6-9, 10-11
Time, 51-53, 57, 58, 59-60, 63
Time Effort, 89, 90
    distinct from time as duration, 56
    Sudden, 56
    Sustained, 56
Tongan dances, 168
Topaz, Muriel, 218
Total body, awareness and use of, 7-8
Total therapy, 6-9, 10-11
Touch, as therapist's tool, 150
Transformation Drives, 57, 61-63
    Spaceless (Passion), 57, 61, 202
    Timeless (Spell), 57, 61, 198-200, 203,
        204, 227
    Weightless (Vision), 57, 62, 200-02

Van Zile, Judy, 176
Venable, Lucy, 171
Vision Drive. *See* Transformation Drives:
    Weightless
Volutes, 35, 80, 92, 122

Walking, 74-75, 205-13
    as beginning of dance, 208
    forms of, 208
    gait, 205, 207
        cultural patterns of, 210-13
    Labananalysis observations of, 206-07,
        210
        crosscultural gait study, 211-13
    other skills as elaborations, 207
    range of (in railroad station), 208-10
        adolescent clowning, 209
        concentration, 210
        couple dancing while waiting, 209-10
        fragmented, 209
        porter at work, 209
        preoccupation, 209
        without purpose, 209
Weidman, Charles, 79, 228
    "Lynchtown," 79
Weight, 51-53, 57, 58, 59-60, 63
    body, 56
Weight (Force) Effort, 89-91
    action in, 56
    Light, 55
    Strong, 55
White, Elissa, 14
Whitehouse, Mary, 143
Willard Parker Hospital, 3-6
Wisconsin, University of, 169
Wolz, Carl, 168

Yaqui Indian Eastern Ceremony, 174-75
Yoga, 143, 169
    misuse of, in terms of Labananalysis,
        147-48, 194-95
Youngerman, Suzanne, 196

Zwerling, Israel, 9, 14

289